The American Medical Ethics Revolution

THE AMERICAN MEDICAL ETHICS REVOLUTION

How the AMA's Code of Ethics Has
Transformed Physicians' Relationships
to Patients, Professionals, and Society

EDITED BY

ROBERT B. BAKER, PH.D.

ARTHUR L. CAPLAN, PH.D.

LINDA L. EMANUEL, M.D., PH.D.

STEPHEN R. LATHAM, J.D., PH.D.

The Johns Hopkins University Press

Baltimore and London

Chapter 8. © Arthur Isak Applbaum
Chapter 20. © George J. Annas
© 1999 The Johns Hopkins University Press
All rights reserved. Published 1999
Printed in the United States of America on acid-free paper

9 8 7 6 5 4 3 2

The Johns Hopkins University Press
2715 North Charles Street
Baltimore, Maryland 21218-4363
www.press.jhu.edu

Library of Congress Cataloging-in-Publication Data
will be found at the end of this book.
A catalog record for this book is available from
the British Library.

ISBN 0-8018-6170-5

Contents

Appendixes

AMA Codes and Principles of Medical Ethics, 1847–1997

Preface

This volume arises from the vision of three organizations: the Center for Bioethics of the University of Pennsylvania, the College of Physicians of Philadelphia, and the Institute for Ethics of the American Medical Association. The sesquicentennial of the AMA's Code of Ethics provided a unique opportunity to contemplate the present and future prospects for American biomedical ethics from the perspective of medical ethics past.

Facilitating this opportunity was a chance encounter and a serendipitous joint appointment. The encounter was at the fifth annual Bioethics Summer Retreat in Taos, New Mexico, in 1993. After meeting Bob Baker, David Orentlicher invited him to serve as an adviser to James Stacey and others at the AMA who were planning the upcoming sesquicentennial celebrations. Serendipitously, Baker was appointed Visiting Scholar at the Center for Bioethics and Wood Institute Fellow of the College of Physicians of Philadelphia in 1996. As it happened, the College of Physicians and the University of Pennsylvania had cosponsored the Philadelphia conference at which the AMA was founded in 1847. After a meeting among the leaders of these organizations, it seemed appropriate for these same institutions to commemorate the founding of the AMA by cosponsoring a sesquicentennial conference, "Ethics and American Medicine: History, Change, and Challenge," in Philadelphia, March 14–15, 1997. Papers delivered at the conference became the basis for this volume.

The conference was a collaborative effort. Nancy Dickey, Daniel Johnson, Kirk Johnson, Charles Plows, and William Mahood gave addresses. Charles Bosk and Herbert Rakatansky chaired sessions. Working behind the scenes to ensure that everything ran smoothly were Lewis Crampton, Vicky Novesel, Jill O'Mahoney Stewart, Katherine Rouse, and Linda Stepanich (of the AMA); Janice Clinkscales, Porsha Simmons, and Roseann Thompson (of the Center for Bioethics of the University of Pennsylvania Health System); Alfred Fishman, Marc S. Micozzi, Thomas Horricks, Gretchen Worden, and Antonia Oberthaler Palmer (of the College of Physicians of Philadelphia).

We are also indebted to the contributors who, after presenting a superlative set of talks, stayed the course, converting oral to written discourse. Wendy Harris of Johns Hopkins University Press was a wonderful editor, deftly and diplomatically guiding the transformation of a collection of talks into a cohesive scholarly volume. Assisting her were the perceptive readers whom she chose to critically review the manuscript, as well as Sarah Cline and Barbara Lamb. We are also grateful to Jonathan Bynum for preparing the index; to Elizabeth Yoder for meticulous copy editing; and to Marianne Snowden for secretarial assistance; and to Emily DeSantis and Victoria Hargreaves for their eagle-eyed proofreading.

Contributors

George J. Annas, J.D., M.P.H., Edward R. Utley Professor and Chair, Health Law Department, Boston University School of Public Health, Boston, Massachusetts

Arthur Isak Applbaum, Ph.D., Associate Professor of Public Policy, John F. Kennedy School of Government, Harvard University, Cambridge, Massachusetts

Robert B. Baker, Ph.D., Professor, Department of Philosophy, Union College, Schenectady, New York

Chester R. Burns, M.D., Ph.D., James Wade Rockwell Professor of Medical History, Institute for the Medical Humanities, University of Texas Medical Branch, Galveston, Texas

Arthur L. Caplan, Ph.D., Trustee Professor of Biomedical Ethics and Director, Center for Bioethics, University of Pennsylvania, Philadelphia, Pennsylvania

Alexander Morgan Capron, J.D., University Professor of Law and Medicine, University of Southern California, Los Angeles, California

Christine K. Cassel, M.D., Professor and Chair, Department of Geriatrics, Mount Sinai Medical Center, New York, New York

Linda L. Emanuel, M.D., Ph.D., Vice President for Ethics Standards, American Medical Association, Chicago, Illinois

Eliot L. Freidson, Ph.D., Visiting Professor of Social and Behavioral Sciences, University of California, San Francisco, California; Professor Emeritus of Sociology, New York University, New York, New York

Albert R. Jonsen, Ph.D., Professor and Chair, Department of Medical History and Ethics, University of Washington School of Medicine, Seattle, Washington

Stephen R. Latham, J.D., Ph.D., Visiting Assistant Professor, Northwestern University School of Law, Chicago, Illinois

Susan E. Lederer, Ph.D., Associate Professor, Department of Humanities, Pennsylvania State College of Medicine, Hershey, Pennsylvania

Florencia Luna, Ph.D., Professor of Philosophy and Applied Ethics, University of Buenos Aires, Buenos Aires, Argentina

Edmund D. Pellegrino, M.D., John Carroll Professor of Medicine and Medical Ethics, Center for Clinical Bioethics, Georgetown University Medical Center, Washington, D.C.

Charles E. Rosenberg, Ph.D., Janice and Julian Bers Professor and Chair, Department of History and Sociology of Science, University of Pennsylvania, Philadelphia, Pennsylvania

Mark Siegler, M.D., Lindy Bergman Professor of Medicine and Director, MacLean Center for Clinical Medical Ethics, University of Chicago, Chicago, Illinois

Rosemary A. Stevens, Ph.D., Professor, Department of History and Sociology of Science, University of Pennsylvania, Philadelphia, Pennsylvania

Robert M. Tenery Jr., M.D., Chair, Council on Ethical and Judicial Affairs, American Medical Association

Robert M. Veatch, Ph.D., Professor of Medical Ethics and Director, Joseph and Rose Kennedy Institute of Ethics, Georgetown University, Washington, D.C.

John Harley Warner, Ph.D., Professor of the History of Medicine and Science and of American Studies, Yale University, New Haven, Connecticut

Paul Root Wolpe, Ph.D., Visiting Assistant Professor of Sociology and Senior Faculty Associate, Center for Bioethics, University of Pennsylvania, Philadelphia, Pennsylvania

Introduction

Few things seem less radical than the successful revolutions of yesteryear. Success breeds familiarity, and familiarity domesticates novelty. Today everyone—accountants, advertisers, architects, bankers, brokers, engineers, financial planners, insurance agents, personal consultants, public officials, realtors, even zookeepers—seems to aspire to self-regulation through formal codes of ethics. The notion of professional self-regulation seems anything but revolutionary. Yet if one peruses the appendix to the *Encyclopedia of Bioethics* (Spicer 1995) or some compendium of nonmedical codes of professional ethics (Gorlin 1990), it quickly becomes evident that no code of professional ethics promulgated by *any* national or international professional organization predates the 1847 American Medical Association Code of Ethics.

The 1847 AMA Code of Ethics is the world's first national code of *professional* ethics, the world's first national code of *medical* ethics, and the ancestor of all professional codes of ethics, medical or nonmedical. In its time, the AMA Code of Ethics was a revolutionary document that was thought to be comparable to the Declaration of Independence.

Before 1847—that is, before what might be called the American medical ethics revolution—members of certain "gentlemanly" occupations—most notably clergy, lawyers, and medical practitioners—differentiated themselves from members of virtually all other occupations by the fact that, when acting in their occupational roles, they considered themselves bound by special role-related duties that preempted the moral requirements of everyday life. The special nature of these role-related duties was symbolized by their professional oaths, which, in medicine, were thought to be descendants of the classic Hippocratic Oath. Indeed, the very word *profession* is literally Latin for 'bound by an oath.'

Oaths embody a distinctive form of ethics. They are activated by the performative utterance "I swear" and are couched in the first person singular. All these features make them inherently personal. Codes, by contrast, are collaborative. The transition from the personal ethics of oaths to the professional ethics of codes thus marks a radical transition from personally interpreted "gentlemanly" ethics to collaboratively interpreted professional ethics—a transition so radical that it is properly described as revolutionary. As it happens, the professional medical ethics revolution was conceived in Britain and born in America.

Doctor Thomas Percival's Revolutionary Proposal

In the eighteenth century British colleges, guilds, and other professional institutions were relatively unconcerned with moral matters; moreover, the legal regulation of medical practice was minimal to nonexistent. Practitioners and the public alike thus took it for granted that the personal character of an individual practitioner served as the principal guarantor of a practitioner's conduct. Indeed, many believed that the only effective constraint on a medical practitioner's conduct was the practitioner's honorable and virtuous character. Not unnaturally, therefore, eighteenth-century medical educators like John Gregory of Edinburgh (1724–73) and his American protégé Benjamin Rush of Philadelphia (1745–1813) focused as intently on forming the character of their medical students as they did on informing their intellect. They lectured to their students at length—typically at the beginning or the end of a course of lectures on a medical subject—about the specific duties that practitioners owed to their patients and about how to develop the qualities, virtues, and personal character suitable to someone practicing medicine as a profession. These moral lessons were illustrated with edifying homilies, narrative tales in which the honorable and virtuous character of successful practitioners were contrasted with the scandalously dishonorable character of practitioners whose vices had ruined their careers. In general, eighteenth-century medical educators strove to instill in their students a sense of the identity of personal and professional honor (chap. 1, this volume; Haakonssen 1997; McCullough 1998a, 1998b).

Although the pervasive identification of the personal with the professional —of personal integrity with professional integrity, of personal honor with professional honor—created lofty standards for personal and professional conduct, it became problematic at the end of the eighteenth century as British practitioners attempted to collaborate with each other in newly expanded medical institutions such as asylums, clinics, dispensaries, infirmaries, and hospitals. In these environments the identification of the personal with the professional converted professional disagreements into personal disputes about gentlemanly honor and integrity; these, in turn, often culminated in "affairs of honor," "pamphlet wars," and even duels (Baker 1993; 1996; Fissell 1993; Harley 1993).

In 1792 one such affair closed the Manchester Infirmary's Fever Hospital in the midst of an epidemic. This extraordinary institutional failure spurred the infirmary's trustees to action. They directed the most eminent physician in their community, Dr. Thomas Percival (1740–1804), leader of the Manchester Philosophical Society, world-renowned author of moral parables, and one of the infirmary's founders, to head a committee charged with drafting institutional regulations that would prevent any recurrence of the fiasco of 1792. The committee drafted the needed regulations, which appear to have effectively pacified personal-professional rivalries at the infirmary (Pellegrino 1985; Pickstone and Butler 1984).

Percival, however, did not leave matters there. For reasons that are largely unexplained (since most of Percival's personal papers were destroyed during the bombing of Manchester in World War II), the disastrous closure of the Manchester Fever Hospital prompted him to draft and circulate in 1794 a tract, *Medical Jurisprudence or a Code of Ethics and Institutes Adopted to the Professions of Physic and Surgery*, that offered the two core medical professions of physic and surgery a "code of ethics" in the form of specific codified duties with respect to patients and fellow practitioners.

There was nothing unique about Percival's contention that physicians and surgeons had duties toward their patients and toward each other—this was standard eighteenth-century medical school material, developed in the lectures of professors like Samuel Bard (1742–1821), Benjamin Rush, and, most influentially, John Gregory. Even the relatively novel idea of presenting these duties as a code—no doubt a function of Percival's own experience in drafting a code for the Manchester Infirmary—was not Percival's invention. As he himself notes, he was influenced by the codified format of Thomas Gisborne's *An Enquiry into the Duties of Men in the Higher and Middle Classes of Society in Great Britain Resulting from Their Respective Stations* (Gisborne 1794), which also codified the professional duties of physicians and surgeons (Baker 1993; Haakonssen 1997). What was unique and fundamentally revolutionary about Percival's code was that, unlike anything written previously, it severed the connection between personal and professional morality.

In *Medical Jurisprudence*, Percival reconceptualized the source of professional obligation, not deriving it from the individual practitioner's prickings of conscience; or from their personal sensibilities about duty and honor; or from the authority of the lay administrators, governors, and trustees of medical institutions. Instead, he grounded professional obligation in the *profession's* fiduciary responsibility for "the ease, the health, and the lives of those committed to their charge" (Percival 1794, sec. I, art. I; 1803, chap. 1, art. 1). Even the cultivation of professional virtues such as "skill, attention, and fidelity" and professional character traits such as "humanity and steadiness" were seen as deriving from the *profession's* prime imperative to serve those "committed to their charge" (Percival 1794, sec. 2, art. 2; 1803, chap. 2, art. 1). Professional ethics was thus to be promulgated by, interpreted by, and enforced by, the medical profession itself. Medicine's moral mandate, the duty of caring for the sick—which had been vested in the character and honor of the *individual* practitioner from the time of the Hippocratic Oath through the teachings of Bard, Gregory, and Rush—was now, for the first time ever, to be considered a *collective* rather than an individual responsibility, a responsibility owed by one group to another.

Perhaps more controversially, Percival claimed that the moral authority of the medical profession—acting collectively through consensus—should supersede not only the conscience and sense of honor of individual practitioners but also the authority of lay institutional administrators and trustees. Medicine was to be a morally self-regulating profession answerable primarily to its own interpretation of its mandate to care for "the ease, the health, and the lives of those committed to their charge."

Percival's revolutionary proposal to transform an ethic of personal conduct and honor into a collective professional ethic was undoubtedly inspired by his experiences drafting a code to prevent repetitions of the disaster of 1792. Before this, Percival had been a relatively conventional Enlightenment-virtue ethicist with a knack for popularizing the intricacies of his subject by writing moral tales for the edification of children and their parents (*A Father's Instructions to His Children*, 1775; *Moral and Literary Dissertations*, 1789). The disaster of 1792, however, displayed the dark side of the identification of the professional with the personal. Medical moralists had hitherto identified the two, believing that, since practitioners were deeply concerned about their own personal honor, if they equated professional honor with personal honor, they would naturally be inclined to act honorably in their professional conduct. The closing of the Manchester Fever Hospital, however, suggested to Percival that whatever success this equation may have enjoyed in controlling the conduct of practitioners engaged in the private practice of medicine, it would be unreliable in collaborative contexts like hospitals; for in hospitals the identification of the professional with the personal of necessity meant that professional differences took on all the appurtenances of personal quarrels. In collaborative contexts, the identification of the personal with the professional became a formulary for perpetual feuding—like the feud that had shuttered the Manchester Fever Hospital (Baker 1993).

The institutional regulations drafted by Percival's committee in 1792 responded to this problem by developing professional procedures for collaborative decision making. They envisioned formal clinical rounds, for example, in which opinions were offered in inverse hierarchical order—that is, in which subordinates report *before* their superordinates—alleviating the pressure to conform to their superordinate's opinion, and thus encouraging them to speak their own minds. In rounds, moreover, the decision of the group, made openly and collectively, became binding on everyone, including "the physician in attendance" (Percival 1794, sec. 1, art. 19–22; 1803, chap. 1, art. 21–22; see Baker 1993, 199–208). Thus professional consensus, whether displayed in rounds or in the development of the 1792 code itself, was considered more authoritative than any individual's opinions, no matter how hierarchically prominent that individual might be.

In 1794, when Percival published his system of professionally agreed upon uniform standards of professional conduct—his "medical jurisprudence"— he expanded the rules of conduct that had initially been invented to govern the actions of practitioners attending the sick poor in hospitals so that they would also apply to private practitioners who attended affluent patients in their homes (1794, sec. 2, art. 1; 1803, chap. 2, art. 1). In so doing, however, Percival undermined the original justificatory authority for his code; for a code that extends its authority beyond the gates of the hospital can no longer justify its rules by appealing to the authority of trustees whose powers extend no further than the hospital grounds.

Necessity playing its traditional role as the mother of invention, Percival vested the justificatory authority for the code in a new source—the very process of collaborative professional decision making that his committee had used to draft it. Professional consensus, when forged in the interests of serving patients, was thus treated as self-justifying. The code of ethics proposed in *Medical Jurisprudence* was to be justified solely by the profession's core collective obligation to care for the sick, as interpreted through collaborative processes that culminated in professional consensus.

Percival had other reasons for seeking to ground moral authority in professional consensus. The lay trustees of eighteenth-century hospital charities, rather like the trustees of some twentieth-century corporations and managed-care organizations, were not always trustworthy guardians of the profession's fiduciary responsibility to serve "the ease, the health, and the lives of those committed to their charge." They were sometimes tempted to cut corners by counterproductively failing to provide ventilation for hospitals or by overcrowding wards (Percival 1794, sec. 1, art. 16; 1803, chap. 1, art. 16). Trustees were also tempted, again like their twentieth-century management counterparts, to explore the "cost-saving" strategy of employing cheaper "drugs of inferior quality." After noting that such cost-saving strategies might be counterproductive, Percival argued that, even if they are not, physicians and surgeons had a *professional* obligation "not [to] suffer themselves to be restrained by parsimonious considerations from prescribing . . . drugs even of high price, when required in diseases of extraordinary malignity and danger. . . . No economy of a fatal tendency ought to be admitted into institutions founded on the principles of purest beneficence" (Percival 1794, sec. 1, art. 8; 1803, chap. 1, art. 8).

Percival had come to believe that medicine's traditional moral mandate to care for the sick was unsafe not only in the hands of individual practitioners but also in the hands of nonprofessional administrators and trustees, so he entrusted the mandate to care to collaborative professional consensus. Medical professionals, acting collaboratively on matters on which they had reached consensus, now had a moral mandate to appraise the conduct not only of fellow professionals but also of their nominal superiors and employers—hospital administrators, managers, and trustees—insofar as managerial actions or policies affected "the ease, the health, and the lives of those committed to their charge."

Like most revolutionary visions, Percival's required a new conceptual-linguistic framework to express it. *Medical Jurisprudence* and the Manchester Infirmary Code appear to contain the earliest printed use of the expression "physician in attendance," or "attending physician" (Reiser 1995), as well as the earliest descriptions of "medical rounds" and medical records. *Medical Jurisprudence* also appears to be the earliest printed work to offer consistently a unitary conception of a "patient," extending by language and precept (sec. 2, art. 1) the concept of a patient—which had hitherto been applied only to paying clientele in the middle and upper classes—to the "sick poor" cared for in dispensaries and hospitals. This extension of the term *patient* is the linguistic analogue of Percival's ideal of a unitary standard of care in which the elaborate code of practitioner-patient conduct developed by medical professionals in their relationships with the upper- and middle-class patrons applied, insofar as it was practical, to all patients—rich and poor, paying and nonpaying alike (Baker 1993).

The expression "medical jurisprudence" was also a linguistic innovation.

Unlike Percival's other neologisms, however, it was not well received by his readers. When Percival reissued his code of ethics in 1803, therefore, he coined two new expressions to encapsulate his new idea of collaborative professional self-regulation: "medical ethics" and "professional ethics." Percival used the expression "medical ethics" as title of the 1803 edition of his code and suggested, in his preface to the volume, that the study of "professional ethics" was useful to the formation of the character of a gentleman—a suggestion that cheekily inverts the traditional relationship between the ethics of character and what was now characterized as "professional" ethics. Both the neologisms were accepted into ordinary English, thereby perpetuating Percival's revolutionary conception of professions as collaboratively self-regulating occupations.

A Revolution Snubbed: The British Reception of Percival's Ideas

Ideas, however revolutionary, do not constitute revolutions. It is one thing to propose a radical change in forms of social life, and quite another to actually change them. Although Percival's proposals for pacifying hospital disputes— medical records, medical rounds, and the other tools of collaborative practice—were implemented within the walls of asylums, clinics, dispensaries, and hospitals over the course of the nineteenth century, his revolutionary reconceptualization of medical morality had few followers in Britain. Perhaps the most notable were Michael Ryan (1800–41), a professor of surgery at the University of London who lectured on medical jurisprudence and who was the first academic anywhere to style himself a "professor of medical ethics," and Jukes Styrap (1815–99), who tried repeatedly but unsuccessfully to convince the British Medical Association to adopt a code of medical ethics. Overall, however, Percival's revolutionary proposal for collaborative professional medical ethics had little appeal in his native land.

Percival's proposal presumes a medical profession willing to promulgate and to enforce explicit moral standards, but the Provincial Medical and Surgical Association (founded in 1832 and known after 1856 as the British Medical Association) declined to adopt any formal code of professional ethics, despite reiterated efforts to draft such a code in the 1840s, 1850s, 1860s, and 1880s (Bartrip 1995; Burns 1993). Perhaps the most trenchant expression of the British medical profession's attachment to a conception of morality as essentially a matter of personal character is the General Medical Council (GMC), the body empowered by the Medical Act of 1858 to oversee professional conduct. The act had stipulated not only the conditions under which practitioners could be registered (that is, licensed) to practice medicine in Britain, but also the conditions under which a medical practitioner's name might be "erased" from the register, thereby withdrawing a practitioner's right to practice medicine. Specifically, the GMC was empowered to strike a practitioner's name from the register if the practitioner was either convicted of a crime or "judged by the [GMC] to have been guilty of infamous conduct in any professional respect" (sec. 29, Smith, 206).

In exercising its power to strike names from the register, the GMC followed the precedent set by the British Medical Association by declining to draft any formal code specifying which forms of conduct were "infamous" in a professional. Before 1883 the GMC even refused to state why particular individuals were struck from the register (Smith 1995, 207). After 1883, however, the GMC began to issue notices explaining why a specific case was considered "infamous conduct in a professional respect." Gradually this list of explanations expanded into a system of "Warning Notices," which were ultimately published in a small pamphlet.

In 1903 the GMC received a petition from 133 British practitioners requesting formal guidance so that practitioners might anticipate what would constitute "infamous conduct" without actually committing a transgression. In 1908 the GMC replied that they not only "have no power to legislate or to issue regulations binding upon the profession" but also that "it is not *desirable* to pass a resolution condemning any practice in general terms . . . for the profession" (Smith, 210, emphasis added). The council seemed to believe that insofar as conduct is a function of character, formal codes of conduct are unnecessary to guide the conduct of persons of good character and are thus useful only to persons lacking good character, who would not otherwise know how to conduct themselves properly. Codes of conduct were thus "undesirable" because they were useful only to persons who, lacking decent character, wish to pretend that they had one.

The British GMC system, which remains in force today, is the logical culmination of the identification of professional morality with personal character.

Prelude to a Revolution

American physicians inherited this British conception of medical morality and initially perpetuated it in their medical societies. Yet, with the foundation of the AMA in 1847, they made a decisive and revolutionary break with the

British conception of character-based medical morality. As historian John Haller (1981) observed, the revolutionary nature of this break was recognized at the time: "[F]ollowing publication of the [AMA] code in 1847, articles in medical journals across the country supported and elaborated upon [the code's] principles. . . . Doctors from Massachusetts to Texas drew from the code for innumerable speeches and lectures before their societies, graduating medical classes, and public lyceums . . . [and] enthusiastically claimed the code to be the most noble production of man since the Declaration of Independence" (237–38).

The analogy with the Declaration of Independence is apt. Just as Americans had embraced and implemented the revolutionary political ideals of British philosophers like John Locke, whose theories about natural human rights and civil rights were never implemented in Britain—a nation that still lacks a Bill of Rights—American medicine was to implement the revolutionary medical ethical ideals of Thomas Percival, which were, by and large, ignored in his native land. Moreover, just as American politicians believed that the revolutionary ideas in the Declaration of Independence would change the political world, first in America and then around the globe, American physicians believed that by embedding Percival's revolutionary ideas in a national code of medical ethics, they would change the nature of medical morality, first in America and then around the globe—which, in fact, they did.

The analogy was apt in another respect as well. The American colonies, and later the states, were the laboratories in which Americans experimented with implementing such revolutionary British political ideas as republican government based on the consent of the governed, and in which they explored the notion that status ought to be merited by achievement rather than inherited from one's ancestors. A similar process of experimentation occurred in the American medical ethics revolution. Starting in New Jersey in 1766 and continuing into the nineteenth century, formally educated medical practitioners founded medical societies to keep abreast of European medical developments and to fortify themselves against untrained competitors. The constitutions of these societies often echoed European medical oaths, reflecting the received European equation of personal and professional integrity and honor. Thus the first article of the Instruments of Association and Constitution of the New Jersey Medical Society (1766) echoes the Hippocratic-style oaths then fashionable in Europe, asserting that "we will never enter any house in quality of our profession, nor undertake any case, either in physick or surgery, but with the purest intention of giving the utmost relief and assistance that our art shall enable us, which we will diligently and faithfully exert for that purpose." In 1808 the New York Medical Society required that all its members swear a Hippocratic-style oath based on a version of the oath then popular in Edinburgh. Enforcing these oaths were officials known as "censors," who, like their counterparts in British medical societies, censured immoral conduct and recommended the expulsion of physicians of disreputable character (chap. 2, this volume).

After nationhood was achieved, as formally trained physicians tried to develop a medical infrastructure of asylums, clinics, dispensaries, hospitals, infirmaries, and medical colleges comparable to those they had experienced while they were being educated in Europe, they began to appreciate that, as Percival realized in 1792, the identification of the personal with the professional, especially in matters of duty and honor, was essentially a formula for contention and dispute. Censors found, moreover, that in increasingly egalitarian and democratic America they needed formal standards to justify specific acts of censorship and recommendations for expulsion. Thus in 1808, when the Boston Medical Society and its allied branches throughout the Commonwealth of Massachusetts attempted, with the sanction of the state legislature, to develop rules for self-regulation—a "Medical Police"—they copied, for the most part word for word, some of the consensus-generating procedures that Percival had proposed in the last version of his code, *Medical Ethics* (1803). They also proffered a justification for imposing these procedures on their members by copying, again word for word, chapter 2, article 23 of Percival's *Medical Ethics*.

Conduct for the Support of the Medical Character

The *esprit de corps* is a principle of action, founded in human nature, and, when duly regulated, is both rational and laudable. Every man, who enters into a fraternity, engages, by a tacit compact, not only to submit to the laws, but to promote the honour and interest of the association, so far as they are consistent with morality and the general good of mankind. A physician, therefore, should cautiously guard against whatever may injure the general respectability of the profession, and should avoid all contumelious representations of the faculty at large, all general charges against their selfishness or improbity, or the indulgence of an affected or jocular scepticism, concerning the efficacy and utility of the healing art. (Association of Boston Physicians 1808, 44; Percival 1803, chap. 2, Article 23. N.B. this passage does not appear in *Medical Jurisprudence*.)

In hindsight, read in the context of the American medical ethics revolution, this passage marks a pivotal transition—the point at which American medical societies begin to part company from their British counterparts (Baker 1995, 25–39; for an opposing view, compare Chapman 1984, 86). Before this, American medical societies had treated practitioners' duty "to maintain harmony and brotherly affection" as a matter of personal "medical character" (New Jersey Medical Association 1766, art. 4), employing "censors" to censure bad conduct and to recommend the expulsion of practitioners whose character was found to be flawed—what we today call the "bad apples." Like its descendant, the GMC, the censor system presupposes that morality is inherently a question of character; however, the Association of Boston Physicians, drawing on Percival's original metaphor of "medical jurisprudence" was asserting that professional conduct was not a function of personal character; it was rather a set of "laws" stipulated by the society to which practitioners were bound by "tacit compact . . . to submit." The move from an ethics of character to one of conduct was thus an extension, in the social sphere of medicine, of the American ideological commitment to egalitarian democracy; for it meant that all persons were treated as moral equals.

The Boston Medical Police set a precedent with which other American medical societies soon began to experiment. They issued codes in which Percivalean ideals of professional ethical self-regulation were articulated, albeit ambivalently juxtaposed next to statements preserving the language and often the morality of personal character (see chap. 2, this volume). Slowly, through decades of experimentation by dozens of municipal, county, and state medical societies, the stage was being set for the entrance of the first entirely Percivalean code of medical ethics, the AMA's 1847 Code of Ethics.

Founding the American Medical Association

The American Medical Association was founded in response to a crisis, but not a crisis that was in any direct way related to ethics; rather, it was a crisis over professionalism and professional standards. From 1649 on, first colonies and later states sought to protect patients from fraudulent claims of medical expertise through a system that would permit patients to distinguish between trained and untrained medical practitioners. The usual mechanism was a system, inherited from the British, that required untrained practitioners to serve a reasonably extensive apprenticeship with "trained" practitioners and then to pass some form of qualifying examination, which was usually administered by the censors of the medical societies.

Problems arose after 1803, when Massachusetts altered this route to qualification by permitting a Harvard medical diploma to substitute for qualifying through apprenticeship and examination. Other states followed Massachusetts' precedent, and soon any M.D. degree sufficed to exempt aspirants from the apprenticeship system. Since qualification by degree was cheaper, quicker, and more prestigious than the older method, it soon became the preferred route; and the number of medical schools in America increased exponentially to satisfy this demand (Shryock 1967, chap. 1).

Substituting educational achievement for qualifying examinations would not in itself have been problematic. At the time, however, accreditation requirements were weak. In some states literally anyone could claim to be a medical educator and issue a medical degree that would automatically entitle the holder to practice medicine. In such a context, bad medical education began to drive out good.

Worse yet, piecemeal reform seemed impossible. No single state could reform its system without a parallel reform in the others. Since medical degrees are eminently portable, were any single state to raise educational standards within its borders, it would merely create a competitive advantage for schools operating beyond its borders. Medical educational reform would either have to be done by everyone everywhere, or no one could successfully implement it anywhere.

Reflecting back, Dr. Nathan Smith Davis (1817–1904), who was later to be lauded as the "father of the AMA," recalled how this Gresham's Law scenario led him to propose the national medical convention, precipitating the chain of events that ultimately culminated in the formation of the AMA:

> The college degree of M.D., being almost everywhere accepted as authority to practice without other examinations, the college that offered to confer it after attendance on the shortest annual courses of instruction and the lowest college fees could generally draw the largest class.
>
> Under these conditions and tendencies the annual courses of medical college instruction were progressively shortened from six months, as required by the first colleges in Philadelphia and New York, prior to 1800, to sixteen weeks or less; all semblance of a requirement of suitable preliminary education was omitted; and before the middle of the century had been reached the number of medical colleges had increased from four to forty, and the annual aggregate number of medical graduates from fifteen to more than one thousand. By nominally studying medicine for three years, including the two annual repetition courses of medical college instruction of less than four months each, the student could obtain a diploma entitling him to practice, which was easier and more economical than to study with a pre-

ceptor four years and pass an examination by the censors of a county or state society.

. . . At the annual meeting of the New York Medical Society in February, 1844, I, then a young delegate . . . presented a series of resolutions "declaring in favor of the adoption of a fair standard of general education for students before commencing the study of medicine; of lengthening the annual course of medical college instruction to at least six months with the grading of the curriculum of the studies; and of having all examinations for license to practice medicine conducted by State Boards, independent of the colleges." . . . At the next meeting, [in] 1845 . . . during a free discussion it was urged with much force that the requirements of a fair standard of education . . . in New York State alone, would only cause the student to abandon her colleges for those of Pennsylvania or the New England States.

This caused [me] to offer the following preamble and resolutions:

"Whereas, it is believed that a National Convention would be conducive to the elevation of the standard of medical education in the United States, and

"Whereas, there is no mode of accomplishing so desirable an object without concert of action on the part of the medical societies, colleges, and institutions of all the states, therefore

"Resolved, That the New York State Medical Society earnestly recommends a National Convention of delegates from medical societies and colleges in the whole Union, to convene in the City of New York on the first Tuesday in May, 1846, for the purpose of adopting some concerted action on the subject set forth in the foregoing preamble." (Davis 1903, 142–43)

The 1846 convention convened by Nathan Smith Davis and other New Yorkers to set national standards was a magnificent failure. On May 5, 1846, 122 delegates—the largest group of American physicians ever assembled—convened at the medical department of the University of the City of New York (which is today know as New York University). By the second day it had become evident that the convention was deadlocked on the central question before it: education. Unable to develop a set of educational standards acceptable to both medical colleges and medical societies, the New York convention was about to dissolve in failure when Dr. Isaac Hays (1796–1879), editor of the *American Journal of the Medical Sciences*, asked Davis whether he would be willing to endorse a proposal for a second convention to be held in Philadelphia the following year to establish a National Medical Society that would be dedicated not only to the reform of medical education but also to the reform of American medical science, medical ethics, and public health. Davis seconded Hays's proposal, and Hays put the following six motions to the convention:

1st. *Resolved,* That it is expedient for the Medical Profession of the United States, to institute a National Medical Association, for the protection of their interests, for the maintenance of their honour, and respectability, for the advancement of their knowledge, and the extension of their usefulness.

2nd. *Resolved,* That a committee be appointed to report a plan of organization for such an Association, at a meeting to be held in Philadelphia, on the first Wednesday in May, 1847.

3rd. *Resolved,* That a committee . . . invit[e] . . . delegates. . . .

4th. *Resolved,* That it is desirable that a uniform and elevated standard of requirement for the degree of M.D. should be adopted by all the Medical Schools in the United States, and that a Committee be appointed to report on this subject [at the national meetings].

5th. *Resolved,* That it is desirable that young men before being received as students of Medicine, should have acquired a suitable preliminary education; and that a Committee [to be appointed, etc.].

6th. *Resolved,* That it is expedient that the Medical Profession in the United States should be governed by the same code of Medical Ethics, and that a Committee . . . be appointed to report a code for that purpose. (National Medical Convention 1846)

Hays's six resolutions were passed unanimously, for good reason. By incorporating and transcending Davis's initial concern with education, the resolutions provided the convention with a raison d'être.

The first three resolutions boldly envision a permanent national medical organization that could address not merely matters of medical education but anything affecting the interests, honor, reputation, or usefulness of the medical profession, or the advancement of medical knowledge. This was so self-evidently a fitting, even if initially unintended purpose for the first national medical convention, that the first three resolutions passed without debate. Resolutions four and five addressed education and were more controversial. In the end, two committees were set up to address Davis's original concerns about medical and premedical education. Resolution six introduces a subject separate and distinct from anything contemplated by Davis and his fellow New Yorkers—a national code of medical ethics. It too passed unanimously.

The American Medical Ethics Revolution

The national code of medical ethics was to be written by a committee of seven, chaired by Dr. John Bell of Philadelphia (1796–1872), with his fellow Philadelphian Isaac Hays acting as editor and secretary and the other members as commentators (chap. 2, this volume). The 5,283-word document that Bell and Hays drafted, which passed unanimously at the 1847 meeting that was to found the AMA, was initially the crowning achievement of the American Medical Association. It committed all affiliated medical societies; all affiliated medical colleges; and all affiliated asylums, clinics, dispensaries, infirmaries, and hospitals and their members to the first unambiguously Percivalean code of ethics adopted anywhere.

The need to assert consensual professional authority had been a dominant theme running through a variety of medical reform movements that had appeared in America, starting with the 1820s movement to develop a standardized pharmacopoeia (in which Bell played a role), through the various educational and licensing reform movements of the 1840s (in which Davis was a prime mover). In general, however, these movements had succumbed to regional parochialism and to an almost inveterate American individualism. No one had found a formula that would make individual clinicians accept collective professional authority. Not even Percival's code of ethics provided a justification for professional authority over individual practice and practitioners that was acceptable to practitioners.

The authors of the AMA Code of Ethics, however, found a formula that made the collective professional authority palatable—the principle of reciprocity—which Bell defined as follows:

> Every duty or obligation implies, both in equity and for its successful discharge, a corresponding right. As it is the duty of a physician to advise, so has he a right to be attentively and respectfully listened to. Being required to expose his health and life for the benefit of the community, he has a just claim, in return, on all its members, collectively and individually, for aid to carry out his measures, and for all possible tenderness and regard to prevent needlessly harassing calls on his services and unnecessary exhaustion of his benevolent sympathies. (Bell 1847, see Appendix B, 317)

Bell's principle gave practitioners a moral right to demand respect and assistance not only from their fellow practitioners but also—and here is the point at which Bell extends the scope of the Percivalean model—from society at large, since, as a matter of reciprocity, society was obligated to reward doctors who perform their professionally defined duties as trustees of science and almoners of benevolence and charity.

Bell's principle thus legitimated a reform agenda in which internal moral and educational reform—collective action by practitioners toward *themselves*—became the basis on which practitioners could demand reciprocal recognition both from the public and from their own patients. But to earn public and patient respect, the profession had to put its own house in order. It had to drive out quacks from its own ranks and to reestablish scientific medical education. The profession also had to treat patients with "attention, steadiness, humanity," delicacy, and discretion. It could never "abandon a patient because the case is deemed incurable" or overcharge vulnerable patients. To earn the respect of the public, moreover, the profession pledged *always* to recognize "poverty . . . as presenting valid claims for gratuitous service" (chap. 1, art. 1, 2, 5) and to accept that "when pestilence prevails" they were "duty [bound] to face the danger, and to continue their labors for the alleviation of suffering, even at the jeopardy of their own lives" (chap. 3, art. 1–3).

Never before had physicians voluntarily subscribed to a code of conduct this demanding. The specific obligations that the AMA physicians had unanimously imposed upon themselves far exceeded earlier rather vague Hippocratic and character-based commitments to help patients and to try to avoid harming them. It set a new moral standard in medicine not only for America but also for the world. American physicians fervently embraced the AMA covenant. It was heralded at college lecterns, lauded at medical societies, and incorporated into the rules of hospitals and asylums. It was praised as a major medical ethical reform in both the medical and the popular press and, as we noted earlier, was heralded as the most significant document to be written in America since the Declaration of Independence. The 1847 Code of Ethics was reprinted by medical societies in Berlin, London, Paris, Vienna, and around the world.

The grand moral vision inscribed in the 1847 Code of Ethics established the newly founded American Medical Association as the preeminent moral and political voice of American medicine. Throughout the rest of the nineteenth century, the AMA's Code of Ethics was the most commonly printed medical document in the English language. In 1855 the AMA reiterated that its Code of Ethics was binding upon all allied municipal, state, and county medical societies, as well as allied asylums, clinics, dispensaries, infirmaries, hospitals, and medical schools, and upon all of their members. This declaration led local societies to clean house by expelling members who performed abortions, who advertised, who publicly endorsed secret nostrums, who patented medicines or medical products, or who consulted with homeopaths and other unscientific practitioners. The AMA also began a campaign to reform medical and premedical education by requiring extensive training in laboratory sciences and in hospital practice.

Over a half-century later, in the first decades of the twentieth century, virtually all the reforms envisioned by Bell, Chapman, Davis, Hays, and the other founders of the AMA had been achieved: the states had implemented new licensing laws; the federal government had founded the Food and Drug Administration, charging it with assuring the safety and efficacy of all drugs sold in America; there were extensive arrangements for the treatment of the poor in hospitals and in private practice; and last but not least, after the publication of the Flexner Report, American medical education had become rigorous, resting on a firm foundation of laboratory science and hospital experience. Ironically, however, the very generation of laboratory-science-educated, hospital-based doctors envisioned by the founders of the AMA rebelled against the moral constraints of the 1847 Code of Ethics.

Revolt and Restoration: From Codes to Principles, 1847–1997

In the 1880s the Medical Society of the State of New York withdrew from the AMA, protesting that its so-called Code of Ethics was a monopolistic, illiberal "etiquette" masquerading as ethics. The rebels took as their motto the question "Why is my liberty judged by another's conscience?" and urged a new conception of American medical practitioners as scientifically trained entrepreneurs. They argued that, since professionals could be trusted to treat their patients honorably, the sole function of medical associations ought to be promoting science. The rebels, in short, were attempting to rescind the Percivalean revolution of 1847 and to reestablish ethics as an extension of personal character (chap. 3, this volume).

The nominal issue over which the rebellion of the 1880s was fought was the consultation clause (chap 2, art. 4, sec. 1), which prohibited members of the AMA from consulting with any practitioner "whose practice is based on an exclusive dogma and of the aids actually furnished by anatomy, physiology, pathology and organic chemistry." Among the "dogmas" excluded was homeopathy, whose central doctrines were incompatible with the laws of chemistry. In metropolitan areas like Boston and New York, surgeons and other specialists protested that the consultation clause was inconsistent with the moral principle of putting patients first, since the clause obligated them to deny quality medical care to those patients who happened to have consulted a homeopath. Defenders of the code were quick to respond, however, that these same specialists did a profitable business in referrals from homeopaths.

As often happens when moral principles align with pocketbooks, the battle over the consultation clause became extraordinarily heated. Physicians who believed that ethics was essentially a matter of character rather than of codes reasserted their beliefs, openly calling for replacing the code with a British-style system. Researchers and specialists generally aligned themselves with the "no code" faction; defenders were, for the most part, general practitioners. The struggle for the heart of the American medical profession soon left the profession heartbroken, as specialists bolted from the AMA, forming colleges that focused on science and eschewed the formulation of codes of professional ethics (chap. 4, this volume).

Eventually the rebels triumphed within the AMA itself. In 1902 John Allen Wyeth (1845–1922), president of the AMA, called for the repeal of the consultation clause. At a 1903 AMA meeting in New Orleans, the anticode faction almost succeeded in repealing the code altogether. Instead, a compromise code, renamed the "Principles of Medical Ethics," was hammered out: the AMA rescinded the 1855 ruling that made its code binding on all member societies; the AMA's enforcement body, the Ethical and Judicial Council was disbanded; the section on the duties of patients to physicians was deleted; and the nominal cause of the revolt, the consultation clause, was repealed. Furthermore, the new Principles of Ethics were merely to be *advisory*, not mandatory.

Despite these setbacks, in some respects the Principles improved on the 1847 Code: they prohibited fee-splitting, and they distinguished secret nostrums (still prohibited) from patent medicines (now permitted). They also introduced the notion of change. The 1847 Code of Ethics was a social contract modeled, in many ways, on the U.S. Constitution. Yet, because the provisions of the contract were seen as *ethical* rather than legal, no provision had been made for amendment. As Albert Jonsen observed, rather like the Ten Commandments, the code seemed to represent immutable moral truths protecting the integrity of the profession; it could not be altered (chap. 17, this volume). Inflexibility, however, rendered the code so brittle that after the relatively short span of fifty years it snapped under the pressure of social change. In a perverse way, therefore, the more flexible conception of ethics embedded in the Principles was ultimately to assure the survival of the AMA's Code of Ethics.

In other respects, of course, since the Principles lacked mechanisms of enforcement, they represented a significant retreat from the Percivalean ideal of a professional ethical self-regulation. The retreat, however, proved remarkably short-lived; the AMA's experiment with laissez-faire ethics lasted less than a decade. The AMA found that without a binding and enforceable code of ethics, it was unable to resolve intraprofessional conflicts or to address pressing moral issues. In 1908 Joseph C. Bryant (1845–1914), president of the AMA, called for a restoration of the code and the Judicial Council; in 1910 George Simmons (1852–1937), editor of the *Journal of the American Medical Association*, led a campaign to restore the Judicial Council. The Judicial Council was restored in 1911, and the Principles were revised in 1912 to give the council the authority that it needed to address and resolve disputes and to respond to so-cial change. It also explicitly recognized and accepted the role of specialists in the profession and strengthened the prohibitions against fee-splitting, com-missions, and contract practice.

Through all of these changes the Principles retained much of the structure and many of the precepts of the original Percivalean code adopted in 1847. All that changed in 1957, when, on the 110th anniversary of its Code of Ethics, acting on recommendation of its Judicial Council, the AMA abandoned the remnants of the Hays-Percival format altogether. In its stead the council rec-ommended the format still used by the AMA: the articulation of a few basic principles (originally ten), supplemented by extensive commentary and advi-sory rulings on specific subjects.

In 1997, on its sesquicentennial, the AMA Code of Ethics had come to consist of four parts. The first two, which form the foundation of the code, con-sist of seven short Principles of Medical Ethics (last revised in 1980), supple-mented by a statement setting out the Fundamental Elements of the Patient-Physician Relationship (added in 1990), which recognize the bioethics revolution (chap. 9, this volume). A third element in the code is the Opinions of the AMA's Council on Ethical and Judicial Affairs (CEJA). CEJA's Opin-ions, currently created at a rate of about eight a year, treat specific facets of medical ethics; together with annotations noting their use by courts and aca-demic journals, they fill over two hundred pages. The rationales behind Opin-ions are traditionally published in detailed CEJA Reports, which may be con-sidered the fourth portion of the code. Since 1984 over seventy CEJA Reports have been published, filling over six hundred pages. Considered as a single body, the four parts of the AMA Code constitute the most comprehensive and influential statement of medical ethics extant. Moreover, despite ongoing de-bates about various principles, fundamentals, opinions, and reports, practi-tioners and the public—courts and regulators alike—treat these CEJA Opin-ions and Reports as authoritative and thus accept as appropriate and proper the idea that the medical community should regulate itself though an organi-zation like the AMA. In this sense, the Percivalean revolution that commenced with the founding of the AMA and the passage of its Code of Ethics remains surprisingly vital.

Reassessing the AMA Code of Ethics on Its Sesquicentennial

Bioethics is sometimes represented as a revolt against traditional medical ethics—particularly against the ethics of Percivalean codes—including the various codes and principles issued by the AMA from 1847 to the present (see chap. 9, this volume). Professional medical ethics, it is said, focuses narrowly on *physicians' duties;* whereas bioethics, in contrast, focuses on *patients' rights.* It is undeniably true that bioethics opened the realm of discourse about the nature and interpretation of medicine's moral mandate to the public and to ethics professionals, yet the focus on patients' rights is properly Percivalean—at least in the American context. For as John Bell argued in his introduction to the 1847 AMA Code of Ethics, "Every duty or obligation implies, both in equity and for its successful discharge, a corresponding right" (Appendix B, 317). Just as it is logically impossible to assert a doctrine of patients' rights without implying a doctrine of physicians duties, it is also logically impossible for the AMA to have consistently asserted codes and principles of physicians' duties for the past century and a half without implicitly endorsing patients' rights. Insofar as American bioethics really is a patients' rights movement, it would appear to be the logical outgrowth of the Percivalean revolution embedded in the AMA's 1847 Code of Ethics and its successors—which, not coincidentally, would explain why the second medical ethics revolution, the bioethics revolution of the 1970s, took place in America, the country first to embrace the Percivalean revolution.

Indeed, if we look at the basic achievements of the bioethics movement, they echo Percivalean precedents. Ethics consultation and ethics committees draw on the process of rounds consultation that Percival first proposed in 1792 and reiterated in his codes of 1794 and in his 1803 work, *Medical Ethics* (Baker 1993); institutional review boards to protect the human subjects of medical research (IRBs) were first proposed by Percival in 1794—as the great whistle-blower Dr. Henry Beecher (1904–1976) himself acknowledged (Beecher 1970, 12, 215, 218). Consensus statements and other formally codified standards of professional conduct—even though issued by quasi-nongovernmental organizations of professionals like the National Institutes of Health—are also preeminently Percivalean. It was, in the end, the AMA's implementation of the Percivalean ideal of professional self-regulation through collaboration, consensus, and codification that made America, and America alone, the natural birthplace of bioethics.

A Living Code: The Sunbeam Case

On the 150th anniversary of the Code of Ethics, the AMA itself showed its appreciation of its Percivalean heritage in three rather distinctive ways. It organized the sesquicentennial conference that provided the material for the present volume; it announced the formation of a new Institute for Ethics at the American Medical Association to provide professional ethical research and advice to CEJA and to the AMA on questions of medical ethics; and it accepted the resignation of several of its executives.

The issue that provoked these resignations was something as seemingly trivial as selling an imprimatur. As the United States nears the end of the twentieth century, the landscape is dominated by names, trademarks, and "logos." Everyone's name seems to be for sale: former presidents, senators, athletes, celebrities, movie stars, even academic institutions sell their names. Visit any college bookstore in the United States (including those at Union College and the University of Pennsylvania) and the staff will happily sell you almost anything with the institutional name on it. Names are a commodity, bought and sold like any other. Nonprofit organizations, moreover, commonly bolster their bottom line by selling their names. "American Medical Association" is a name, and so the Sunbeam corporation attempted to purchase the name to use on medical related equipment. Viewed simply as a commercial transaction, this was a profitable and unproblematic venture.

The AMA name, however, represents more than a trade association. It represents professional standards and professional self-regulation. Unlike its British counterpart, the American Medical Association had committed itself to a formal code of ethics. The 1847 Code of Ethics stated unequivocally that "it is derogatory to the dignity of the profession, to resort to public advertisements. . . . These are the ordinary practices of empirics, and are highly reprehensible in a regular physician" (chap. 2, art. 3). Today's code states in numerous places that it is impermissible for physicians to promote their own financial interests if those interests conflict with the patient's interest in receiving quality health care. Had the AMA's deal with Sunbeam been implemented, the AMA would have profited from recommending Sunbeam products, even though the AMA had not tested and was not qualified to test these products. Moreover, the deal would have given the AMA a financial interest in the successful sale of Sunbeam health-related products that might have prevented the AMA from promoting superior products from competing manufacturers. On reflection, it became apparent that what might initially have appeared to be a routine commercial transaction was incompatible with the principles embodied in the AMA's own Code of Ethics. The AMA was acting, corporately, in a manner that violated the principles that governed its members individually: the very same principles that prohibit physicians from placing their own financial interests into potential conflict with their patients' interests also prohibit a professional medical association from placing its financial interests into conflict with those of the public whose health it is committed to promoting. The corporate body thus found itself on the wrong side of an ethical boundary and, to its credit, withdrew its offer to sell its name and accepted the resignation of a number of its officers.

This incident attests to the continuing power of the Percivalean conception of professional ethics as a set of publicly stated standards of conduct that everyone—including the public at large—can use to assess professional mistakes. Percival did not think of character as something fixed. He recognized the inevitability of error—moral as well as medical—in a complex world. When one encountered such errors, Percival believed, one needed to review them "with scrupulous impartiality." "If errors of omission or commission are discovered," he held, "it behooves that they should be brought fairly and fully to . . . view. Regrets may follow, but criminality will thus be obviated; for good intentions . . . cannot anticipate the knowledge that events alone disclose." Percival added one proviso, one condition essential to obviating error—that "the failure be made conscientiously subservient to future wisdom and rectitude in professional conduct" (Percival 1803, chap. 2, art. 28). To err is human; forgiveness, however, is contingent on altering one's conduct to prevent future repetitions of the error. The AMA could and did publicly acknowledge its error. This recognition, and the role played by the AMA's own Code of Ethics—which it makes available to the public electronically and in print—attests to the viability of Percival's ideals and those of the American medical ethics revolution on the 150th anniversary of the AMA's Code of Ethics.

Marking the Sesquicentennial:
A Conference and a Book

As we remarked earlier, to celebrate the sesquicentennial of the 1847 Code of Ethics, the American Medical Association, working in collaboration with the Center for Bioethics of the University of Pennsylvania—an independent bioethics center that strives for the integration of bioethics and the social sciences, including history—invited independent scholars to join with the AMA's leadership in convening a conference, Ethics and American Medicine, in Philadelphia on March 14 and 15, 1997. The purpose of the conference was to reassess not only the AMA's Code of Ethics and its historical significance but also the status of professional ethical self-regulation 150 years after Percival's revolutionary idea was first implemented by the founding of the AMA.

The essays that form the chapters of this volume were all originally presented at the conference. They are collected in four sections. In Part I leading historians of medical ethics analyze and reassess the history of the AMA Code of Ethics: *Chester Burns* sets the stage by analyzing the conception of medical morality developed by Benjamin Rush and other eighteenth- and early nineteenth-century physicians; *Robert Baker* develops the case for reading the 1847 Code of Ethics as a revolutionary paradigm shift in the nature of medical morality, critiquing, in the process, many received readings of the 1847 Code and of American medical ethics; *John Harley Warner* analyzes the anticode movement of the 1880s; and *Rosemary Stevens* assesses the challenge to medical ethics posed by the emergence of specialty practice medicine at the end of the nineteenth century. Closing this section of the book is an essay by historian *Susan Lederer* analyzing the perception of medical ethics in the nineteenth and twentieth centuries, not from a professional's perspective, but through the lens of the popular media.

In Part II some of the leading scholars currently writing about the medical profession and medical professionalism today—*Arthur Applbaum, Alexander Capron, Linda Emanuel, Eliot Freidson, Stephen Latham, Edmund Pellegrino, Mark Siegler, and Robert Veatch*—use the 150th anniversary of the AMA's attempt to implement Percival's notion of a collaboratively self-regulating profession to reevaluate the relevance and viability of this ideal in America today. This debate leads directly to Part III, in which historian *Charles Rosenberg,* sociologist *Paul Root Wolpe,* and geriatrician *Christine Cassel* join with *Robert Tenery* of the American Medical Association to discuss current challenges to American medical ethics: the traditional challenge of alternative medicine, the challenge of providing access to medical care in a world of limited resources, and the challenge of managed care.

Underlying many of the essays in this volume is a sense of moral crisis precipitated by the shift from a system of fee-for-service medicine to a system of fee-for-system medicine, better known as "managed care." It is clear to everyone thinking about codes of medical ethics in 1997 that in an effort to contain the burden of three decades of explosive medical costs, Americans, skeptical of the ability of the profession and government to arrive at a solution, turned to the free market to find one. The market did as asked, and in the 1980s healthcare costs, measured in terms of both inflation and overall expenditures, fell significantly. Yet it is also clear that the fundamental paradigm shift from fee-for-service to fee-for-system has taken place in the context of a market economy that has, to this point, shown little interest in preserving the sanctity of the doctor-patient relationship. The virtues of fidelity, humanity, steadfastness, tenderness, confidentiality, and integrity that loom so large in the original AMA Code of Ethics, and that the AMA has defended for over a century and a half, are rarely invoked in the corporate boardrooms and stockholder meetings where many of today's crucial health decisions are being made. Profits threaten to preempt the personal, the professional, and more fundamentally still, the ethical dimension of the patient-physician relationship. Most of the conference presenters and participants believed that the main challenge facing medicine in 1997 was that of ensuring that free-market medicine remains moral medicine and that medical ethics rises to the challenge of preserving medicine's moral mandate within the context of managed care.

Part IV turns from the present to the future. It opens with a futurological analysis firmly rooted in an understanding of the history of medical ethics offered by one the founders of bioethics, *Albert Jonsen*. Another philosopher with an eye on the future, *Arthur Caplan*, then discusses the ability of bioethics to cope with challenges posed by the genetic revolution. The section on the future of bioethics closes with a discussion of bioethics in the developing world by Argentine bioethicist *Florencia Luna* and with an analysis of the internationalization of bioethics by *George Annas*.

Part of the power of Percivalean codes lies in their formal and public nature. Appendixes contain all of the major formulations of the AMA's codes of ethics, starting with the 1847 Code of Ethics (published here with John Bell's Introduction, and Isaac Hays's Note to the Convention). The three major revisions of the AMA's Principles (1903, 1912, and 1957) are reprinted along with the current version of the Principles of Medical Ethics (last revised in 1980) and the Fundamental Elements of the Patient-Physician Relationship. Although the editors decided not to include the more than two hundred pages of Opinions and Reports current in 1997, we include some sample Opinions by the AMA's Council on Ethical and Judicial Affairs, and some sample CEJA Reports, which state the rationales behind the Opinions. This is, as we noted earlier, the largest single body of medical ethical commentary extant; it is the living heritage of Percival, of his American disciples Bell and Hays, and of the American medical ethics revolution.

References

American Medical Association. 1847. *Code of Ethics.* Minutes of the Proceedings of the National Medical Convention held in the City of Philadelphia in May 1847, 83–106. See Appendix C.
Association of Boston Physicians. 1808. The Boston Medical Police. In *The Codification of Medical Morality: Historical and Philosophical Studies of the Formalization of Medical Morality in the Eighteenth and Nineteenth Centuries.* Vol. 2, *Anglo-Amer-*

ican Medical Ethics and Medical Jurisprudence in the Nineteenth Century, ed. Robert Baker, 41–46. Dordrecht: Kluwer, 1995.

Baker, Robert. 1993. Deciphering Percival's Code. In *The Codification of Medical Morality: Historical and Philosophical Studies of the Formalization of Western Medical Morality in the Eighteenth and Nineteenth Centuries.* Vol. 1, *Medical Ethics and Etiquette in the Eighteenth Century*, ed. Robert Baker, Dorothy Porter, and Roy Porter, 179–212. Dordrecht: Kluwer.

———. 1996. Resistance to Medical Ethics Reform in the Nineteenth Century. *Malloch Room Newsletter of the New York Academy of Medicine* 13 (Spring).

———. 1997. The Kappa Lambda Society of Hippocrates: The Secret Origins of the American Medical Association. *Fugitive Leaves*, Third Series, Vol. 11, No. 2, College of Physicians of Philadelphia.

Baker, Robert, ed. 1995. *The Codification of Medical Morality: Historical and Philosophical Studies of the Formalization of Medical Morality in the Eighteenth and Nineteenth Centuries.* Vol. 2, *Anglo-American Medical Ethics and Medical Jurisprudence in the Nineteenth Century.* Dordrecht: Kluwer.

Baker, Robert; Porter, Dorothy; and Porter, Roy, eds. 1993. *The Codification of Medical Morality: Historical and Philosophical Studies of the Formalization of Western Medical Morality in the Eighteenth and Nineteenth Centuries.* Vol. 1, *Medical Ethics and Etiquette in the Eighteenth Century.* Dordrecht: Kluwer.

Bartrip, Peter. 1995. An Introduction to Jukes Styrup's *A Code of Medical Ethics* (1878). In *The Codification of Medical Morality: Historical and Philosophical Studies of the Formalization of Medical Morality in the Eighteenth and Nineteenth Centuries.* Vol. 2, *Anglo-American Medical Ethics and Medical Jurisprudence in the Nineteenth Century*, ed. Robert Baker, 145–48. Dordrecht: Kluwer.

Beecher, Henry K. 1970. *Research and the Individual: Human Studies.* Boston: Little, Brown.

Bell, John. 1847. Introduction to the Code of Medical Ethics. *Minutes of the Proceedings of the National Medical Convention held in the City of Philadelphia, in May 1847*, 83–92. See Appendix B.

Burns, Chester. 1993. Reciprocity in the Development of Anglo-American Medical Ethics, 1765–1865. In *The Codification of Medical Morality: Historical and Philosophical Studies of the Formalization of Western Medical Morality in the Eighteenth and Nineteenth Centuries.* Vol. 1, *Medical Ethics and Etiquette in the Eighteenth Century*, ed. Robert Baker, Dorothy Porter, and Roy Porter, 135–44. Dordrecht: Kluwer.

Chapman, C. 1984. *Physicians, Law, and Ethics.* New York: New York University Press.

Davis, Nathan S. 1903. *History of Medicine, with the Code of Medical Ethics.* Chicago: Cleveland Press.

Fissell, Mary E. 1993. Innocent and Honorable Bribes: Medical Manners in Eighteenth-Century Britain. In *The Codification of Medical Morality: Historical and Philosophical Studies of the Formalization of Western Medical Morality in the Eighteenth and Nineteenth Centuries.* Vol. 1, *Medical Ethics and Etiquette in the Eigh-*

teenth Century, ed. Robert Baker, Dorothy Porter, and Roy Porter, 19–46. Dordrecht: Kluwer.

Gisborne, Thomas. 1794. *An Enquiry into the Duties of Men in the Higher and Middle Classes of Society in Great Britain Resulting from Their Respective Stations, Professions and Employment.* London: B. and J. White.

Gregory, John. 1772. *Lectures on the Duties and Offices of a Physician.* London: W. Straham and T. Cadell.

Gorlin, Rena. 1990. *Codes of Professional Responsibility.* Washington, D.C.: Bureau of National Affairs.

Haakonssen, Lisabeth. 1997. *Medicine and Morals in the Enlightenment: John Gregory, Thomas Percival, and Benjamin Rush.* Amsterdam: Ridopi.

Haller, J. 1981. *American Medicine in Transition, 1840–1910.* Urbana: University of Illinois Press.

Harley, David. 1993. Ethics and Dispute Behavior in the Career of Henry Bracken of Lancaster: Surgeon, Physician, and Manmidwife. In *The Codification of Medical Morality: Historical and Philosophical Studies of the Formalization of Western Medical Morality in the Eighteenth and Nineteenth Centuries.* Vol. 1, *Medical Ethics and Etiquette in the Eighteenth Century,* ed. Robert Baker, Dorothy Porter, and Roy Porter, 47–73. Dordrecht: Kluwer.

McCullough, Laurence. 1998a. *John Gregory and the Invention of Professional Medical Ethics and the Profession of Medicine.* Dordrecht: Kluwer.

———. 1998b. *John Gregory's Writings on Medical Ethics and Philosophy of Medicine.* Dordrecht: Kluwer.

National Medical Convention. 1846. *Minutes of the Proceedings of the National Medical Convention, held in the City of New York, 1846.* New York.

New Jersey Medical Association. 1766. *Instruments of Association and Constitution.* New Brunswick, N.J.

Pellegrino, Edmund D. 1985. Thomas Percival's Ethics: The Ethics Beneath the Etiquette. In Thomas Percival, *Medical Ethics,* 1–52. Birmingham, Ala.: Classics of Medicine Library.

Percival, Thomas. 1794. *Medical Jurisprudence or a Code of Ethics and Institutes Adopted to the Professions of Physic and Surgery.* Manchester, UK, privately circulated.

———. 1803. *Medical Ethics; Or, A Code of Institutes and Precepts, Adapted to the Professional Conduct of Physicians and Surgeons.* London: J. Johnson.

———. 1807. *The Works, Literary, Moral and Medical of Thomas Percival.* London: J. Johnson.

Pickstone, John. 1993. Thomas Percival and the Production of Medical Ethics. In *The Codification of Medical Morality: Historical and Philosophical Studies of the Formalization of Western Medical Morality in the Eighteenth and Nineteenth Centuries.* Vol. 1, *Medical Ethics and Etiquette in the Eighteenth Century,* ed. Robert Baker, Dorothy Porter, and Roy Porter, 161–78. Dordrecht: Kluwer.

Pickstone, John, and S. V. Butler. 1984. The Politics of Medicine in Manchester, 1788–1792. *Medical History* 28:227–49.

Reiser, Stanley. 1995. Creating a Medical Profession in the United States: The First

Code of Ethics of the American Medical Association. In *The Codification of Medical Morality: Historical and Philosophical Studies of the Formalization of Medical Morality in the Eighteenth and Nineteenth Centuries.* Vol. 2, *Anglo-American Medical Ethics and Medical Jurisprudence in the Nineteenth Century,* ed. Robert Baker, 89–104. Dordrecht: Kluwer.

Shryock, Richard Harrison. 1967. *Medical Licensing in America, 1650–1965.* Baltimore: Johns Hopkins University Press.

Smith, Russell G. 1995. Legal Precedent and Medical Ethics: Some Problems Encountered by the General Medical Council in Relying upon Precedent when Declaring Acceptable Standards of Professional Conduct. In *The Codification of Medical Morality: Historical and Philosophical Studies of Medical Morality in the Eighteenth and Nineteenth Centuries.* Vol. 2, *Anglo-American Medical Ethics and Medical Jurisprudence in the Nineteenth Century,* ed. Robert Baker, 205–18. Dordrecht: Kluwer.

Spicer, Carol. 1995. Appendix: Codes, Oaths, and Directives Related to Bioethics. In *Encyclopedia of Bioethics,* ed. Warren T. Reich, 5:2599–842. New York: Macmillan.

I

American Medical Ethics:
Historical Reflections

1

Setting the Stage

Moral Philosophy, Benjamin Rush, and Medical
Ethics in the United States before 1846

CHESTER R. BURNS, M.D., PH.D.

In 1792 Benjamin Rush (1746–1813), a distinguished physician in Philadelphia, told a class of medical students: "I object to its [moral philosophy's] being made a part of academical education. It was originally introduced into Christian colleges from pagan schools and has constantly tended to impress a belief of the independence of morals upon religion. A course of lectures upon the evidences, doctrines, and precepts, of Christianity, will not only supply its place, by legitimating its objects, but will expand the mind of our pupil by fixing it upon the most elevated subjects of human contemplation" (Rush 1811, 174–75). Rush's objection epitomized the beliefs of Protestant Reformers who thought that the study of moral philosophy was unnecessary for a virtuous Christian; indeed, they thought it dangerous because of its heretical implication that human reason, unaided by God's revelation, could discover the foundations of good and evil conduct. Rush urged doctors to honor Christian ideals, but he did not situate their professional ethics in Protestant beliefs. Ironically, he instead became America's first systematic philosopher of medicine by modifying the legacies of British moral philosophy and medical ethics.

British Moral Philosophy and British Medical Ethics

The Catholic moral theology and philosophy fashioned during medieval times and the secular ethics of Plato, Aristotle, and Cicero, as they had been resurrected by Renaissance humanists, challenged the sixteenth-century Protestant Reformers who designed the curricula of modern universities. Some

Protestants wished to reject both Catholic moral philosophy and classical ethics. These were the Calvinists and Lutherans, who insisted upon God's sovereignty, human sinfulness, and the human need for salvation as the path to the highest good. Other Protestants wished to reject Catholic traditions but not philosophical inquiry. They wanted to design rationalist and naturalist systems of ethical inquiry that would not be in conflict with Protestant religious beliefs.

During the seventeenth and eighteenth centuries, British clergy, professors, and scholars created models of the new moral philosophy. English authors read by colonial Americans included Henry More, Thomas Hobbes, John Locke, William Wollaston, Joseph Butler, Richard Price, Lord Shaftesbury (Anthony Ashley Cooper, the third earl), and William Paley (Fiering 1969; Willey 1964). Though the English scholars were influential, the eighteenth-century Scottish professors—at Glasgow, Edinburgh, and Aberdeen—were even more influential in the colonies and the early American republic (Bryson 1945). These Scottish authors, including Francis Hutcheson, David Hume, Adam Smith, Thomas Reid, Adam Ferguson, Dugald Stewart, and David Fordyce, wrote books about moral philosophy that were used by college students and professors in Great Britain and the United States for many years.

Francis Hutcheson (1694–1746) was an especially dynamic teacher of moral philosophy at the University of Glasgow between 1730 and 1746. Hutcheson lectured in English instead of in Latin, always hoping "to direct men to that course of action which tends most effectually to promote their greatest happiness and perfection" (Sher 1990, 97). A professor of moral philosophy at the University of Edinburgh between 1764 and 1784, Adam Ferguson (1723–1816) displayed great similarities to Hutcheson's style and, as Richard Sher noted, placed "the reputation of the Edinburgh chair on a par with the chair at Glasgow" (Sher 1990, 121). Both Hutcheson and Ferguson believed that moral philosophy would help transform teenage boys into virtuous gentlemen, benevolent Christians, and loyal British citizens.

Attending, but not graduating from, the University of Edinburgh, David Hume (1711–76) became a central figure among the Scottish thinkers. He found a place for both feeling and reason in ethical theory. Though the universal sentiment of sympathy was essential for motivating the quest for goodness and justice, Hume believed that reason could be used to shape and modify passions, thereby fusing virtuous motives with behaviors that would win public approval (Beauchamp 1993, 110–16).

A close friend of Hume, Adam Smith (1723–90) was professor of moral philosophy at Glasgow between 1752 and 1764 (Ross 1995). In *A Theory of Moral Sentiments*, published in 1759, Smith reconstructed Humean sympathy. Smith agreed with Hume that sympathy with the motives of a virtuous person allows humans to judge a deed as proper or right. However, he did not agree with Hume that usefulness was the principal criterion for determining the propriety of an act. A judgment of propriety itself could be sufficient for assigning righteousness to a specific behavior. Hume and Smith agreed that judgments about right and wrong were always determined within social contexts. Placing oneself in the predicament of another, either by robust feelings of sympathy or by judgments of propriety, permitted a social assessment (Beauchamp 1993, 117–18).

The systems of moral philosophy designed by individual thinkers differed in ways that are important to the development of Scottish moral philosophy. However, the framework of fundamental assumptions that guided most Scottish moral philosophers appears to have been far more important to Anglo-American physicians than the nuances of their ideological differences. The Scottish savants championed methodical and logically systematic thinking grounded in introspection and observation. Each human possesses an innate capacity for making moral choices. Fashioning reasons as preludes to these choices is important but not sufficient, because these choices are motivated by feelings that are universal for all humans. Each person has the capacity to blend reasons, feelings, and actions into habitual patterns of public service that also reward self-interest. The criteria enabling such habits of goodness can be discovered and learned. Individuals who exercise these habits achieve happiness and success; groups that honor such habits develop public policies that result in civilized progress for all. By opening the moral adventure to everyone, and by insisting on a process of discovery by each person and group, these moral philosophers invited reflective humans to rethink and reform criteria used by established authorities, whether churchmen, political leaders, physicians, or others.

A demonstrable link between Scottish moral philosophy and British medical ethics occurred in the lectures of John Gregory (1724–73). Except for four years of medical studies at Edinburgh and Leyden, Gregory spent the early years of his life in Aberdeen, where he was born. He practiced medicine, taught mathematics and natural philosophy, and served as professor of medicine at the university. He was an active member of the Wise Club, a local philosophical society that included his cousin, Thomas Reid (1710–96), who in 1752 became professor of philosophy at King's College in Aberdeen (Lawrence 1984, 254–55). In 1764 Reid succeeded Adam Smith as professor of moral philosophy at Glasgow, and Gregory moved his medical practice to Edinburgh. In the following year, Gregory became professor of medicine at the University of Edinburgh.

Gregory and other physicians regularly associated with moral philosophers and others designated by Richard Sher as the "Moderate Literati" in Edinburgh, central figures in the Scottish Enlightenment during the latter decades of the eighteenth century (Sher 1985). Though Gregory acknowledged that "enquiries that relate to man in his moral, political, or religious capacity" were "foreign" to the medical profession, he journeyed into that territory with a series of introductory lectures during the 1760s that were published as six chapters in 1772 and are generally acknowledged as the earliest definitive analysis of medical ethics by a modern British doctor (Gregory 1772, 111).

In his first two chapters (70 pages), Gregory explicitly discussed the virtues and duties of physicians. Larry McCullough argues that Gregory's approach was grounded in Hume's notion of sympathy (McCullough 1993). Though Gregory devoted three pages to the importance of sympathy (1772, 19–21), he also included "patience, good-nature, generosity," and "compassion" among the "gentler virtues that do honour to human nature" (8–9) and "patience, attention, discretion, secrecy, and honour" as specific moral obligations for physicians (12). Gregory did not reduce a physician's morality to any one virtue.

Moreover, no "gentler virtues" could substitute for the scientific and clinical knowledge that improved therapeutic outcomes. Gregory dealt with the education of a physician and with medicine as a science in the other four chapters (168 pages). An uneducated, unscientific doctor could not be morally virtuous.

Thomas Percival (1740–1804) was the other British physician who exerted a major formative influence in shaping modern Anglo-American medical ethics. Percival studied medicine at Edinburgh for two years but received his degree from Leyden in 1765. After practicing in his hometown of Warrington, England, for two years, he moved to Manchester, where he continued as a general physician until his death in 1804. In 1792 the trustees of the Manchester Infirmary asked Percival to prepare a set of rules that could be used to govern practice at the infirmary. Percival circulated a draft two years later, but the final book, with the title *Medical Ethics, or a Code of Institutes and Precepts, Adapted to the Professional Conduct of Physicians and Surgeons,* was not published until 1803. Percival's book displayed a form of the new moral philosophy that exerted even more influence on doctors than had Gregory's lectures (Pellegrino 1986).

Percival knew the writings of several moral philosophers, including Paley, Price, Hutcheson, and Smith. But he decided to offer his moral values as a set of maxims, not as a book of speculative philosophy.[1] He divided medical ethics into four dimensions. One involved a physician's character; the other three, a physician's relationships with other doctors, with patients, and with the public at large. He composed ninety-two maxims reflecting judgments about ethical propriety within each dimension, and he arranged these into four chapters that addressed professional conduct in hospital practice, professional conduct in general practice, conduct of physicians toward apothecaries, and conduct of physicians in cases involving a knowledge of the law (Baker 1993, 179–211; see chap. 2 of this volume for further discussion of these maxims).

For both Gregory and Percival, the character of a gentleman determined a physician's moral propriety. Imbued with notions of personal honor, a gentleman physician was virtuous because he was a person who exhibited the virtues of prudence, compassion, and benevolence as he served patients, families, and community institutions. These were the medical ethics transmitted to Benjamin Rush as he listened to the lectures of Gregory when he studied at Edinburgh between 1766 and 1768, and as he corresponded extensively with Percival between 1786 and 1801 (Corner 1948, 43; Butterfield 1951, 406).

Benjamin Rush as a Moral Philosopher of Medicine

Rush's objection to moral philosophy was a reflex of the New Side Presbyterianism that suffused his earliest years. Rush was tutored by an uncle, Samuel Finley, whose academy at Nottingham, Maryland, was the brightest educational star for the New Side Presbyterians, who cherished holy affections and personal conversions and who spearheaded much of the Great Awakening of the mid-eighteenth century (Sloan 1971, 55–62). While still a teenager, however, Rush became acquainted with moral philosophy as part of the curriculum at the College of New Jersey (now Princeton) from which Rush graduated in 1760. After serving five years as an apprentice to John Redman, a prominent Philadelphia doctor, he studied medicine at Edinburgh, receiving an M.D. in 1768.

After visits to London and Paris, Rush returned to Philadelphia in 1769 to become one of that city's most distinguished citizens: a member of the Continental Congress and signer of the Declaration of Independence, a doctor in the Continental Army, a founder of Dickinson College and public advocate for other educational institutions, and a physician who regularly attended the sick poor, mentally ill persons, and prisoners (Goodman 1934; Fox, Miller, and Miller 1996).

After practicing medicine for two decades, the forty-four-year-old doctor gave his first lecture on medical ethics in February 1789 (Rush 1818, 254–64). In subsequent years he gave at least seven lectures on different aspects of medical ethics, all introductory orations in various courses. The sixty-eight-year-old doctor gave the last one in 1812, five months before his death. Viewed together, these lectures reveal not only the influences of Gregory and Percival but also the originality of Rush's adaptation of Scottish moral philosophy to the moral predicaments of American doctors. Just as the philosophers had fashioned an image of a morally acceptable citizen by systematically connecting virtues, duties, and feelings with economic success and social justice, Rush fashioned an image of a morally acceptable physician by systematically relating virtues, duties, and feelings with business success and legal expectations.

Rush used three words to capture the values he deemed most sacred: piety, humanity, and patriotism (Rush 1811, 120–40). Sustaining the ancient Stoic virtues that were so important to the Scottish philosophers, these words symbolized one's relationship to God, to other humans as individuals and groups, and to a community or nation as a public entity. Though Rush mentioned prayer and reading of Christian scriptures as examples of *piety*, he focused on patriotism and humanity in fashioning a host of moral imperatives for doctors.

By honoring civic and forensic duties, doctors displayed their *patriotism*. Sustaining Percival's link between ethics and jurisprudence, Rush urged doctors to share medical knowledge when it was needed during civil and criminal investigations and trials associated with such matters as deaths caused by wounds and poisons; rape, abortion, and child murder; and assessments of mental illness that could affect the validity of wills, rights of witnesses, and outcomes of trials (Rush 1811, 363–95). Rush also urged doctors to use their knowledge in fulfilling public health duties associated with sanitation and control of epidemic diseases. A truly virtuous physician welcomed the legal and social duties associated with a community's quest for justice.

Examples of *humanity* included studies to improve medical knowledge, proper respect for other doctors, sympathy and compassion toward patients, and gratuitous services to the sick poor. Doctors who wanted to make improvements in medical science, for example, were obligated to perform autopsies to determine the causes of death and to keep records about epidemics and cases of chronic disease (Rush 1811, 141–65). Doctors who wanted to improve their profession were obligated to establish professional societies that would render each physician "more respectable in the eyes of the public" (Rush 1812, 36).

Respectable physicians who fulfilled their duties would enjoy many worthwhile feelings (Rush 1811, 210–31). If physicians practiced as tradespeople, however, pains would predominate over pleasures. Such tradespeople usually relied only on book knowledge, flattered the rich and neglected the poor, failed to add a single improvement to medicine, did not relate to the joys and sorrows of their patients, and did not behave in a friendly manner toward colleagues. Tradespeople were neither virtuous nor happy.

Rush emphasized causally reciprocal relationships between the virtues and duties of physicians, the pleasures of a medical career, and the honorable methods of acquiring business and reputation. Honorable methods included diligent studies, fidelity and punctuality with patients, polite manners, sympathy with the sick, attending the poor, decent dress, respect for religion and public worship, and cures of difficult diseases.

Dishonorable methods included character assaults on other physicians, performing cures with disguised remedies, taking undue advantage of physicians during consultations, publishing accounts of cases that never existed or cures that never occurred, and reducing professional fees to lure patients from fellow physicians (Rush 1811, 232–55). Other vices included careless or superficial examination of sick persons; harsh answers to questions posed by patients; refusal to attend patients at night; desertion of old patients during an epidemic; extravagant fees; and a fondness for public amusements at clubs and theaters. Failure to discharge one's duties confirmed vices, created pains, and produced business failures.

Employing honorable methods and avoiding professional vices did not, however, eliminate all pains from a doctor's life. Some patients did not take their prescriptions or complained about the effects of particular medicines. Others would dismiss doctors if their prescriptions did not produce a cure or if the doctor held unpopular religious or political opinions, wrote poetry, or wore shoes that made offensive noises (Rush 1811, 253–54).

As a way of dealing with these vexations and depicting the moral "rights" of doctors (without using "rights" language per se), Rush delineated a host of moral duties for patients (Rush 1811, 318–39). Patients should prefer physicians whose "habits of life" were regular and who were not devoted to pleasure at "the theater, the turf, the chase." They should choose educated doctors, and each family should designate one physician with responsibility for the care of the entire family. Patients should send for the physician in the morning but be ready to receive him at any time of the day. They should not oppose the clinical judgments of their doctors, and they should obey the doctor's advice about prescriptions. They should speak well of a doctor's services and pay fees promptly. Though such imperatives for patients appear presumptuous today, they resonated with the values of early nineteenth-century American doctors who searched for moral authority and respect (Haber 1991, 45–66).

Rush became America's first systematic moral philosopher of medicine by adapting the basic tenets and methods of the British philosophers to the moral challenges of American physicians. The moral philosophers offered comprehensive analyses of an individual's social obligations, categorizing these as duties to God, to oneself, and to others in specific situations. Rush offered a comprehensive analysis of a doctor's obligations, categorized as duties to God, to oneself, to other physicians, to patients, and to the public at large. Like his British mentors who championed a moral law binding all humans, Rush forged a rigorous causal reciprocity between ideals and conduct, ethics and etiquette. Honoring the ideals produced virtuous behaviors, which, in turn, validated the ideals. Together, they assured social status and beneficial outcomes.

Moral Philosophy and Medical Ethics in the United States

Benjamin Rush played another extremely influential role in the transfer of Scottish moral philosophy to the United States. As a medical student at Edinburgh, Rush had been directly responsible for persuading Mrs. John Witherspoon to leave Scotland so that her husband could accept the presidency of Princeton (Corner 1948, 50–51). Witherspoon (1723–1794) served as professor of moral philosophy and president for twenty-six years, from 1768 to 1794 (Sloan 1971, 103–45).

By 1830 prominent teachers of moral philosophy at Northern and Southern schools had included Charles Morton (1627–98) and Levi Hedge (1766–1844) at Harvard; Samuel Johnson (1696–1792), John Daniel Gros (1738–1812), and John McVickar (1787–1868) at Columbia; Witherspoon and Samuel Stanhope Smith (1750–1819) at Princeton; Thomas Upham (1799–1872) at Bowdoin; Francis Wayland (1796–1865) at Brown; Philip Lindsley (1786–1855) at Cumberland in Nashville; and Jasper Adams (1793–1841) in Charleston (Rand 1928; Howe 1970; Meyer 1972; Fiering 1981). These teachers sanctified the new moral philosophy and its methods as fundamental cultural foundations for educated American gentlemen. Their courses became the capstone of education for every student who graduated from an American college or university before the Civil War.

Though expressed in varying ways, the central themes of their courses were piety, humanity, and patriotism (Smith 1956, 16–21). Formally educated gentlemen could be trusted to blend piety, humanity, and patriotism in consciences that prompted virtuous behaviors. Studies of moral philosophy helped students learn how to keep their intentions authentic and how to nurture their "gentler" virtues. They also learned the importance of displaying these intentions and virtues in public behaviors that improved the lives of fellow humans and championed the moral standards of the new American nation.

Similar hopes motivated those American physicians who, like Rush, exhorted their colleagues and students with orations about medical ethics, and those who, like some of Rush's many students, created and adopted codes of medical ethics (Burns 1995, 3:1610–16). During the late colonial years and the early decades of the American republic, clergy used their pulpits to bring parishioners closer to a Christian model, and doctors used classrooms and meeting halls to bring students and colleagues closer to a professional model. In a politically free nation, persuasion of this sort was the path to personal conviction, and personal conviction was the bedrock of each individual's conscience.

Voluntary assent, catalyzed by the persuasive powers of a physician orator, could be strongly reinforced when a group of physicians transformed the private authority of an individual physician's conscience into the public authority of a professional society's conscience. By 1800 physicians had organized societies in New Jersey, Massachusetts, New York, Connecticut, South Carolina, Pennsylvania, Delaware, New Hampshire, and Maryland. Some of these groups included explicit standards of professional conduct in their bylaws. The New Jersey physicians agreed that they should discourage quacks, participate readily in all consultations, and treat the poor without charge. Rush enthusiastically supported the establishment of the College of Physicians of Philadelphia, whose members adopted a set of bylaws that included specific rules for consultations (1788). Several societies explicitly prohibited the use of secret remedies (Burns 1969, 95–98).

These physicians believed that right and wrong professional conduct would be determined by honoring specific moral standards. The doctor who was unwilling to consult honestly with other reputable physicians was practicing irresponsibly. Dispensing secret remedies was a moral affront to other physicians. Medical quacks harmed patients and devalued honest professionals. Morally adequate physicians provided medical care for any patient who needed such care, regardless of financial status. Physicians believed that these bylaws were binding by the voluntary agreement of those who became members of a particular society.

American doctors continued to organize new professional societies during the first half of the nineteenth century. Some separated certain standards from the bylaws and gave them special attention as codes of ethics. Before 1846 the most important of these were adopted in Boston, New York, and Baltimore.

In March 1808 members of the Boston Medical Association adopted a set of rules called the *Boston Medical Police.* The nine sections of this code included rules that addressed consultations, interferences with another doctor's practice, arbitration of differences between doctors, quack medicines, professional respectability, fees, practicing for a sick or absent doctor, and seniority among practitioners (Baker 1995).

A committee of three doctors, John Warren (1753–1815), Lemuel Hayward (1749–1821), and John Fleet (1766–1813), prepared this code. Although they acknowledged the writings of Gregory, Percival, and Rush, the committee selected all of the precepts in the *Boston Medical Police* from the second chapter of Percival's *Medical Ethics.* This *Boston Medical Police* became the model for codes of medical ethics adopted by at least thirteen societies between 1810 and 1842 (Burns 1969, 102–4).

Three New York physicians, James Manley, Felix Pascalis (1750–1833), and John Steele, worked for two years before presenting a code to fellow members of the New York State Medical Society, who adopted it in 1823. These doctors understood Percival's entire viewpoint and did not limit their code's maxims to those in Percival's second chapter. They addressed issues of personal character as well as the legal context of medical practice. They urged fellow doctors to honor their obligations to courts and other legal officials in matters of forensic medicine and public health. This code reflected a grasp of medical ethics not present in previous American codes.

Designing a truly American code also seemed to be the goal of Eli Geddings (1799–1878), Thomas H. Wright, John Fonerden (1804–69), Henry Willis Baxley (1803–76), and John Graves, whose code was adopted by fellow members of the Medico-Chirurgical Society of Baltimore in 1832. These doctors studied the writings of Gregory, Percival, and Rush as well as the codes adopted in Connecticut and New York. After a brief introduction, they subdivided their code into five major divisions, addressing such topics as consultations, quackery, fees, and the duties of patients toward their physicians. The last section was a vintage summary of Rush's duties for patients.

The adoption of these codes in New York City and Baltimore had not gone unnoticed in Philadelphia. In 1839 the College of Physicians of Philadelphia asked Benjamin Coates (1797–1881), John Otto (1774–1844), and Thomas Hewson (1773–1848) to rewrite the college's "Regulations to Promote Order." The new rules, adopted in 1843, addressed the conduct of physicians toward patients, the conduct of physicians toward their professional brethren, consultations, quack medicines, and fees. These new rules were Percival's precepts, very slightly rephrased (Burns 1969, 113–15). What might be viewed as reactionary conservatism could also be interpreted as a strong desire to sustain a British legacy that sanctified the gentlemanly elitism cherished by the Philadelphia doctors, who were reeling from the social and professional changes of the Jacksonian era.

But the New York and Baltimore doctors were hardly rejecting the gentlemanly beliefs of Gregory, Percival, Rush, or their Philadelphia colleagues. They embraced the social environment of the New World more openly, and they understood that Percival's vision of professional ethics could not be reduced to physician-physician etiquette. Moreover, the Baltimore doctors used Rush's ideas about the obligations of patients to emphasize a feature of moral philosophy that had created and justified a new political order for the world. Moral obligations implied moral rights. An acceptable social contract between doctors and patients in a new democratic republic would acknowledge the rights and duties of both groups. American doctors were obliged to discover and proclaim these duties and rights as basic components of their moral contract with the publics they served.

The urges to codification among American doctors coincided with the prominence of moral philosophy in the colleges. More than one of the physician orators, and at least six of the doctors who prepared the previously described codes, had graduated from an American college.[2]

Certainly not every physician orator and codifier had experienced an undergraduate course in moral philosophy, but not a few understood the congruence between the moral views taught in American colleges and the professional ethics advocated by the doctors. Honoring the rules of the codes and the maxims of the orators would enable conscientious physicians to be virtuous, benevolent, just, happy, and successful practitioners. Rush's hopes would be fulfilled.

To appreciate the import of moral philosophy for medicine, American doctors did not need to experience a formal course in moral philosophy, however. Gregory and Percival had already married these cultural legacies, and the offspring of Percival's codes provided appealing templates for those American doctors who celebrated a fundamental tenet of British moral philosophy: the power of ancestors who had discovered timeless moral values. American doctors embraced the tenets and methods of British moral philosophers and

British medical ethicists because they believed in their veracity and in their appropriateness as moral foundations for truly professional physicians.

Notes

1. In an introduction to a reprint of Thomas Percival's *Medical Ethics*, published in 1975, I emphasized that Percival's views of professional ethics were far more than the narrow viewpoint of professional etiquette that had been attributed to him by Chauncey Leake and others (see Burns 1977, 284–97).

2. The six are Lemuel Hayward (Harvard), John Warren (Harvard), John Fleet (Harvard), Henry Baxley (St. Mary's in Baltimore), Thomas Hewson (College of Philadelphia), and John Otto (Princeton). The source of information for Hayward was Thacher 1828 (1977), 286–88. The source for the others was Kelly and Burrage 1928: Baxley (75), Fleet (413), Hewson (564), Otto (925), and Warren (1260).

References

Baker, Robert. 1993. Deciphering Percival's Code. In *The Codification of Medical Morality: Historical and Philosophical Studies of the Formalization of Western Medical Morality in the Eighteenth and Nineteenth Centuries.* Vol. 1, *Medical Ethics and Etiquette in the Eighteenth Century,* ed. Robert Baker, Dorothy Porter, and Roy Porter. Dordrecht: Kluwer.

———. 1995. An Introduction to the Boston Medical Police of 1808. In *The Codification of Medical Morality: Historical and Philosophical Studies of the Formalization of Western Medical Morality in the Eighteenth and Nineteenth Centuries.* Vol. 2, *Anglo-American Medical Ethics and Medical Jurisprudence in the Nineteenth Century,* ed. Robert Baker. Dordrecht: Kluwer.

Beauchamp, Tom L. 1993. Common Sense and Virtue in the Scottish Moralists. In *The Codification of Medical Morality: Historical and Philosophical Studies of the Formalization of Western Medical Morality in the Eighteenth and Nineteenth Centuries.* Vol. 1, *Medical Ethics and Etiquette in the Eighteenth Century,* ed. Robert Baker, Dorothy Porter, and Roy Porter. Dordrecht: Kluwer.

Bryson, Gladys. 1945. *Man and Society: The Scottish Inquiry of the Eighteenth Century.* Princeton: Princeton University Press.

Burns, Chester R. 1969. Medical Ethics in the United States before the Civil War. Ph.D. diss., Johns Hopkins University.

———. 1977. *Legacies in Ethics and Medicine.* New York: Science History Publications.

———. 1995. Colonial North America and Nineteenth-Century United States. In *Encyclopedia of Bioethics,* ed. Warren Reich. New York: Macmillan.

Butterfield, L. H. 1951. *Letters of Benjamin Rush.* Princeton: Princeton University Press.

Corner, George W. 1948. *The Autobiography of Benjamin Rush.* Princeton: Princeton University Press.

Fiering, Norman Sanford. 1969. Moral Philosophy in America, 1650–1750, and Its British Context. Ph.D. diss., Columbia University.

————. 1981. *Moral Philosophy at Seventeenth-Century Harvard: A Discipline in Transition.* Chapel Hill: University of North Carolina Press.

Fox, Claire G.; Miller, Gordon L.; and Miller, Jacquelyn C. 1996. *Benjamin Rush, M.D.: A Bibliographic Guide.* Westport, Conn.: Greenwood Press.

Goodman, Nathan G. 1934. *Benjamin Rush: Physician and Citizen, 1746–1813.* Philadelphia: University of Pennsylvania Press.

Gregory, John. 1772. *Lectures on the Duties and Qualifications of a Physician.* London: W. Strahan and T. Cadell.

Haber, Samuel. 1991. *The Quest for Authority and Honor in the American Professions, 1750–1900.* Chicago: University of Chicago Press.

Howe, Daniel Walker. 1970. *The Unitarian Conscience Harvard Moral Philosophy, 1805–1861.* Cambridge: Harvard University Press.

Kelly, Howard A., and Burrage, Walter R. 1928. *Dictionary of American Medical Biography.* New York: D. Appleton.

Lawrence, Christopher John. 1984. Medicine as Culture: Edinburgh and the Scottish Enlightenment. Ph.D. diss., University College, London.

McCullough, Laurence B. 1993. John Gregory's Medical Ethics and Humean Sympathy. In *The Codification of Medical Morality: Historical and Philosophical Studies of the Formalization of Western Medical Morality in the Eighteenth and Nineteenth Centuries.* Vol. 1, *Medical Ethics and Etiquette in the Eighteenth Century,* ed. Robert Baker, Dorothy Porter, and Roy Porter. Dordrecht: Kluwer.

Meyer, D. H. 1972. *The Instructed Conscience: The Shaping of the American National Ethic.* Philadelphia: University of Pennsylvania Press.

Pellegrino, Edmund D. 1986. Percival's Medical Ethics: The Moral Philosophy of an Eighteenth-Century English Gentleman. *Archives of Internal Medicine* 146: 2265–69.

Rand, Benjamin. 1928. Philosophical Instruction in Harvard University from 1636 to 1906. *Harvard Graduates' Magazine Association* 37:29–49, 188–200.

Ross, Ian Simpson. 1995. *The Life of Adam Smith.* Oxford: Clarendon Press.

Rush, Benjamin. 1811. *Sixteen Introductory Lectures to Courses of Lectures upon the Institutes and Practice of Medicine, with a Syllabus of the Latter.* Philadelphia: Bradford and Innskeep.

————. 1812. Introductory Lecture upon the Duties of Physicians to Each Other. 2 November 1812. Unpublished manuscript, Library, Historical Society of Pennsylvania.

————. 1818. *Medical Inquiries and Observations.* Philadelphia: M. Carey & Son.

Sher, Richard B. 1985. *Church and University in the Scottish Enlightenment: The Moderate Literati of Edinburgh.* Princeton: Princeton University Press.

————. 1990. Professors of Virtue: The Social History of the Edinburgh Moral Philosophy Chair in the Eighteenth Century. In *Studies in the Philosophy of the Scottish Enlightenment,* ed. N. A. Stewart. Oxford: Clarendon Press.

Sloan, Douglas. 1971. *The Scottish Enlightenment and the American College Ideal.* New York: Teachers College Press.

Smith, Wilson. 1956. *Professors and Public Ethics: Studies of Northern Moral Philosophers Before the Civil War.* Ithaca: Cornell University Press.

Thacher, James. 1828. *American Medical Biography.* New York: Milford House, 1977 reprint.

Willey, Basil. 1964. *The English Moralists.* New York: W. W. Norton.

2

The American Medical
Ethics Revolution

ROBERT B. BAKER, PH.D.

Both the title and the central premise of this volume contradict the two most commonly accepted views of the origins and nature of the American Medical Association (AMA) and its Code of Ethics. One rather cynical view, which is widely shared by scholars, laypersons, and even some members of the organization itself, holds that the AMA is essentially a trade organization founded to serve the interests of orthodox medical practitioners. In this view, the AMA's forays into "medical ethics" are simply public relations exercises designed to pacify the public and to gull legislators into supporting orthodox medicine's monopolizing proclivities. Alternatively, there is the patriarchal account, sustained by the AMA's own sense of its history, which treats the AMA as the child of a single founding father, Nathan Smith Davis, who founded the organization to serve the public by defending American medicine against the incursions of shoddy educators and quacks of all stripes. Since Davis himself had little interest in medical ethics in the early years of the AMA, those who view Davis as the organization's founder see little that is revolutionary in the code of ethics adopted by the AMA in 1847. In their reading, the 1847 AMA Code of Ethics merely parrots a code of ethics that had been published by the English physician Thomas Percival in 1803—a code that had, moreover, been copied by many other American medical societies previously. In either reading there was nothing "revolutionary" about the founding of the AMA or the drafting of its code of ethics.

This essay challenges these interpretations. I argue that they were originally convenient myths that were accepted to unify the organization during periods of turmoil and to distance the organization from a divisive and controversial code of ethics. Later these myths were perpetuated by scholarly critics of the

AMA, who used them to debunk the organization and its pretensions to morality. A better picture of the AMA and its code of ethics emerges, I argue, if the organization is seen as the product of a radical reformist vision of American medicine that was wedded from the beginning to eminently practical concerns about protecting the profession from undereducated and unorthodox competitors. In this essay, I review the mundane details of the minutes of forgotten meetings to try to recapture both the radical vision and the practical concerns that led to the formation of the AMA. I show how and why various myths about the origins of the AMA developed and why it became politic to dismiss an ethical revolution as mere "professional etiquette." The essay closes with an analysis rejecting the received interpretation of the AMA Code of Ethics and proposing a more historically accurate alternative.

The Founder and the Parrot: Received Accounts of the AMA's Founding and Its Code of Ethics

In 1947, to celebrate the centennial of its founding, the American Medical Association commissioned one of its most eminent members, Dr. Morris Fishbein (1889–1976), former editor of the *Journal of the American Medical Association* (*JAMA*), to write a history of the organization. In this history, Fishbein accorded the title "founder of the AMA" to a single individual, opening the volume with his biography and using his portrait as a frontispiece. The "founder" so honored was Nathan Smith Davis, a Christian gentleman born in a log cabin in upstate New York on January 9, 1817, who later went on to become the founding editor of *JAMA*, founding chair of the Judicial Council, and president of the AMA. Davis's claim to being the "founder" lay in the fact that as a young man of twenty-nine he had proposed a conference on medical education reform, which, in turn, proposed founding a national medical organization, later called the AMA, and had chaired the committee from which this proposal emanated. An anonymously published tract, *History of the American Medical Association,* underscored these facts, and in 1875 the AMA struck a medal recognizing Davis's signal contributions. At its semicentennial or "jubilee" meeting held in Philadelphia in 1897, the AMA formally heralded "Father" Davis as the organization's founder. In 1903 Davis publicly acknowledged this title in his *History of Medicine with the Code of Medical Ethics,* and on Davis's death in 1904, the title "founder of the AMA" was mentioned in most eulogies and memorial notes.

Thus the official tale of the founding of the AMA unfolded first at the AMA's jubilee meeting in 1897 and was later retold in a more scholarly fashion in Fishbein's 1947 book celebrating the AMA's centennial. The tale not only extols the leadership of Davis but also downplays the importance of the organization's Code of Ethics. Inattention to the Code of Ethics was politic at both the jubilee and the centennial celebrations because on both of these occasions the Code of Ethics was controversial and would, in fact, soon be radically revised. Moreover, at the time of the 1947 centennial, inattention to the code seemed appropriate since the leading scholar of the document, Chauncey Leake, contended that it was merely a code of professional etiquette that parroted the language of an English physician, Thomas Percival of Manchester (Leake 1927). Fishbein accepted Leake's parroting thesis: "When Isaac Hays presented the report of his committee to the convention of 1847, he . . . decided that little improvement could be made on the principles as set forth by Thomas Percival" (Fishbein 1947, 36). It was thus the Englishman Percival, not the American Hays, who deserved whatever credit—or blame—might be associated with the AMA's Code of Ethics.

The tales constructed for the AMA's jubilee and centennial celebrations allocate responsibility to some—to Nathan Smith Davis of Binghamton and Chicago for founding AMA and to Thomas Percival of Manchester, England, for penning the words parroted by his American disciples—and deny responsibility to others—specifically to Hays as author of the AMA's Code. Yet while these are ideal jubilee and centennial tales—evoking a great leader whose portrait could conveniently serve as the frontispiece of a centennial volume—they are more appropriately treated as institutional myths than as history. In what follows I argue that the AMA was founded, not by a single heroic individual, Nathan Smith Davis, but by hardworking committees and conferences, and that, moreover, Davis did not play a pivotal role in the key decisions that led to the foundation of the AMA. If one had to single out one individual as pivotal to the process, the honor would most properly be accorded to a figure who has traditionally been portrayed as the honest scrivener of a moral code dictated decades earlier by Percival: Isaac Hays. Yet—and this is the second point on which I shall challenge the received view—the code of ethics that Hays and his fellow Philadelphian John Bell offered to the founding convention of the AMA in 1847 was a radically innovative document that transformed and transcended Percival's ideas, providing the foundation for what is best described as "the American medical ethics revolution."

Reassessing Davis's Title as "Founder of the AMA"

Fishbein credits Davis with the role of founder of the AMA because Davis was so honored at the jubilee celebration, because Davis chaired two important committees and served on a third, and because Davis proposed the conference on medical education that, in turn, proposed founding a national medical association. Yet even on the received reading of the record, the founding of the AMA is as much about committees and conferences as it is about individuals. Davis's concerns about education would have had no effect, for example, had they not been acted upon by the Medical Society of the State of New York. As Fishbein himself remarks, it was actually Davis's older colleague, Dr. Alden March of Albany, who proposed the idea of a second national conference on educational reform (Fishbein 1947, 6), and it was the society, not Davis, that convened the conference. Moreover, the conference, which was held at the University of the City of New York (now New York University) in 1846, was organized by Dr. Edward Delafield of New York City, not by the young Dr. Davis of Binghamton—although Davis chaired the ten-person committee on educational reform out of which the proposal to found the AMA emanated.

Does all this conference action and committee work justify the claim that some one individual founded the AMA? One is tempted to object that surely Davis was credited with founding the AMA, not because he served on some committees, but because he was the first to conceive the idea of a national medical organization and was its foremost champion. In fact, the minutes of the founding convention—which are preserved with Isaac Hays's papers in the libraries of the American Philosophical Society and the College of Physicians of Philadelphia—indicate that Davis played no such role.

Perhaps the pivotal question about the origins of the AMA should be this: Why did a committee commissioned to develop a series of proposals about educational reform proffer instead proposals on an entirely different subject, the foundation of a national medical organization? The answer would appear to be that the committee found itself at an impasse. The twenty-nine-year-old reformer Davis proposed that medical schools be subject to external accreditation. Medical school faculties, however, were unwilling to forego autonomy as the price of educational reform. Isaac Hays of Philadelphia brokered a compromise by referring this question to a committee that could pursue these and similar issues on an ongoing basis. Thus, reading between the lines in the minutes, it would appear that since referring a controversy to a committee requires some ongoing organization to which the committee can report—in a remarkable instance of a tail wagging a dog—a national medical society, the AMA, was invented to create an organization that would receive the ongoing reports of the education reform committee.

What the actual lines penned in the minutes reveal is that, on a motion from Dr. Lewis Bush, the committee's mandate was broadened from educational reform to "all subjects proper." Bush's motion opened the possibility of dealing with issues beyond medical education. The minutes also indicate that the committee then agreed to hold a second convention to found a national medical society. Four cities were considered as the site for a successor convention: Albany, Alden March's city; New Haven, home of the convention's president, Jonathan Knight; New York City; and Philadelphia, home of vice president Bell and also of Hays. Philadelphia was ultimately chosen. Although the minutes do not indicate why, one suspects that since the 1846 convention had almost been dissolved on the grounds that the South and the West were underrepresented, it was probably because Philadelphia, in addition to being the largest medical center in the United States, was also the most southwestern of the cities on the list. It is important to appreciate the difficulty of long cross-country trips in the prerailroad era. Nathan Smith Davis recalled that his trip to the 1847 convention "by the old stage coach . . . took longer to get from the village of Binghamton [New York] to Philadelphia . . . than it does to go [by railroad, in 1897] from Chicago to San Francisco" (Danforth 1907, 75–76).

On Wednesday, May 6, 1846, the resolutions involving the founding of a national medical society were presented to the conference as a whole. This was the moment at which the idea for the national organization that was to become the AMA was first formally proposed. It is noteworthy, therefore, that the proposal was put before the convention, not by Nathan Smith Davis, the young Broome County educational reformer from the village of Binghamton, New York, but by Isaac Hays, the fifty-year-old editor of the leading medical journal of his day, the *American Journal of the Medical Sciences*, and a leading member of the Philadelphia medical establishment. Yet Davis had chaired the education committee. Since in all other cases it was committee chairs who presented the findings of their committees to the conference, the fact that it was Hays, not Davis, who proposed a national medical society is probably significant. (So too is the fact that the proposal was written in Hays's hand and is preserved with Hays's papers.)

Why did Davis not present the proposal to found a national medical society? Perhaps the young Davis lacked the stature necessary to make such a proposal; perhaps the idea was originally Hays's. Certainly the committee's report would embarrass Davis, since it confessed his committee's failure to agree upon measures for educational reform—which, after all, was Davis's issue and the raison d'être not only for the committee but for the conference itself. Worse yet, one of the resolutions on education represented a defeat for Davis's own plan to make the educational establishment accountable by establishing independent review and licensing boards. An ambiguous remark in Hays's notes suggests that Davis, realizing that his conference had failed, permitted Bell,

Bush, Hays, and unnamed others to transform the Davis-Delafield-March conference into an occasion for founding a national medical organization—thereby snatching a victory, of sorts, from the jaws of defeat. We do not know exactly what transpired. Yet Davis was not called upon to chair any of the committees responsible for forming the new national medical society—not even the education committee. Since Davis's claim to the title "founder of the AMA" is based on his proposal to hold the 1846 education conference, then by the same criterion, since Hays was the person who actually proposed founding a national medical society and a conference to found it, Hays would seem to have a greater claim to the title "founder" than Davis.

The penchant for naming individuals as "founders," however, should not obscure the deeper point that, despite the noteworthy contributions of individuals like Davis and Hays, it was ultimately committees and committee work that founded the AMA. The three committees charged with forming the new medical society were chaired by Bell, Hays, and Watson, respectively. Hays's committee had the all-important responsibility of organizing the Philadelphia convention, of assuring attendance by a geographically representative body of delegates—and of garnering a stellar array of medical luminaries to launch the new medical society. As editor of the leading medical journal of his day, Hays was extremely well-connected, but the correspondence indicates that he called upon the services of the entire Philadelphia medical establishment, including his influential mentor Nathaniel Chapman, to attain the desired attendance.

In 1847 Hays welcomed some 268 delegates from twenty-two states to the convention held at the Great Hall of the Philadelphia Academy of Natural Science, more than triple that of the 1846 conference (which registered 119 delegates, although only 80 actually attended). There were also twice as many medical institutions and societies, and nearly double the number of states represented. As anticipated, the southern and the western states had adequate representation. The American medical elite, moreover, attended in force. Among the luminaries were Josiah Bartlett, Nathaniel Chapman, Alonzo Clark, Austin Flint, Oliver Wendell Holmes Sr., Jonathan Knight, Alden March, Edward Phelps, and George Wood.

Hays's work would have come to naught, however, had not Watson's committee (on which Davis served) brought to these delegates an organizational plan that they could accept as the constitution for a national medical organization and had not Bell's committee given the new association a raison d'être beyond technical questions of education—a code of medical ethics that embodied the vision of the ideal physician that would guide the American medical profession triumphantly into the twentieth century. It is difficult to review these events or to read the minutes of the series of meetings that took place in New York and Philadelphia from 1844, when Davis first brought his educational concerns to the attention of the Medical Society of the State of New York, through 1847, when the AMA was actually founded, and attribute the formation of the AMA to any one individual. The spark was undoubtedly Davis's drive for educational reform, but it was Alden March who conceived the idea for a national conference, it was the parliamentary acumen of Lewis Bush that allowed a committee that found itself deadlocked to turn its attention elsewhere, and it was Hays's diplomatic talents that resolved the impasse by creating the proposal for a national medical society. Hays's organizational skill culminated in a successful, truly national meeting at which the constitution drafted by Watson's committee and the code of ethics put forth by Bell's committee were accepted.

Constructing the Myth of "Father Davis"

Why then was Nathan Smith Davis given all the credit for founding the AMA at the jubilee celebrations of 1897? There appear to have been four factors, over and above the proclivity to simplify complex events by creating "heroes": senescence, assertiveness, reticence, and divisiveness. When the semicentennial jubilee meeting was held in 1897, only four people who had attended the 1847 founding conference were still alive: Nathan Smith Davis, Alfred Stillé, John Johnson, and David Atwater. Of these only two—Alfred Stillé of Philadelphia, secretary at the 1846 and 1847 meetings, and Nathan Smith Davis—had attended both meetings. Thus when Davis, an eminent physician and an important member of the AMA, laid claim to the title of "founder," no one, except for Stillé, was in a position to challenge the claim—and Stillé declined to attend the jubilee celebrations, even though they were held in his home city of Philadelphia.

Complementing Davis's assertiveness was the reticence of the other key players, most notably, Bell and Hays. By the time of the jubilee, Bell was a forgotten man. He had died in 1872 and was only dimly remembered as the editor of the long-defunct *Eclectic Journal of Medicine*. Bell's once-brilliant career had faded when he left Philadelphia in 1848 after a bitter public dispute over his failure to receive a professorship at the University of Pennsylvania. After he left Philadelphia, Bell played virtually no role in the national medical organization he had helped to found, and although the AMA continued to publish its code of ethics, Bell's introduction was never reprinted.

Hays, in contrast, remained active in AMA affairs until his sixties, serving as treasurer until 1852 and chairing the committee that edited and published the AMA's official journal, *Transactions*, until 1853. However, Hays never claimed the title of editor of *Transactions*. His reluctance to do so reflects a life-long tendency. In 1827 Hays became founding editor of the *American Journal of the Medical Sciences* (*AJMS*)—an expanded national version of Nathaniel Chapman's *Philadelphia Journal of the Medical Sciences*. Yet unlike Bell, Chapman, and other Philadelphia editors of the period, for almost a decade Hays did not put his name on the cover or the editorial page—even though John Shaw Billings and other cognoscenti referred to the *AJMS* as "Hays's journal." Gradually, however, Hays proclaimed his editorship, first in small print on the inner cover and finally in larger letters on the outer cover. Hays's entire life was a maze of backdoor entries (for example, into the University of Pennsylvania indirectly, through Chapman's private institute), of professorships and public speaking engagements declined, of unsigned articles and editorials. As the anonymous editor of *AJMS* he perfected the art of editorial ventriloquism, putting his own ideas into the words of others. Hays's action at the 1846 convention—stepping forward in a public forum to propose a national medical society—was strikingly uncharacteristic. Hays almost always preferred to act through the agency of others; he instinctively avoided the public stage.

Why did Hays prefer to act discretely offstage, as treasurer or secretary, or working in relative anonymity as an editor? In a memorial minute written for the *Transactions of the College of Physicians of Philadelphia* in 1881, Alfred Stillé remarks on Hays's characteristic diffidence and concludes the memorial notice with the seemingly unrelated remark that Hays was "by birth a Hebrew, [who] through long life adhered to the ancient faith; but while fixed in his own views he was entirely liberal to those of others, often quoting Pope's lines: 'For modes of faith let graceless zealots fight: / His can't be wrong whose life is in the right'" (Stillé 1880, 36).

"Graceless zealots" is as good a description of anti-Semites as any other. It would seem that Hays, a Sephardic Jew, was reluctant to speak in his own voice in public fora because he had been bothered by "graceless zealots." Privately, in Philadelphia's medical and scientific circles (most notably the American Philosophical Society), Hays was a respected and influential figure—as he was within the inner circles of the AMA. Yet in public fora, where zealotry might make itself evident, he was circumspect and often self-effacing—except in 1846 when he uncharacteristically played a public role by proposing the founding of a national medical association and the drafting of a national code of medical ethics.

But collective senescence, coupled with Davis's assertiveness and Hays's reticence, were not the only factors underlying the AMA's enthusiastic embrace of the myth that Nathan Smith Davis had single-handedly founded the organization. In 1897 the AMA needed a unifying figure around whom the organization could rally. As John Harley Warner and Rosemary Stevens discuss in detail in chapters 3 and 4 of this volume, in the 1880s the AMA was being torn apart by the controversy over its Code of Ethics and, more generally, over the tension between specialists and generalists. The specialists wanted a scientific society that would leave medical and ethical standards to the individual practitioner; the generalists wanted a medical society that would develop common medical and ethical standards. In the end, the specialists began to bolt the organization and the AMA was in danger of dissolving. Davis played a key role in holding the organization together. Wherever possible he brokered compromises to woo the dissident breakaway New York medical society and the specialists back into the AMA. Thus Davis's *JAMA* became a more scientific journal, closer to the ideals of specialists than Hays's *Transactions*. Davis stood for scientific progress, for educational reform, and for a reasonable code of ethics. He represented everything to which the AMA aspired. Davis may have aggrandized his role as founder, but as "Father Davis" he was empowered to play the unifying role that the AMA desperately needed. Had Davis not existed, the AMA would have needed to invent him. But there he was, in the fatherly flesh, laying a seemingly impeccable historical claim to being the founder of the AMA, even as he acted as a unifying figure during the organization's hour of need. Not unnaturally, his claims to being the founder were enthusiastically embraced by a grateful organization.

New Wine, Old Bottles: Bell, Hays, Percival, and the 1847 Code

In the 1870s, as the AMA's Code of Ethics became increasingly more controversial, its defenders found it ever easier to attribute its content to the eminent and eminently English Manchester physician Thomas Percival. The collaboration between two of the founders of the AMA, the now-forgotten teetotaling Protestant abolitionist John Bell and the elusive Sephardic Jew Isaac Hays, was ignored—except for the incident of a note that Isaac Hays, characteristically reticent to appear on a public platform, had John Bell read to the convention. This note underpins the "parroting Percival" interpretation of the Code of Ethics offered by Leake, Fishbein, and almost all later scholars of the code.

The members of the Convention, [Hays] observed, would not fail to recognize in parts of it, expressions with which they were familiar. On examining
a great number of codes of ethics adopted by different societies in the United
States, it was found that they were all based on that by Dr. Percival, and that
the phrases of this writer were preserved, to a considerable extent, in all of
them. *Believing that language that had been so often examined and adopted,
must possess the greatest of merits for a document such as the present, clearness
and precision, and having no ambition for the honours of authorship, the Committee which prepared this code have followed a similar course, and have carefully preserved the words of Percival wherever they convey the precepts it is
wished to inculcate. A few of the sections are in the words of the late Dr. Rush,
and one or two sentences are from other writers.* But in all cases, wherever it was
thought that the language could be made more explicit by changing a word,
or even a part of a sentence, this has been unhesitatingly done; and thus there
are but few sections which have not undergone some modification; while,
for the language of many, and for the arrangement of the whole, the Committee must be held exclusively responsible. (Isaac Hays, Note to Convention; see Appendix A, this volume. Italics added.)

The italic section—quoted by Fishbein (1947, 35) and relied on by almost all
interpreters—emphasizes parroting. Yet the sentence that follows suggests extensive modification, innovation, and editing, "unhesitatingly done," since all
but a few sections have "undergone some modification." The committee also
claims responsibility "for the language of many [sections] and for the arrangement of the whole." Thus, although Hays claims that the committee (primarily Bell and Hays[1]) "preserved the words of Percival," he is also claiming to
have edited, modified, extended, and reorganized them. The parroting thesis,
in effect, emphasizes the first claim but ignores the second claim entirely.

   The parroting thesis also ignores Bell's lengthy introduction to the Code of
Ethics—a document that is never mentioned by commentators on the code,
perhaps because it was never officially reprinted by the AMA. In his introduction, Bell characterizes the Code of Ethics as a form of "medical deontology,"[2] asserting what is now known as "the applied ethics model"—that is, Bell
claims that "as a branch of general ethics, medical ethics must rest on the basis of religion and morality" (Appendix B, 317). According to Bell, the specific
moral-religious principle that was applied to generate the 1847 Code of Ethics
was the principle of reciprocity: that "every duty or obligation implies, both
in equity and for its successful discharge, a corresponding right" (317). This
principle entails that insofar as a community believes that the physician is "required to expose his health and life for the benefit of the community, [the

physician, in reciprocity] has a just claim . . . on all [the community's] members, collectively and individually for aid to carry out his measures" (317). The practical implication of Bell's analysis was that if physicians were "true to themselves, by a close adherence to their duties, and by firmly yet mildly insisting on their rights" (322), society was obligated to reciprocate by granting their demands.

Bell's political strategy was exhilarating, but the new conceptual framework was a convention politician's nightmare. The AMA had been conceived out of intellectual gridlock. One could not reasonably expect that the always contentious, preeminently practical physicians at the AMA's founding convention would immediately endorse such innovative but "highfalutin'" notions as applied ethics, "medical deontology," or "the principle of reciprocity." Bell's innovations thus presented an extraordinary challenge, even to someone with Hays's gifts as a "convention floor politician." Hays's response, for which he was well suited from a lifetime's practice in editorial ventriloquism, was to pour the heady new wine of Bell's applied ethical reforms into older Percivalean bottles. He did this by means of an exceptional bit of stagecraft—the note that he had Bell read to the convention. By having the eminently Protestant Bell read the note, while he himself remained offstage, Hays deftly avoided unsettling questions about the right of a Jew to dictate ethics to an assemblage of Christians. This brilliant convention-floor strategy was further reinforced by the central claim of the note that "having no ambitions of authorship, the Committee which prepared this code . . . have carefully preserved the words of Percival . . . [adding some] words of the late Dr. Rush" (Appendix A, 315). The claim not only obviated potential objections from "graceless zealots" on the convention floor but also, by grounding the code in the "familiar" words of Percival and Rush—ostensibly the common source material for earlier American codes of ethics—headed off debates about Bell's innovative ideas and potentially fractious disputes over the actual wording of specific sections of the code.

Hays's strategy worked. On Friday morning, May 7, 1847, the founding convention of the organization soon to be called the American Medical Association discussed Bell and Hays's code. After a motion to amend one of the articles failed, Dr. Lewis C. Bush of Delaware—the same Dr. Bush who had made the parliamentary motion that paved the way for the formation of the AMA at the 1846 convention—called for the question. The motion to approve the code passed unanimously, and the American Medical Association had a code of ethics (see Baker 1995 for details).

Fishbein misreads the drama and import of these events, actually commending Hays for ingenuously admitting a form of plagiarism that had been duplicitously concealed by the authors of earlier codes: "Isaac Hays stated clearly that the code had been derived from that of Percival and thus neatly reprimanded the New York and Baltimore societies which adopted these codes without giving credit to Percival" (Fishbein 1947, 37). Yet the authors of the 1823 New York System of Ethics—James Manley, Felix Pascalis, and John Steele—and of the 1832 Baltimore System of Ethics—E. Geddings, Thomas Wright, John Fonerden, H. Willis Baxley, and John Graves—fully documented their sources, giving Percival credit, wherever credit was due him. If they gave even more credit to John Gregory than to Percival, it was because their debt to Gregory was deeper. Thus if we ignore, for the moment, the fact that, unlike Hays, these earlier codifiers always claimed authorship of the codes they produced, the most significant difference between these earlier codes and Bell and Hays's AMA Code is that the earlier codes drew extensively from the work of Gregory, while Bell and Hays's code virtually eliminates Gregorean influences.

As Table 1 indicates, a detailed analysis of the three sections of the 5,283-word AMA Code shows that approximately two-thirds of the material in the 1847 Code of Ethics derives primarily from *Extracts from Percival's Medical Ethics* (1826), while the remaining third is almost evenly divided between original material (some borrowed from earlier American codes) and material borrowed primarily from Rush. There is virtually no material from Gregory. With the exception of the 1808 *Boston Medical Police*, no earlier American code of ethics incorporated Percival's words so extensively or exclusively; and no earlier code had so utterly abandoned Gregory. Thus while Hays was entirely truthful in proclaiming that the 1847 Code, like its precursors, derived from Percival, he neglected to point out that, unlike its precursors, it was not Gregorean. To suggest that the 1847 Code was innovative, however, would have been impolitic. Hays, as always, was politic to a fault.

It is important to appreciate that the major source for most of the words in the 1847 Code is not Percival's *Medical Ethics* itself but, as Leake (1922) noted, the *Extracts from Percival's Medical Ethics*, published by the Philadelphia branch of the Kappa Lambda Society of Hippocrates in 1826. This observation is important, not only because the various Kappa Lambda editions of Percival Americanize Percival's very British status-conscious hospital-oriented code of ethics, adapting it to private-practice medicine in egalitarian America (Baker 1993), but also because the editors of the 1826 edition of the *Extracts* were none other than John Bell and Isaac Hays (Baker 1997). In 1846, when Bell and Hays accepted the roles of chair and secretary of the code of ethics

Table 1. Major Sources of the 1847 Code of Ethics

	Words in 1847 Code		
Code Section	*No.*	*%*	*Major Source*
Chap. I, Art. I	767	14.5	Kappa Lambda edition of Percival
Chap. I, Art. II	977	18.5	Rush via 1832 Baltimore Code
Chap. II	2870	54	Kappa Lambda edition of Percival
Chap. III	699	13	Original material
Total	5283	100	

Note: A major source is the source of more than half of the words in a section. Many phrases have multiple sources (e.g., a phrase from Gregory, reiterated in Percival, that is echoed in the Boston Medical Police and preserved in the Baltimore Code).

drafting committee, they were reprising the roles they had played twenty years previously as publisher and editor of the 1826 Kappa Lambda edition. Thus, the "carefully preserved words of Percival" reiterated in the 1847 Code were those that Bell and Hays had trimmed and salted for American consumption two decades earlier.

American Egalitarianism and the Tragedy of Kappa Lambda

In many ways the most significant feature of the code of ethics that Bell and Hays prepared for the AMA was that it broke with precedent by excluding Gregorean influences. Why did Bell and Hays craft a non-Gregorian code of ethics? To appreciate their reasons it is helpful to review the series of events that Leake calls the "tragedy" of Kappa Lambda. The Kappa Lambda Societies of Hippocrates were secret societies, probably founded in Britain in the late nineteenth century, dedicated to reforming medicine by recruiting honorable, learned, and talented persons into the medical profession, while excluding all others (Baker 1997; van Ingen 1945). The notion of recruiting the talented and honorable, while excluding the untalented and dishonorable, is a natural extension of the prevalent British belief that medical success was a function of inherited talent and that medical morality was an extension of the moral character of the person into the practice of medicine. From this perspective, the only way to improve medical practice was to improve the quality of medical practitioners. (The English physician Thomas Beddoes [1760–1808] proposed a similar reform in 1802, although there is no evidence that he was a member of Kappa Lambda; see Beddoes 1802; Porter 1993.)

This very British understanding of moral reform in medicine was challenged in 1820 by the American physician Samuel Brown (1769–1830), a professor of medicine who became head of the local chapter of the Lexington, Kentucky, chapter of Kappa Lambda. Brown was a Percivalean who believed that moral reform in medicine should address doctors' conduct. To implement Brown's views, the Lexington chapter of the Kappa Lambda Society published the first American edition of Percival's code of ethics, *Extracts from Medical Ethics* (1821), and sought to establish new chapters of Kappa Lambda, whose membership would pledge itself to adhere to the precepts of Percival's code. Brown's ideas found an enthusiastic adherent in Dr. Samuel Jackson (1787–1872), professor of medicine at the University of Pennsylvania, who founded a Percivalean branch of the society in Philadelphia in 1823. In 1826 the Philadelphia society commissioned two of its members—John Bell and Isaac Hays—to publish a revised edition of *Extracts from Percival's Medical Ethics*. In the same year the Philadelphia society began to publish the *North American Medical and Surgical Journal* (1826–29).

These noticeably public activities put the newer code-oriented Percivalean branches of the Kappa Lambda Society in Lexington and Philadelphia at odds with the older oath-oriented secret societies in New York and Washington, D.C. A heated correspondence ensued in which the oath-oriented branches strove to preserve the secrecy of the society, while the code-oriented branches pressed for publicity. The issue was taken out of the hands of the membership in 1830, when an anonymous whistle-blowing letter to the Medical Society of the State of New York revealed the existence of a "Secret Medical Society" that controlled senior appointments at New York Hospital and at the Lying-in Hospital. A special investigative committee found that the members of the New York Kappa Lambda Society controlled "an unjust monopoly of the emoluments and honors of the profession" and charged it with usurping the name of Hippocrates to put a patina of honor on the shameless pursuit of personal advantage. It also advised all men of honorable character to resign from Kappa Lambda.

Not everyone took their advice; secret Kappa Lambda societies continued in New York and elsewhere for at least another thirty years. The Philadelphians, however, took the censure of the investigative committee seriously and dissolved their branch of the Kappa Lambda Society of Hippocrates on February 5, 1835. (For a full account, see Baker 1997.)

At the core of the Kappa Lambda controversy lay a fundamental question about the nature of medical morality: Was it primarily a function of character or of conduct? If morality was essentially a matter of character, then the oath-oriented secret societies (and the British institutions from which they were descended) were right to exclude the unworthy from positions of authority and power. But if morality was a matter of conduct, then positions of authority and power should be open to anyone and everyone who conducted themselves properly. Nineteenth-century British society was elitist and inegalitarian and thus readily accepted the idea that ethics was inherently a matter of personal character. After the election of Andrew Jackson as president in 1828, however, American society took a decidedly egalitarian anti-elitist turn. Elites and elitist organizations were deemed incompatible with American democratic ideals of an open, socially egalitarian society based on achievement—that is, on conduct—rather than presumptions of elevated character. Elitist organizations everywhere were under attack, and formal statements of conduct—ethical codes—began to supplant the earlier ethics of character and gentlemanly honor. The tragedy of Kappa Lambda taught Bell and Hays that the ethics of character was ultimately elitist and thus incompatible with the Jacksonian egalitarian ideals. This lesson would inform the Percivalean code of conduct that they would draft for the AMA sixteen years later.

Gregorian and Percivalean Codes: A Comparison

Gregorian ethics of character and Percivalean codes of conduct and deportment differ significantly. Bard, Gregory, Rush, and other medical educators tended to focus on questions of character because they addressed their lectures to medical students in their formative years, when their moral character might still be molded. Percival, however, had to deal with fully qualified physicians working in acute care institutional settings whose character was, for better or worse, fully formed. Unable to influence physicians' underlying character, Percival naturally focused on something that he could hope to influence, their conduct and deportment. Consequently, his codes were designed to guide the conduct and deportment of whomever happened to play the role of physician or surgeon. The emphasis on conduct also permitted Percival to focus on the procedures for moral problem solving and for developing a professional consensus on appropriate conduct, subjects that were largely ignored in the earlier character-focused literature.

Before 1847 almost all American medical societies subscribed to codes predicated on a fundamentally Gregorian ethics of character, which were overlaid with a few Percivalean strictures on conduct usually concerning consultation. Consider, as an illustrative example, the two codes singled out by Fishbein: the 1823 New York *System of Ethics* and the 1832 Baltimore *System of Ethics*. Both codes open with a properly Gregorian discussion of the "Personal

Character of Physicians." The earlier 1823 New York *System of Ethics* opens as follows:

> It would be difficult to determine which of the three learned professions in society requires the most virtue, or the most purity or perfection of personal character. . . .
> 1. A physician cannot successfully pass through his career without the aid of much fortitude of mind, and a religious sense of all his obligations of conscience, honor, and humanity. His personal character should therefore be that of a perfect gentleman, and above all, be exempt from vulgarity of manners, habitual swearing, drunkenness, gambling, or any species of debauchery, and contempt for religious practice and feelings. (Medical Society of the State of New York 1823, 7)

The later 1832 Baltimore *System of Medical Ethics* opens with an even lengthier discussion of the character of the physician:

> No situation in life can exact a more rigid adherence to the principles of virtue, integrity, benevolence and humanity, than that of the physician. Indeed, the very nature of his profession renders it requisite that he should possess the utmost purity of character; for to medical men are confided the dearest and most important interests of human nature. Not only are they the guardians of health, and the ministers whose duty it is to soften the pillow of sorrow and affliction, but to them also are entrusted the lives, the honor, and the reputation of their patients. As therefore, all ranks and conditions of society are subject to the diseases and the casualties which embitter existence, all are alike dependent upon them for the exercise of their skill and benevolence. . . . The couch of splendor and the squalid cot are alternatively the scenes of their benevolent actions; and the calls of distress, from whatever quarter they emanate, are obeyed with alacrity, regardless of all personal considerations of comfort, fortune, health or even life. They restring the severed chords of mind; encourage and animate drooping spirits; fortify the resolution; temper the perverted judgment; dispel the withering phantoms which dethrone the powers of intellect; pluck out the strings of affliction and mollify the poignancy of grief and despair. In their bosom, too, we find a safe depository for our cares and our confidence, and in their sympathies and friendly admonitions, a mitigation of many of the ills and troubles of existence.—Confident in their virtue and integrity, we can unbosom to them our most secret thoughts and reflections—expose our faults and our foibles—our vices and delinquencies, and while we are encouraged by them to firmness under affliction, and to probity and virtue in our actions,

we are secure against any violation of our confidence, or exposures of our faults or infirmities. For all these acts then, how great are the obligations of the community to the medical profession, and how well earned the high and unlimited respect and confidence which it has at all times secured wherever its duties have been expressed with honor, integrity and humanity!—To merit and preserve this esteem and confidence, the Father of Physic exacted of all his disciples a solemn oath enjoining the practice of every virtue. It has, indeed, been a custom in civilized communities, with enlightened and honorable physicians, to establish, and religiously observe, certain rules of etiquette, calculated to maintain its honor and dignity inviolate, and to cherish and preserve a sentiment of good feeling amongst its members. A departure from these rules should be considered as a degradation of the medical character, and a flagrant violation of the principles of honor. (Medico-Chirurgical Society of Baltimore 1832, 5–7)

These Gregorian discussions of the character of the physician serve as the moral platform underlying both the New York and the Baltimore codes. The New York *System* states that a physician's "personal character should be that of a gentleman," for it is a gentlemanly "fortitude of mind," and a gentlemanly acceptance of "obligations of conscience, honor and humanity" that, when extended into medicine, form the basis of the system of ethics enumerated in the code. The Baltimore *System* also opens with the claim that physicians "should possess the utmost purity of character." "Enlightened and honorable physicians" thus naturally follow the precedent set by "the Father of Physic," Hippocrates, by swearing "a solemn oath enjoining the practice of every virtue." In "civilized communities," they also "establish, and religiously observe, certain rules of etiquette, calculated to maintain its honor and dignity inviolate, and to cherish and preserve a sentiment of good feeling amongst its members."

Notice that the Baltimore *System* represents itself as a set of "rules of etiquette" that virtuous and honorable medical gentlemen in civilized societies agree upon to regulate their interactions *with each other.* This claim is mirrored in the structure of the Baltimore *System of Ethics,* which opens with a discussion of the "Duties of Physicians to each other" and continues with "Duties of the Faculty in relation to quackery," "Conduct to be observed in relation to consultations," and "Duties of Physicians relative to the pecuniary compensation for their services." Only in the fifth and last section does the Baltimore *System* turn to patients, and then in a way antithetical to modern expectations—the section is about "Duties of Patients towards their Physician."

The contrast between these earlier medical society codes of gentlemanly honor and etiquette and Bell and Hays's 1847 AMA Code of Ethics is striking.

The first and most arresting difference is that, unlike the New York and Baltimore *Systems*, the AMA Code opens, as we today would expect a proper code of medical ethics to open, with a discussion of the physician's duties toward patients:

> Chapter One. Of the Duties of Physicians to Their Patients, and of the Obligations of Patients to Their Physicians
> Art. I. Duties of Physicians to Their Patients
> 1. *A physician should not only be ever ready to obey the calls of the sick, but his mind ought also to be imbued with the greatness of his mission, and of the responsibility he habitually incurs in its discharge. Those obligations are the more deep and enduring, because there is no tribunal other than his own conscience, to adjudge penalties for carelessness or neglect.* Physicians should, *therefore,* minister to the sick with due impressions of the importance of their office; reflecting that the ease, the health, and the lives of those committed to their charge, depend on their skill, attention and fidelity. They should study, also, in their deportment, so to unite tenderness with firmness, and condescension with authority, as to inspire the minds of their patients with gratitude, respect and confidence.
> 2. Every case committed to the charge of a physician should be treated with attention, steadiness and humanity. Reasonable indulgence should be granted to the mental imbecility and caprices of the sick. Secrecy and delicacy, when required by peculiar circumstances, should be strictly observed; and the familiar and confidential intercourse to which physicians are admitted in their professional visits, should be used with discretion, and with the most scrupulous regard to fidelity and honor. The obligation of secrecy extends beyond the period of professional services—none of the privacies of personal and domestic life, no infirmity of disposition or flaw of character observed during professional attendance, should ever be divulged by him except when he is imperatively required to do so. *The force and necessity of this obligation are indeed so great, that professional men have, under certain circumstances, been protected in their observance of secrecy by courts of justice.* (Appendix C, 324)

In reading this code, it is important to distinguish the 94 words (here in italics) that were added in 1846–47 by Bell and Hays from the 188 words taken directly from the 1826 Kappa Lambda edition of *Extracts from Percival's Medical Ethics,* which Bell and Hays had edited twenty years earlier.[3] The italic words added by Bell and Hays, in striking contrast to the earlier *Systems,* open the AMA code with a statement of physicians' duties to their patients, not with a discussion of the physician's own character. Thus the AMA Code, which refers to itself unambiguously as a code of medical ethics, looks beyond physicians' solipsistic concerns with personal virtue to focus on their mission and their professional duties—treating as first among their professional duties, their duties to their patients.

The transformation from a virtue ethic to a professional ethic resonates in details of language and construction. The Baltimore *System* employs the term *virtue* four times in the opening passage alone, whereas the AMA Code employs the term only once in the entire code. In contrast, the term *professional* is used four times in the opening passage of the AMA Code and thirty-three additional times in the text. The New York *System of Ethics* quotes a line from Gregory—that "there is no tribunal other than [a physician's] own conscience, to adjudge penalties for carelessness or neglect" (Medical Society of the State of New York 1823, 7)—to establish the need for the "purity and perfection of [the] *personal* character" of the physician (emphasis added). Bell and Hays appeal to the same line to make the case for physicians' professional "obligations." Thus, the italic *therefore* in the passage quoted above transforms a traditional Gregorian appeal to the purity and perfection of character into a Percivalean argument for physicians' professional obligations. Throughout the AMA Code, moreover, Gregorian virtues—attention, authority, condescension, fidelity, firmness, humanity, skill, steadiness, tenderness—are systematically converted into Percivalean duties of deportment.

The 1847 AMA Code is also revolutionary in marrying Percivalean ethics to Jacksonian egalitarianism and anti-elitism. This wedding is evident in the italic words with which Bell and Hays open the code. Their first words do not parrot anything in Percival; they state, in new non-Percivalean language, a non-Percivalean duty—albeit a duty that had been central to the American traditions of medical morality from the colonial period onward—the duty to "obey the calls of the sick." This duty, a natural artifact of the frontier experience, is discernible in American codes of moral conduct as early as the New York Midwives Oath of 1715 and was reiterated in both the 1823 New York and the 1832 Baltimore *System*(s).[4] It requires that physicians make emergency calls when summoned by anyone who is sick, irrespective of social status or wealth. Before 1847, however, a physician's responsibility for making emergency calls to everyone, including the poor, had been construed as accouterment of gentlemanly character. Thus, the authors of the New York *System of Ethics* note that failure to "afford some attention to the poor" would be "proof of [a physician's] selfishness [and] want of humanity"; while the authors of the Baltimore *System of Ethics* remark that gentlemen do not "exercise unfeeling rigor in the collection of fees" (Medico-Chirurgical Society of Baltimore

1832, sec. IV, art. V, p. 15). The AMA Code, in contrast, converts this gentlemanly virtue into a professional duty: "Poverty . . . should always be recognised as presenting valid claims for gratuitous service . . . [which] should always be cheerfully and freely accorded" (chap. III, art. I, sec. 3).

The 1847 American Medical Ethics Revolution

The 1847 AMA Code of Ethics thus represents a twofold revolution: the revolutionary transformation of an ethics of character into an ethics of conduct, and the substantive moral transformation of Percival's status-sensitive morality into an egalitarian ethic acceptable to Jacksonian America. These two revolutions transform an earlier ethic of gentlemanly virtue, which had been based on notions of status and prerogative, into an egalitarian professional medical ethics based on ideals reciprocity; and these, in turn, transform the underlying logic of American medical ethics into that of a social contract.

To appreciate the logical underpinnings of these revolutionary transformations, it is important to analyze the way in which the actual text of the code was constructed. The text appears to have been edited almost entirely by Hays, who used the editorial process, specifically the insertion of titles and subtitles, to reconfigure *Extracts from Percival's Medical Ethics* to conform to Bell's principle of reciprocity. Hays's chapter titles are as follows: chapter 1, "Of the Duties of Physicians to Their Patients, and of the Obligations of Patients to Their Physicians"; chapter 2, "Of the Duties of Physicians to Each Other and to the Profession at Large"; and chapter 3, "Of the Duties of the Profession to the Public, and of the Obligations of the Public to the Profession." Although these titles do not in themselves change a line of Percival's text, by parsing the duties later enumerated as reciprocal duties that each of the four named parties— physicians, patients, profession, and public—owe to each other, the titles and subtitles restructure the code as a quadrilateral social contract. Thus, simply by adding titles and subtitles, by modifying the "arrangement of the whole"— an act for which Hays, or at least his "committee [accepts] exclusive responsibility"—Hays made Percival's words conform to Bell's principle of reciprocity. The effect of this technique, which Hays had no doubt honed to perfection through a lifetime of editorial ventriloquism, was to reconfigure the code into a quadrilateral social contract between physicians, patients, profession, and the public without changing a single line of text.

Yet Hays's contractarian "arrangement of the whole" had significant implications for the interpretation of the words in the text. As historian Stanley Reiser (1995) observed, "What will strike the modern mind as a great point of difference between present-day codes and the 1847 code is the burden the 1847 code placed on patients' relationships to physicians" (89–90). In Britain, this burden had been justified by the inferior status of the hospital patient. American egalitarianism allowed no such presumption, so American physicians needed an alternative justification.

The Americanization of the status-based British concept of patient gratitude commenced with an 1808 lecture that Dr. Benjamin Rush delivered to his students at the University of Pennsylvania, in which Rush justifies the patient's gratitude as a form of nonmonetary compensation for the sacrifices of physicians. Rush's lecture, as it happened, was reprinted in 1831 as an appendix to the American edition of Michael Ryan's *Medical Jurisprudence,* and in that form it provided source material for section 5 of the Baltimore *System of Ethics*—the section on patients' duties to their physicians.

The authors of the Baltimore *System* observe that section 5 states what physicians "certainly have a right to require and expect" from their patients, since physicians make "so many sacrifices of comfort, ease, and health, for the welfare of those who employ them."

> IX. A patient should, after recovery, allow his physician due credit, and not, as is too often the case, forget his services as soon as there is no longer any occasion for them. He should also feel it his duty to remunerate him properly for these services. To qualify him for the exercise of the service he has rendered, [his physician] has spent his youth in painful, and in some instances, disgusting studies. He has, perhaps, visited foreign countries, and either at home or abroad, expended the whole of his patrimonial property in acquiring a knowledge of his profession. To enable him to get into business, he has passed the first seven or ten years of his life in laboring for nothing among the poor, and in deriving from fortuitous business only a bare subsistence. From the deduction of the time that has been mentioned and from the premature death or old age induced by his labors, the years in which it is possible for him to accumulate property, are reduced to a small number. His whole life during these years is one continued stream of labor, self-denial, and solicitude. (Medical-Chirurgical Society of Baltimore 1832, 22–23)

Compare the above passage with the comparable passage in the 1847 AMA Code:

> 10. A patient should, after his recovery, entertain a just and enduring sense of the value of the services rendered him by his physician; for these are of

such a character, that no mere pecuniary acknowledgment can repay or cancel them. (327)

Notice that the pathos is absent. No litany of personal sacrifices was enumerated to justify the patient's duty of giving the physician his due in the AMA Code. Why? Because in the AMA Code, reciprocity is not grounded in the personal sacrifice of physicians but upon Bell's ethical principle of reciprocity—which Hays had converted into a social contract.

Like any other contract, Hays's social contract involves a *quid pro quo* between each of the four parties, including physicians and patients. Thus, since physicians undertake professional duties of deportment and conduct toward their patients (detailed in chap. I, art. I), patients owe their physicians reciprocal duties of deportment and conduct (detailed in chap. I, art. II). Consequently, Hays's social contract requires that each of the positive duties that physicians have toward their patients—to "obey the calls of the sick," to treat every patient attentively, faithfully, skillfully, tenderly, with attention, confidentially, humanity and steadiness—and each of the negative duties—not overcharging and not "abandoning a patient because the case is deemed incurable"—be matched by reciprocal positive and negative duties that patients have toward their physicians. For example, since the primary positive duty of professional physicians is to promptly and immediately "obey the calls of the sick," reciprocity requires that "the obedience of the patient to the prescriptions of his physician should," in turn, "be prompt and implicit" (chap. I, art. II, sec. 6).

Other physician duties also generate reciprocal patient duties: physician confidentiality is to be reciprocated by the patient's free and open communication with physicians; physicians' duties to be formally educated are reciprocated by patients' obligation to take medical advice only from formally educated medical practitioners; the attention and fidelity of the physician to the patient is to be reciprocated by the devotion and fidelity of the patient to the physician; and, since physicians are duty-bound not to abandon their patients and not to overcharge them, patients are held to have the reciprocal negative obligations of not abandoning their physicians and of not ignoring their doctor's bills. As to article 10, it is correlative to the generally transcendent duties of physicians toward their patients. Since physicians are obligated to come when called, irrespective of the prospect of payment, they are entitled, in turn, to an appreciation of "the value of the services rendered," irrespective of the money paid.

Hays's editorial art not only transforms Bell's principle of reciprocity into a fourfold social contract but also gives patients implicit demand rights against physicians. None of the earlier noncontractarian systems of ethics contains a statement of physicians' duties to their patients. In contrast, the AMA Code of Ethics, by virtue of its contractarian structure, vests patients with specific reciprocal rights that they can demand from their physicians. Patients have the right to be attended to immediately in medical emergencies, and "individuals in indigent circumstances" have a right to "professional services . . . cheerfully and freely accorded" (chap. III, art. I, sec. 3). These demand rights revolutionize the patient-physician relationship. For the first time in the history of medical ethics, patients could demand conduct from their physicians as a matter of right, irrespective of the physician's aspirations toward virtue at any particular moment.

Ironically, this revolutionary reconceptualization of the patient-physician relationship tends to be overlooked today because reciprocal demand rights seem weak by comparison with the more absolute rights that were later to be vested in human research subjects by the 1947 Nuremberg Principles, and in patients by the 1973 American Hospital Association's Patients' Bill of Rights. By adopting Bell and Hays's code of ethics in 1847, however, the American medical profession became the first to envision their relationship with their patients and with the public in terms of a social contract, and thus the first to recognize that patients had demand rights exercisable against individual physicians and that the public had rights against the profession more generally.

The latter is also an often-overlooked landmark in the history of medical ethics. It is significant, however, that the contractarian structure of the 1847 Code of Ethics gives the public specific demand rights against the medical profession. These are developed in the one chapter that consists of entirely new material written by Bell and Hays, chapter 3, "Of Duties of the Profession to the Public, and of the Public to the Profession." In the earlier codes, physicians were envisioned as offering community service as a mark of gentlemanly character. Thus, the preamble to the Baltimore *System* states that physicians, acting from "benevolence," may "point out salutary instructions by the adoption of which mankind may be secured against the incursions of disease and death, and by which, health . . . may be preserved. By their benevolent admonitions they warn us of the dangers that surround us, and devise means for their avoidance or removal." Chapter 3 of Bell and Hays's social contract converts this personal virtue into a professional obligation:

Article I. *Duties of the Profession to the Public*
1. As good citizens, it is the duty of physicians to be ever vigilant for the welfare of the community, and to bear their part in sustaining its institutions and burdens: they should also be ever ready to give counsel to the public in relation to matters especially appertaining to their profession, as on subjects of medical police, public hygiene, and legal medicine. It is their province to enlighten the public in regard to quarantine regulations . . . and in regard to measures for the prevention of epidemic and contagious diseases; and when pestilence prevails, it is their duty to face the danger, and to continue their labors for the alleviation of the suffering, even at the jeopardy of their own lives. (Appendix C, 333)

The transformation from virtue to duty is particularly striking in the case of duties during epidemics. Whereas the Baltimore *System* had encouraged physicians to display their virtuousness by healing and consoling amidst "the darkness of pestilence," the AMA Code of Ethics obligates physicians to attend to the sick during epidemics as a matter of public duty. Attending the epidemic-stricken sick was not optional but virtuous conduct; it was a form of mandatory duty. No previous statement of medical morality had ever made refusal to treat the epidemic-stricken sick a censurable offense. This is a tough standard even in the context of today's heightened moral standards. What makes it more remarkable, however, is that in 1847, with the single exception of smallpox, physicians had no vaccines or other means of protecting themselves against infectious disease. There is thus no hyperbole in the line in the AMA Code that states that exercising the duty to "alleviate the suffering" of the epidemic-stricken would jeopardize physicians' lives.

Since the duties enumerated in the AMA Code of Ethics were reciprocal, article 2 of chapter 3 stated three reciprocal obligations of the public to physicians: "a just appreciation of medical qualifications," "a proper discrimination between true science and the assumption of ignorance and empiricism," and finally, "no longer to allow the statute books to exhibit the anomaly of exacting knowledge from physicians, under liability to heavy penalties, and of making them obnoxious to punishment for resorting to the only means of obtaining it." This last reference was to statutes criminalizing the dissection of cadavers—which was especially important at the time because the new knowledge of anatomy made possible new methods of treating trauma (e.g., setting compound fractures and treating wounds) that represented the most significant advances in mid-nineteenth-century medicine. These seem to be relatively modest requests, at least by comparison with the reciprocal duties undertaken by physicians—to treat the public even in epidemics and to treat the poor gratis. Yet, as we shall see in the next section, read in conjunction with chapter 2, article 4, section 1, they form the basis of the most common scholarly misreading of the AMA Code of Ethics.

Reinterpreting the American Medical Association's Code of Ethics

The myths created by the AMA about its origins were intended to insulate the organization from controversies over its Code of Ethics; however, by distancing the organization from its code, they naturally raise questions about the code's actual function, thereby laying the foundation for what was to become the received scholarly interpretation of the code. In 1927 Chauncey Leake, a medical reformer in the muckraking tradition, adduced the first scholarly analysis supporting the claim that the code was merely a set of "trade union rules" designed to protect an AMA monopoly on medical practice. In his introduction to a new edition of Percival's *Medical Ethics* (1927), Leake asserted that Percival had made a fundamental semantic error, erroneously applying the label "medical ethics" to rules of medical etiquette. Thus, since Hays's Note to the Convention clearly established that the code merely parroted Percival's words and ideas, Leake concluded that the AMA had perpetuated Percival's semantic misnomer in its so-called Code of Ethics—undoubtedly finding it convenient to give their "trade union rules" the honorific title "medical ethics."

Leake's debunking analysis was soon the received scholarly view—Fishbein even accepted it in his 1947 centennial history. A few decades later, sociologist Jeffrey Berlant was to use Leake's analysis as the basis for his delegitimating Weberian critique of professional prerogative and power in his 1975 monograph *Profession and Monopoly*. In the process, Berlant modernized Leake's semantic analysis of the ethics-etiquette "error" (the height of scholarly fashion in the twenties, but hopelessly dated in the seventies) by providing a socioeconomic analysis designed to show that the AMA was parading Percival's "etiquette" to disguise its true intent—"monopolizing" the medical marketplace by driving out homeopaths and other irregular practitioners. Sociologist-historian Paul Starr incorporated this analysis into his monumental *Social Transformation of American Medicine* (1982), arguing that "while monopoly was doubtless the intent of the AMA's program, it was not the consequence; the irregulars thrived" (91). The Leake-Berlant-Starr analysis has since been reiterated in virtually all of the more recent histories of nineteenth-century American medicine (Haller [1981] being a notable exception), and it is now the received scholarly interpretation of the AMA's 1847 Code of Ethics.

Yet while claims of "semantic confusion" and "monopolization" sound wonderful in reformist polemics, they rest on remarkably shaky historical premises. Leake's semantic confusion hypothesis, for example, has no basis whatsoever in the actual texts of *Medical Ethics*. It is true that Percival coined the expression "medical ethics," but it is also true that he appears to have been the first writer to use the term "etiquette" in a medical context. Both expressions, moreover, are used in the modern sense. Thus Percival characterizes *medical ethics* as "moral rules of conduct prescribed towards . . . patients" (chap. II, art. I), and he uses *etiquette* in remarks like the following: the "amicable intercourse and co-operation of the physician and apothecary, if conducted with the decorum and attention to etiquette . . . will add to the authority of the one, the respectability of the other, and to the usefulness of both" (chap. III, art. III). It is clear from this passage that Percival equates etiquette with decorum, and not with the "moral rules of conduct prescribed towards patients" (i.e., not with "medical ethics"). The man who coined the expression "medical ethics" clearly intended his coinage to be used in the way that we still use it today; there simply is no textual evidence suggesting otherwise (see Baker 1993; Haakonssen 1997; McCullough 1998; Pellegrino 1985; Pickstone 1993).

By contrast, the charge that the AMA Code of Ethics is "monopolistic" has a clear textual basis in chapter II, article IV, section 1 of the Code of Ethics (which, in turn, is based on chap. I, art. XI of Percival's *Medical Ethics*). I reproduce it below. The italic text indicates material Bell and Hays added to their 1826 Kappa Lambda edition of *Extracts from Percival's Medical Ethics* in 1847 and represents original new text.

ART. IV. *Of the duties of Physicians in regard to consultations*
1. A regular medical education furnishes the only presumptive evidence of professional abilities and acquirements, *and ought to be the only acknowledged right of an individual to the exercise and honors of his profession. Nevertheless,* as in consultations, the good of the patient is the sole object in view, and this is often dependent on personal confidence, *no* intelligent *regular* practitioner, *who has a license to practise from some medical board of known and acknowledged respectability, recognised by this association, and who is in good moral and professional standing in the place in which he resides,* should be fastidiously excluded from fellowship, *or his aid refused in consultation when it is requested by the patient. But no one can be considered as a regular practitioner, or fit associate in consultation, whose practice is based on an exclusive dogma, to the rejection of the accumulated experience of the profession, and of the aids actually furnished by anatomy, physiology, pathology, and organic chemistry.*

It is evident from the contrast between the italic and the nonitalic text that Bell and Hays tightened the conditions for consultation significantly in 1847. Moreover, just as critics of the code have charged, the last sentence targets homeopathy. Unlike Leake's charge of semantic confusion, therefore, there *is* textual evidence to support the Berlant-Starr charge of "monopolization."

The text of the 1847 Code, moreover, is consistent with the position that Bell, and more particularly Hays, staked out in their medical journals. Thus in 1843, when Hays began to edit a weekly supplement to the *American Journal of the Medical Sciences* called *Medical News,* he observed that one of *Medical News*'s purposes was to challenge:

> [t]he numerous medical delusions of the day, and the devices resorted to by charlatans to delude the public, [which] will receive due attention and be fully exposed. Quackery never assumed a more audacious front, or appeared in more guises than at present; and with the aid of the powerful auxiliaries it has enlisted, seems to overshadow the whole country, unless proper efforts are made to arrest it, and medical men are furnished with the means of refuting the numerous falsehoods and absurdities daily propagated, and which obtain credence mainly because the truth in regard to them is never made known. (Hays 1843, 1–2)

Notice that Hays, like most commentators of the period, distinguished between "quacks," who were ethically suspect because they fraudulently peddled nostrums that they themselves knew to be fake, and "medical delusionaries," who were scientifically suspect but who nonetheless practiced a form of medicine that they themselves believed to be effective. The groups Hays characterized as "medical delusionaries" would today be called "alternative" or, to use an even more complimentary expression, "complementary" practitioners—botanical healers, Christian Scientists, homeopaths, and so forth. Yet clearly Hays believed that "medical men" were duty-bound to "refute" both willful "quackery" and ethically innocent "delusions," insofar as they were both based on "falsehoods" and "absurdities." The clear intent of chapter II, article IV of the code was to instrumentalize Hays's rejection of "absurdities," "delusions," and "falsehoods" by prohibiting members of the AMA from consulting with alternative practitioners. Prima facie, therefore, the evidence for the received reading of the AMA Code of Ethics as an instrument of "monopolization" seems well documented.

But is this reading coherent? To condemn the AMA for "monopolizing the medical marketplace" is to presuppose the possibility of a free market in medicine; for in the absence of some possible "free market," the expression "monopolization" makes no sense. A market can be said to be free only if there can be multiple buyers and sellers, each of whom is free to buy or sell as they choose and thus to bargain competitively on a level playing field in which, for example, they possess symmetrical access to information. Any artificial or natural monopoly on supply or demand or information undercuts the model of a "free market." Yet it is a commonplace of medical economics, iterated and reiterated with near unanimity by economists (Boulding 1958, 255; Buchanan 1960, 400–401; Enthoven 1988; Ginzberg 1954; Klarman 1965; Light 1997; Samuelson 1955, 122), that the conditions for a free market do not obtain in medicine. Consider, for example, the first and foremost of the duties of the physician toward the patient stipulated in the AMA Code of Ethics, the duty to "obey the calls of the sick." This duty addresses emergency situations in which patients are clearly in no position to bargain or to negotiate a price. Even where there is no emergency, however, there is no level playing field between buyer and seller in medicine. Sellers have a natural monopoly on information, while purchasers are, for the most part, incapable of judging the value of the information or the interventions that they purchase—not only because they are ignorant, but also because placebo treatments have psychological efficacy independent of any physiological action and because most illnesses are self-limiting (e.g., colds tend to abate irrespective of treatment). Once treatment commences, moreover, the purchaser is typically physically unable and psychologically unwilling to terminate a relationship with one provider to commence a relationship with another.

There is no free market in medicine. Medicine is, as economist Kenneth Arrow argued in a classic 1963 essay, a product sold in the most imperfect of markets. To permit market forces to prevail in this context is thus to permit the unmitigated exploitation of purchasers by providers. Arrow conjectured that professional medical ethics can be rationally reconstructed as an effort to rectify the inability of markets to perform their normal functions. Ethical codes protect consumers, even as they insulate those who subscribe to ethical standards from the unfair market practices of less scrupulous rivals. Read from this perspective, the AMA's 1847 Code of Ethics appears to be a systematic attempt to protect physician and patient (provider and purchaser) alike, by substituting ethical constraint for the perils of free-market competition. For example, the first duty of physicians prevents them from extorting money from patients during medical emergencies by requiring them to "obey the calls of the sick," irrespective of the sick person's ability to pay. The code also protects nonemergency patients from extortion. Thus, duties 4 and 5 of the AMA Code of

Ethics prohibit some of the means physicians might use to exploit patients' ignorance in a fee-for-service system: overcharging by making "unnecessary visits" or justifying high fees by "making gloomy prognostications" that "mag-
nify the importance of [the physician's] services in the treatment and cure of
disease."

The most noteworthy antimarket stance taken by the AMA Code is chapter II, article I, section 3, which prohibits advertising as "derogatory to the dignity of the profession." Specifically prohibited are "promising radical cures
. . . boast[ing] of cures and remedies, adduc[ing] certificates of skill and success" and so forth. At the same time as the code prohibited these practices on
the part of regularly trained professionals, chapter III, article I, section 4 declared open war on all who would treat medicine simply as commodities for
sale in the marketplace: "It is the duty of physicians, who are frequent witnesses of the enormities committed by quackery, and the injury to health and
even destruction of life caused by the use of quack medicines, to enlighten the
public on these subjects, to expose the injuries sustained by the unwary from
the devices and pretensions of artful empirics and impostors."

Were an efficient medical marketplace possible, were the public capable of
judging for itself the competency of practitioners or the efficacy of their wares,
the AMA's prohibition against advertising and the sale of proprietary medicines, its war on "artful empirics and impostors," would undoubtedly count
as a monopolizing constraint on free trade. Yet the public could not and cannot determine either competency or efficacy; consequently, as Joseph G. Baldwin remarked in 1853, unscrupulous traders in the medical marketplace can
and will exploit their ignorance:

> Nobody knew who or what they were, except as they claimed, or as a surface
> view of their characters indicated. Instead of taking to the highway and mag-
> nanimously calling upon the wayfarer to stand and deliver . . . some un-
> scrupulous horse doctor would set up his sign as "Physician and Surgeon"
> and draw his lancet on you, or fire at random a box of pills into your bowels,
> with a vague chance of hitting some disease, unknown to him, but with a bet-
> ter prospect of killing the patient, whom or whose administrator, he charged
> some ten dollars a trial for his marksmanship. (vii–viii)

Baldwin's demand for constraints on the medical marketplace confirms Arrow's analysis. In 1847 the AMA tried to remedy the imperfections of the medical market by imposing a system of ethical constrains. To now condemn these
constraints as "monopolization" is simply to insist that, contrary to all known

facts, a free medical marketplace is possible. Such insistence rings hollow in an era when the medical market is constrained by licensing and when all drugs are vetted for safety and efficacy by the U.S. Food and Drug Administration—especially if the critics of the AMA Code do not also demand the repeal of the food and drug laws, and the laws on education and licensure.

The monopolization argument has also been extended to ideas. Partisans of the intellectual monopolization claim that, at least in 1847, Christian Science and homeopathy were equal or perhaps even superior to the medicine championed by the AMA. The argument focuses on therapeutics, specifically on the penchant of the "regulars" for dangerous "heroic" practices like blood-letting, and for prescribing purgatives that were often based on mercury (calomel) and other heavy metals. In striking contrast, Christian Science healing and homeopathic dilutions "did no harm" physiologically, while still enjoying the same placebo effects that were the therapeutic mainstay of the "regular" practitioners. Yet had Mary Baker Eddy (1821–1910), Samuel Christian Hanhemann (1755–1843), or Samuel Thomson (1769–1843) and their followers merely been critiquing particular therapeutic practices, not only would they have had eminent allies and supporters in schools of conventional medicine (including John Bell), but also their followers would have been welcome in the AMA. What distinguishes heterodoxy from orthodoxy is not some dispute over the efficacy of this or that therapeutic intervention, but fundamental issues about the nature of health, healing, and healers. For the founders of alternative schools of medicine, the issue was never confined to pragmatic concerns over therapeutics; they sought to challenge orthodox organizational structures, healthcare delivery systems, presumptions of authority and belief, and the very epistemic structures and "science" underlying "orthodoxy" (see Gevitz 1988; chap. 14, this volume).

Nonetheless, the leading figures in the AMA agreed with the heterodox critique of conventional therapeutics. Bell was a pharmacological reformer active in the movement to establish a national pharmacopoeia; he was also a leader of the movement to purge mercurials from commonly prescribed drugs. In their journals Bell and Hays published the latest in French medicine, including the critiques of bleeding and mercurial compounds. Had homeopaths merely been critics of the therapeutics of mid-nineteenth-century America, they would have found staunch allies in Bell and Hays and in such later critics as Oliver Wendell Holmes. Homeopathy and other forms of alternative medicine, however, are complete epistemic systems that, as Hays notes in the code, reject not only the accumulated experience of the profession (a rejection that lies at the core of heterodoxy) but also the evidence of anatomy, physiology, pathology, and organic chemistry. Bell and Hays thus held that—whatever the merits of alternative medicine as a critique of particular therapies and practices—if a heterodox school rejected the applied-scientific model of medicine, it must be excluded from the AMA's educational-moral reform movement.

In the end, Bell and Hays's applied-science conception of medicine won in the marketplace of ideas. Victory was assured, in part, because the applied-science ideal is neutral with respect to particular theories and therapeutics. So-called orthodox medicine was thus capable of absorbing rapid and radical changes in theory and practice, including those from heterodox sources. Within three years of its founding, the AMA endorsed the use of ether in operations, even though the discovery was made by a Hartford Connecticut dentist, Horace Wells (1815–48). Later in the century the AMA endorsed Sir Joseph Lister's (1827–1912) antiseptic system of surgery, and Louis Pasteur (1822–95) and Robert Koch's (1843–1910) germ theories of disease. In striking contrast, the theories and treatments employed by "alternative" schools, like Christian Science and homeopathy, have changed only slightly in the course of 150 years. Ironically, however, the rhetoric of "alternativeness" and "unorthodoxy" seems to assign the role of the innovator to heterodoxy, while assigning the role of conservative to "conventional," "regular," "allopathic," or "orthodox" medicine.

In retrospect, the charge of "monopolization" is intellectually incoherent and inconsistent with the chronological unfolding of events. Yet once we dismiss this charge, we need to develop an alternative interpretation of the AMA's Code of Ethics. Perhaps any new interpretation should start with the proposition that the founders of the AMA and the authors of its Code of Ethics really were moral reformers who, even as they donned the mantle of Percivalean authority, cut and shaped their code to suit the spirit of their age—Jacksonian democracy—by rejecting the older elitist models of Gregorian virtue ethics. The AMA's Code of Ethics was thus originally a coup d'état, a seizure of moral authority by a revolutionary vanguard, but it ultimately became the foundational document for the American medical ethics revolution. The fundamental presuppositions of the 1847 Code—ethics based on reciprocal relationships rather than inherited status; ethics where prerogatives are justified by mutual consent; ethics in which physician and patient, the profession and the public, continually redesign and renegotiate the rules and the rights that regulate their interactions—remain the basis of both American and international bioethics. In one sense, therefore, today's bioethics movement is merely the latest chapter in a medical ethics revolution that dates back to the code of ethics that Bell and Hays convinced the organization that was to become the American Medical Association to adopt in 1847.

Notes

1. The seven-member committees that founded the AMA consisted of a core of three members, living relatively near each other, who actually drafted the text, and four members who served as commentators on the draft. The third member of the drafting committee for the code of ethics was Dr. Gouverneur Emerson (1796–1874) of Philadelphia. Like Bell and Hays, Emerson was an alumnus of the University of Pennsylvania, a member of the American Philosophical Society, of the College of Physicians of Philadelphia, and, perhaps most significantly, of the Philadelphia Chapter of the Kappa Lambda Society of Hippocrates. The other members of the committee were Dr. Richard Dennis Arnold of Savannah Georgia (1808–76), the first secretary of the AMA and vice president in 1851–52; Drs. Alonzo Clark and Theophilus C. Dunn of New York; and W. W. Morris of Delaware. Like Bell, Emerson, and Hays, Clark and Dunn were alumni of the University of Pennsylvania.

The only two members of the committee who claimed credit for authoring the code were Bell and, implicitly, Hays. Morris may have played a role, but there is no evidence indicating that he did, nor are there surviving correspondence, anecdotal accounts, or internal textual evidence to suggest that the non-Philadelphians were involved in developing the code.

Bell and Hays seem to have played the roles implicit in their statements to the AMA convention. Bell forthrightly claimed credit for the underlying conception of the code before the AMA, whereas Hays was implicitly credited with being in charge of the details of editing the code and crafting specific language. This relationship reprises the two men's earlier relationship in creating the Kappa Lambda code and the editorial styles they effected in their respective journals. Bell always appears the bold and literary editorializer, proud of his prose style almost to a point of vanity; Hays, the self-effacing editor, always content to find the words of others to voice his opinion. Bell's introduction thus speaks his views in his own voice and provides the strategy for the 1847 Code, which was implemented with self-effacing and politic politeness by Hays's meticulous editing of the language contributed, for the most part, by others.

2. Bell did not invent the expression "medical deontology"; he borrowed it, with acknowledgment, from Dr. Maximilien-Isidore-Amand Simon's *Deontology Médicale, ou des Devoirs et des Droits des Médecins dans l' État Actuel de la Civilisation* (Paris: J.-B. Bailliere, 1845, Libraire de l'Academie Royale de Médicine). Simon, in turn, borrowed the term *deontology,* with acknowledgment, from the English philosopher Jeremy Bentham. Bell's principle of reciprocity also seems implicit in Simon's work.

3. Even the lines taken from the 1826 Kappa Lambda edition do not simply parrot Percival. They amalgamate material from chapters 1 and 2 of the 1803 edition of

Percival's *Medical Ethics* and, following the precedent set in earlier Kappa Lambda editions, Americanize Percival's text both linguistically and conceptually. Linguistically, as in all Kappa Lambda texts, expressions like "physicians" replace more limited expressions like "hospital physicians." Conceptually, in Bell and Hays's Kappa Lambda edition, Percival's anemic British conception of "secrecy" is supplanted by a more robust America conception of confidentiality (see Baker 1993, 1997; Maehle 1997, 502).

4. Both the New York and Baltimore codes explicitly recognize that the virtuous physician answers the patient's call, but they treat this response as an aspect of the physician's character, not as a duty owed directly to the patient. Thus the New York *System of Ethics* states that "in urgent cases of sickness, or of injury occasioned by accidents, a call for medical or surgical help should be obeyed immediately, unless such compliance be to the detriment of some other sufferer" (div. III, art. XIX); while the Baltimore *System of Ethics* states that honorable physicians should respond to "calls of distress, from whatever quarter they emanate . . . with alacrity" (6).

References

American Medical Association. 1847. Code of Ethics. *Minutes of the Proceedings of the National Medical Convention held in the City of Philadelphia, in May 1847*, 83–106; this volume, 324–34.

Arrow, Kenneth. 1963. Uncertainty and the Welfare Economics of Medical Care. *American Economic Review* 53:941–69.

Baker, Robert. 1993. Deciphering Percival's Code. In *The Codification of Medical Morality: Historical and Philosophical Studies of the Formalization of Western Medical Morality in the Eighteenth and Nineteenth Centuries.* Vol. 1, *Medical Ethics and Etiquette in the Eighteenth Century*, ed. Robert Baker, Dorothy Porter, and Roy Porter, 179–212. Dordrecht: Kluwer.

———. 1997. The Kappa Lambda Society of Hippocrates: The Secret Origins of the American Medical Association. *Fugitive Leaves*, Third Series, Vol. 11, No. 2, College of Physicians of Philadelphia.

Baldwin, J. 1853. Flush Times of Alabama and Mississippi. In *The Formation of the American Medical Profession: The Role of Institutions, 1760–1860*, ed. J. Kett, vii–viii. New Haven: Yale University Press.

Beddoes, Thomas. 1802. *Hygeiia or Plutus: or Essays Moral and Medical, on the Causes Affecting the Personal State of Our Middling and Affluent Classes*. Bristol: J. Mills.

Bell, John. 1847. Introduction to the Code of Medical Ethics. *Minutes of the Proceedings of the National Medical Convention held in the City of Philadelphia, in May 1847*, 83–92; this volume, 317–23.

Berlant, Jeffrey. 1975. *Profession and Monopoly: A Study of Medicine in the United States and Great Britain*. Berkeley: University of California Press.

Boulding, Kenneth E. 1958. *Principles of Economic Policy*. Englewood Cliffs, N.J.: Prentice Hall.

Buchanan, J. W. 1960. *The Public Finances.* Homewood, Ill.: Irwin.

Danforth, Isaac. N. 1907. *The Life of Nathan Smith Davis, A.N., M.D., L.L.D., 1817–1904.* Chicago: Cleveland Press.

Davis, Nathan S. 1903. *History of Medicine, with the Code of Medical Ethics.* Chicago: Cleveland Press.

Enthoven, A. 1988. *Theory and Practice of Managed Competition in Health Care Finance.* Amsterdam: North Holland.

Fishbein, Morris. 1947. *A History of the American Medical Association, 1847 to 1947.* Philadelphia: W. B. Saunders.

Flint, Austin. 1895. *Medical Ethics and Etiquette: The Code of Ethics Adopted by the American Medical Association, with Commentaries.* New York: D. Appleton.

Gevitz, Norman. 1988. *Other Healers: Unorthodox Medicine in America.* Baltimore: Johns Hopkins University Press.

Ginzberg, E. 1954. What Every Economist Should Know About Health and Medicine. *American Economics Review* 44:104–19.

Gregory, John. 1772. *Lectures on the Duties and Offices of a Physician.* London: W. Straham and T. Cadell.

Haakonssen, Lisabeth. 1997. *Medicine and Morals in the Enlightenment: John Gregory, Thomas Percival, and Benjamin Rush.* Amsterdam: Ridopi.

Haller, J. 1981. *American Medicine in Transition, 1840–1910.* Urbana: University of Illinois Press.

Hays, Isaac. 1843. *Prospectus.* Philadelphia: Medical News and Library.

Klarman, H. E. 1965. *The Economics of Health.* New York: Columbia University Press.

Leake, Chauncey. 1922. What Was Kappa Lambda? An Historical Narrative Outlined for the Reader's Amusement, As a Tragedy, According to the Usual Divisions of Dramatic Construction. *Annals of Medical History* (June):192–206.

————. 1927. *Percival's Medical Ethics.* Baltimore: Williams & Wilkins.

Light, Donald W. 1997. From Managed Competition to Managed Cooperation: Theory and Lessons for the British Experience. *Millbank Quarterly* 77:297–341.

Maehle, Andreas-Hogler. 1997. Review of R. Baker, The Codification of Medical Morality, Vol. II. In *Medical History* 41:500–502.

McCullough, Lawrence B. 1998. *John Gregory and the Invention of Professional Medical Ethics and the Profession of Medicine.* Dordrecht: Kluwer.

Medical Society of the State of New York. 1823. *System of Medical Ethics.* New York: William Grattan.

Medico-Chirurgical Society of Baltimore. 1832. *System of Medical Ethics.* Baltimore: James Lucan and E. K. Deaver.

National Medical Convention. 1846. *Minutes of the Proceedings of the National Medical Convention, Held in the City of New York, 1846.* New York.

Pellegrino, Edmund D. 1985. Thomas Percival's Ethics: The Ethics Beneath the Etiquette. In Thomas Percival, *Medical Ethics,* 1–52. Birmingham, Ala.: Classics of Medicine Library.

Percival, Thomas. 1794. *Medical Jurisprudence or a Code of Ethics and Institutes Adapted to the Professions of Physic and Surgery.* Manchester, U.K., privately circulated.

————. 1803. *Medical Ethics; Or, A Code of Institutes and Precepts, Adapted to the Professional Conduct of Physicians and Surgeons.* London: J. Johnson.

Pickstone, John. 1993. Thomas Percival and the Production of Medical Ethics. In *The Codification of Medical Morality: Historical and Philosophical Studies of the Formalization of Western Medical Morality in the Eighteenth and Nineteenth Centuries.* Vol. 1, *Medical Ethics and Etiquette in the Eighteenth Century,* ed. Robert Baker, Dorothy Porter, and Roy Porter, 161–78. Dordrecht: Kluwer.

Porter, Roy. 1993. Plutus or Hygeia? Thomas Beddoes and the Crisis of Medical Ethics in Britain at the Turn of the Nineteenth Century. In *The Codification of Medical Morality: Historical and Philosophical Studies of the Formalization of Western Medical Morality in the Eighteenth and Nineteenth Centuries.* Vol. 1, *Medical Ethics and Etiquette in the Eighteenth Century,* ed. Robert Baker, Dorothy Porter, and Roy Porter, 73–92. Dordrecht: Kluwer.

Reiser, Stanley. 1995. Creating a Medical Profession in the United States: The First Code of Ethics of the American Medical Association. In *The Codification of Medical Morality: Historical and Philosophical Studies of the Formalization of Medical Morality in the Eighteenth and Nineteenth Centuries.* Vol. 2, *Anglo-American Medical Ethics and Medical Jurisprudence in the Nineteenth Century,* ed. Robert Baker, 89–104. Dordrecht: Kluwer.

Samuelson, Paul A. 1955. *Economics,* 3rd ed. New York: McGraw-Hill.

Starr, Paul. 1982. *The Social Transformation of American Medicine.* New York: Basic Books.

Stillé, Alfred. 1880. Memoir of Isaac Hays, M.D. *Transactions of the College of Physicians of Philadelphia,* 3rd series, 5:36.

Van Antwerp, Lee D. 1945. Kappa Lambda, Elf or Ogre. *Bulletin of the History of Medicine* 17:327–35.

Van Ingen, Philip. 1945. Remarks on "Kappa Lambda, Elf or Ogre?"—And a Little More Concerning the Society. *Bulletin of History of Medicine* 18:513–43.

3

The 1880s Rebellion against the AMA Code of Ethics

"Scientific Democracy" and the Dissolution of Orthodoxy

JOHN HARLEY WARNER, PH.D.

During the 1880s the American Medical Association's Code of Ethics came under vigorous attack from within the regular medical profession, and the code fashioned in 1847 to be an instrument of solidarity became one of division. Professional leaders squared off in what they publicly framed as a battle of right against wrong, good against evil, but which some privately recognized for what it largely was: the emergence among American physicians of incommensurable belief systems, divergent notions of how moral values and ethical behavior in the profession should be defined and upheld. The battles of the 1880s, which created intellectual and institutional rifts that would last into the twentieth century, marked the contested ascendancy in American medicine of a new ideal of science, one that posited fundamentally new relationships between science and medical practice, professional identity, and professional integrity.

Understanding the rebellion against the AMA Code of Ethics means making sense of what to our eyes might seem a paradox. Those who led the assault on the code and its use to maintain professional standards often were the very same physicians who were seeking to make scientific standards in medicine more rigorous. As a group, these were the physicians who most energetically championed the new experimental sciences and the optimistic belief that the laboratory would transform clinical medicine—bringing to therapeutics, for example, an exact method and approach to certainty. Yet their confidence in a new ideal of science and its place in medicine went hand in hand with their opposition to the Code of Ethics as a professional embarrassment. Among the most vocal opponents of the AMA Code were physicians who believed that the advancement of science had rendered it obsolete, and who looked to the experimental sciences as a new source of authority and of more reliable criteria for integrity (Rosenkrantz 1985; Warner 1991). Evoking the premise that, as one New York specialist put it in 1883, "ethics must vary with time and place" (Ely 1883, 23), critics declared that the AMA Code was "no longer a living power" and that "the day of its usefulness has passed" (F.R.S. 1883, v, vii).

This is the line of interpretation I want to follow here. The uprising against the code, I will argue, signaled a movement to redefine what counted as professionally correct behavior. At the same time, it was part of a larger revolt against the ideology of medical orthodoxy and the constraints on professional conduct that it sustained, a revolt that called for wide-ranging social, intellectual, and behavioral changes.

The chief target in vilifying the 1847 Code was the prohibition against consulting with unorthodox or irregular physicians on the grounds that they were medically and morally unfit. The section in the article of the code that addressed the "duties of physicians in regard to consultations" was worded thus:

A regular medical education furnishes the only presumptive evidence of professional abilities and acquirements, and ought to be the only acknowledged right of an individual to the exercise and honours of his profession. Nevertheless, as in consultations the good of the patient is the sole object in view, and this is often dependent on personal confidence, no intelligent regular practitioner who has a license to practice for some medical board of known and acknowledged respectability, recognized by this association, and who is in good moral and professional standing in the place in which he resides, should be fastidiously excluded from fellowship, or his aid refused in consultation, when it is requested by the patient. But no one can be considered as a regular practitioner, or a fit associate in consultation, whose practice is based on an exclusive dogma, to the rejection of the accumulated experience of the profession, and of the aids actually furnished by anatomy, physiology, pathology, and organic chemistry. (Code 1848, 18–19, see Appendix C, 329)

The reference to practitioners who adhered to "an exclusive dogma" applied to all those derisively termed "sectarians" or "quacks." But the leading concern was homeopathic physicians, adherents of the medical system founded in the late eighteenth century by the German physician Samuel Hahnemann

(1755–1843), practitioners who generally held an M.D. degree and were as well educated as most regulars. Many leaders of the rebellion called for the repeal of all written ethical codes in medicine as unnecessary and antiquated restraints on the freedom of the individual physician, "glad," as one put it, "to leave the subject of medical ethics and etiquette to the personal discretion, justice, honesty, and humanity of each practitioner" (Roosa 1883b, 104). But it was rejection of the consultation clause that became a hallmark of reformers' new identity as liberal professionals and of their dissent from the AMA.

Orthodoxy in American medicine had been created during the second quarter of the nineteenth century, and in that process the most important force was the power and competition of alternative healers. Historians have emphasized how botanic and homeopathic critics fostered change in regular medicine by encouraging a move away from heroic bleeding and purging toward a milder therapeutic course. They have given less attention to the profoundly conservative influence that alternative healers simultaneously worked upon the mentality of the regular profession, engendering a tenacious adherence to tradition that made change difficult and at times professionally suspect. Homeopathy thus fostered not only regular stability but also reaction, and it was the critical element in transforming regular physicians' confidence in their heritage into a dogmatic ideology of orthodoxy. Homeopaths further cemented the language and imagery of sectarianism by labeling regular medicine *allopathy*, a term the newly designated allopaths scorned (see Warner 1987). "You should consider yourself insulted at being called an 'Allopathic,'" one regular medical student wrote in his class notebook, copying his professor's words; "you have a perfect right to avail yourself of all means, wherever found" (Rice 1855). It was orthodoxy, not so much orthopraxy, that mattered in displaying professional regularity.

With the strengthening impulse to orthodoxy, regular physicians sought ways to set themselves apart from heterodox healers and to purify their own ranks. Yet at a time when even the honorific licensing laws that had been in place were being repealed, there was little hope that the state would act as boundary setter. Instead, the growing awareness of orthodox identity after the 1820s was expressed most visibly by the proliferation of voluntary but exclusive orthodox institutions. By the 1840s regular societies and schools had embraced an official policy of discrimination against irregular practitioners. Homeopaths (as well as other irregular physicians such as Eclectics) were barred from regular medical societies, while some members who met with irregulars in consultation were charged with heresy and expelled. Regular schools revoked the diplomas of alumni who took up unorthodox ways, suspended students who associated with homeopaths, and refused to allow students who had apprenticed with homeopaths to attend lectures. In this context, the founding of the AMA in 1847 functioned, as one physician put it in that year, "to draw the line of demarcation between those who are of the profession and those who are not" (C[oventry] 1847, 372). The consultation clause became the most celebrated implement of orthodox purity, an institutional and behavioral boundary that separated and distinguished those faithful to tradition. "To a young physician going forth into a life full of moral conflicts the wearing of this aegis would be one of his surest defenses," one AMA president later asserted: "Next to the holy scriptures, and the grace of God, it would serve most effectually to guard him from evil" (G. B. Wood 1856, 402).

Rhetoric demonizing homeopathy persisted through the final third of the century, as did official policies of discrimination. Yet by the 1870s and 1880s, clear signs had emerged that this ideology of orthodoxy, forged during the antebellum period, was starting to be pulled apart at the seams. A growing number of eminent, often younger regular physicians set out to erode invidious barriers between homeopath and allopath as part of a wider program for reconstructing their own professional identity. In their view, the ideals and apparatus of orthodoxy, far from being the best assurance of the physician's success at the bedside and the profession's success in society, held medicine back, impeding their program to redefine professional identity, authority, and moral legitimacy.

One prominent argument against the consultation clause was that science was the ultimate touchstone of clinical propriety and had rendered distinctions between competing beliefs and practices made on any other grounds meaningless: faith in the authority of science over clinical practice was to be a virtual substitute for the commandments of ethical codes that drew distinctions between orthodox and unorthodox practitioners. As one practitioner in 1883 put it in explaining his opposition to the Code of Ethics, "There can be in medicine no heresy, because there is no orthodoxy" (Hun 1883, 58). The conviction that specialized knowledge would guide effective intervention— the ethical sanction for their program—harmonized with a broader faith that scientific expertise offered a new and more solid foundation for professional identity and integrity.

Indeed, the debate over the Code of Ethics cannot be fully comprehended without recognizing it as part of a larger debate over newly emerging ideals of science and the place science should occupy in a rapidly changing medical world. The controversy that raged in the 1870s and 1880s over the proposition that the new experimental sciences would bring some significant measure of certainty to clinical practice, for example, no less than the proposition that the restrictive stipulations of the consultation clause were indispensable to assuring correct behavior at the bedside, became more and more a lightning rod for divergent pronouncements on the proper relationships among science, practice, and professional responsibility. The intermeshing of the two controversies becomes even more evident when we see that the proselytizers for therapeutics based on experimental physiology allied themselves with the opponents of the Code of Ethics, while some of those who most harshly denounced the program for experimental therapeutics were among the most vocal defenders of the code (see Warner 1991).

This alignment can be illustrated by the positions taken by the authors of four of the most prominent American textbooks on therapeutics and the practice of medicine in the 1870s and 1880s. Horatio C. Wood (1841–1920) and Roberts Bartholow (1831–1904), who looked to experimental physiology as a new foundation for medical therapeutics, both thought the Code of Ethics was outdated. These clinicians made it absolutely clear that in seeking to ground therapeutics on experimental physiology, they were in revolt against clinical empiricism, which leading physicians long had looked to as the only sure pathway to therapeutic progress (Warner 1992). Wood, who was professor of materia medica and therapeutics at the University of Pennsylvania, noted facetiously that empiricism had sanctioned the therapeutic use of camel dung and dried frogs (H. C. Wood 1883–84, 634). Wood and his confreres instead claimed a legitimate place for reasoning from the laboratory to the bedside and claimed, moreover, that there were universal laws in therapeutics, just as there were universal laws in the basic science, physiology, on which they sought to base it (see, e.g., Bartholow 1884; H. C. Wood 1880). Both Wood and Bartholow used the example of experimental therapeutics to sustain their argument that physicians who trusted in the natural laws revealed by experimental science no longer needed the artificial laws embodied in codes of professional ethics. "Homeopathy and allopathy are dreams of a by-gone time," Bartholow, at the time a professor of materia medica at the Medical College of Ohio, proclaimed as early as 1872. "Modern science is indifferent to Hippocrates and Hahnemann. The therapeutics of to-day rejects dogmas, and the therapeutics of the future will accept nothing that can not be demonstrated by the tests of science" (Bartholow 1872, 636). Wood shared this conviction; he used his contribution to a collaborative textbook on practical therapeutics as an opportunity to assail the Code of Ethics and to affirm the liberty of scientific physicians to meet in consultation with whomever they pleased (Wood, 1891–92, 19).

Austin Flint (1812–86) and Alfred Stillé (1813–1900), on the other hand, condemned the notion that therapeutics could be grounded on experimental physiology and unabashedly presented their textbooks as bastions of clinical empiricism (see, e.g., Flint 1879, 54; Stillé 1874, viii). These men were also among the most strident defenders of the Code of Ethics and all it stood for. Flint, who since midcentury had been recognized as one of the most eminent professors of the principles and practice of medicine in the country, denied that precise rules of the sort promised by experimental therapeutics could ever be attained in clinical medicine and made the inescapable uncertainty of therapeutic practice a fundamental premise in pleading the necessity of "rules of conduct adapted to the peculiarities of medicine [that] constitute medical ethics" (Flint 1883b, 3). And just as Wood used an essay spelling out his philosophy of therapeutics as an occasion to lash out against the code, so Stillé used an address professing his very different therapeutic faith as an occasion to defend it. Stillé, a Philadelphia physician who had served as first secretary of the AMA as well as its president in 1871, accused the advocates of experimental therapeutics of seeking to impose their scientific laws "like a new delivery of the decalogue." Several paragraphs later he prefaced his defense of the AMA Code of Ethics by placing it in a tradition he traced back to "that most ancient of moral codes, the Decalogue." In language he might just as well have used in assailing supporters of physiological therapeutics, Stillé went on to denounce those who would overturn the code for what he called their "egotistical materialism." Such a position, he said, "tends to rob man of trust in . . . the established order of things" (Stillé 1884, 435, 436, 437).

The most aggressive and nationally prominent of many local battles was the one waged in New York State (see Appel 1987; Hamstra 1987, 60–85; Kaufman 1971, 125–40; King 1983a; Rosenkrantz 1985; Rothstein 1972, 301–5; Warner 1991). At the 1882 meeting of the Medical Society of the State of New York, a group of elite, science-oriented, urban specialists such as New York City ophthalmologists Cornelius R. Agnew (1830–88) and Daniel B. St. John Roosa (1838–1908) and dermatologist Henry G. Piffard (1842–1910)—supported by its president, Manhattan pediatrician Abraham Jacobi (1830–1919)—pushed through a vote deleting the consultation clause from the society's Code of Ethics. Many of these physicians wanted to abolish the code altogether but compromised with less radical reformers. Their coalition enacted what was called the "New Code," which differed from the "Old Code" of the AMA chiefly in its deletion of the consultation clause. Members were henceforth free to consult any legally qualified medical practitioner—and by this time New York State had enacted licensing laws that legally recognized homeopaths, a trend evident in other states as well.

At its annual meeting a few months later, the AMA refused to seat delegates from the New York medical society. Rather than seeing this as a setback, however, opponents of the consultation clause viewed the move as a reactionary measure that could rally dissidents against both the ideology of orthodoxy and the AMA itself. "The action of the American Medical Association in refusing to admit the New York delegation will, I think, be productive of much good," a Washington, D.C., physician reflected in a letter to the New York activist Agnew. "Only one course can be open to those who value professional integrity, liberty, and advance," he proposed, calling for the formation of a new association on a more "liberal basis" that shunned "ignorant exclusiveness." "You can never restore this dying body, the Am Med Association," he asserted, urging Agnew: "Let us profit from its failures and rear on its ashes an organization free from disease, and clearing away the rubbish, rear a structure devoted to science, firm, broad and as enduring as time" (Bigelow 1882).

During the next two years conservatives—led by Flint, then in his early seventies—waged a vigorous campaign to have the consultation clause restored by the Medical Society of the State of New York. The AMA escalated tensions at its next annual convention by requiring that all delegates sign a pledge to observe the ban on consulting with homeopaths and by naming Flint president-elect. Frustrated in their attempts to restore the AMA Code intact, in 1884 New York conservatives split off to form their own orthodox society, the New York State Medical Association, which ceremoniously restored the consultation clause and was duly recognized by the AMA. Into the early twentieth century, New York had two state medical societies, split by dissension over the consultation clause.

Shortly before the vote that would divide the New York medical society, a private exchange of letters between two leading figures in the opposing factions, Flint and Agnew, made it clear that they recognized the far-reaching implications that the anticode rebellion in New York might have for the institutional and intellectual organization of American medicine. "I trust that you will not think me intrusive if I venture to say that you have now an opportunity to save the American Medical Association," Agnew wrote to Flint, urging that allegiance to the AMA's Code of Ethics should play no role in that organization's embrace of other professional organizations, including not only the dissident New York society but also the specialty bodies that at the time were proliferating. "The Association should be prepared to absorb the various American societies which represent the acknowledged specialties such as the American Ophthalmological Society &c &c. and make them its working sections" (Agnew 1883a). Flint, however, replied in a letter explicitly marked "private" that while he believed that "in the 'new movement' inaugurated by yourself & others, you have acted conscientiously," he was resigned to the fact that no amount of discussion, even by people of good will, could resolve the underlying incommensurability in their outlooks. "A division of the profession seems inevitable," he told Agnew. "I would appeal to you to use your influence to prevent this, were it not that I must suppose you to be as firm in your conceptions of right and duty, as I am in mine" (Flint 1883a).

Defenders of the AMA Code agreed that medicine was scientific but were disturbed by claims that science could be relied upon as an arbiter of professional conduct. In their view it was precisely because science could *not* deliver exact and invariant rules for practice that the physician needed the kind of guidance the Code of Ethics provided. Flint, like others in his camp, linked his support for the code to his dismissal of the notion that experimental science could ever bring therapeutic certainty. As Flint asserted in his book *Medical Ethics and Etiquette,* written in 1883 to defend the code, "The practice of medicine, when contrasted with other pursuits, is peculiar. The medical practitioner does not deal with facts and laws having the exactness of those pertaining to physics" (Flint 1883b, 1–2). The inbuilt uncertainties of medical practice, he argued, were the reason further guides to behavior of the sort established by the Code of Ethics were necessary. Thus, after listening to criticisms of the code at a county medical society meeting in Ohio, one member declared that "what he had heard here in this discussion reminded him of the absurd cry of certain self-styled moral and social reformers, who claimed that the advanced civilization of the nineteenth century had outgrown the Bible" (Clarke County 1875, 161). Medical reformers, in the name of science, were undercutting the moral order of the past that assured the integrity of the regular profession. "It is a sign of decadence in the American social and medical systems," Stillé concluded, "that such laws are treated as obsolete" (Stillé 1884, 437).

The language of physicians who, like Flint, remained faithful to the AMA Code was infused with moral indignation: at issue was the "survival of right over wrong" (Van der Warker [1884], 21), while the annulment of the consultation clause was "a fire-brand of Nihilism in the profession" (Proceedings 1884, 597). For rank-and-file general practitioners, and especially for older professional leaders who remembered the battles they had waged to establish the ideals and institutions of orthodoxy, it seemed a reckless violation of orthodox purity. More concretely, they charged that those who had jettisoned the clause had betrayed orthodoxy for a lucrative alliance with homeopaths. Critics correctly pointed out that the move to overturn the code had been led by urban specialists, a group gaining prominence and power yet still new and somewhat suspect. New York City specialists, prominent physicians in their forties or very early fifties, were the most active opponents of the AMA Code; and their backers came disproportionately from Manhattan, Brooklyn, Albany, and Rochester. These specialists stood to gain the most financially from deleting the consultation clause, for not only did they practice in the urban centers that had the greatest concentrations of homeopaths, but their claims to special expertise meant that they were the physicians most likely to be called into consultation by a homeopath confronted with a perplexing case. Abolition of the consultation clause, one critic put it, "looks like a desperate endeavor on the part of those New York specialists who are itching to consult with all sorts of irregulars in order to increase their income" ("Truth" 1883, 54). According to this appraisal, they had placed socioeconomic interests above professional integrity. "Whatever else may rise or fall in regard to this subject, that School, whose foundations were laid by Hippocrates and his followers, will stand," one self-described "Country Doctor" from upstate New York wrote angrily to Agnew. "As in Christianity so in this, there is 'One faith—one baptism'—we of the Country are amazed by the action of the Roosas, Jacobis and Agnews and others and will not permit ourselves to be led by them for a moment—we do not and *will not trust them*" (Nichols 1882).

The presumption of urban specialists that their claims to expert knowledge placed them above the established professional order drew further assaults from defenders of the AMA Code against such symbols of medical specialism as instruments, which—tellingly—were also regarded as the most visible emblems of experimental science in clinical medicine. In his 1884 presidential address to the first annual meeting of the New York State Medical Association, the group newly organized to reembrace the AMA Code, a physician from Onondaga County urged "conservative progress" in therapeutics and a prudent suspicion of promises of rapid progress or certainty, characteristic features of the program for experimental therapeutics. He particularly warned against "the innumerable instruments of precision, which promise to substitute mathematical accuracy for vague guesses and which are too often used, not to supplement but to supplant other and valuable methods of investigation." There was real danger, he went on, in "all the 'scopes,' all the 'graphs,' and all the 'meters'" for which clinical authority increasingly was being claimed, particularly by specialists. "These rightfully challenge recognition and study, while with unappeasable appetite they devour our substance if we attempt to add them to our *armamentarium*" (Didama 1884, 22). It was perhaps fitting that Flint's last address, published posthumously as *Medicine of the Future*, not only cautioned that "the only solid basis of therapeutics is clinical experience" but also ended by warning against medical specialization as "a dangerous tendency" (Flint 1886, 16, 36).

For their part, those who rejected the AMA Code insisted that the consultation clause was an infringement on the physician's personal liberties. Some no doubt were enticed by the prospect of open interaction with homeopaths and its economic rewards, but other deeply held convictions also informed their stance. As Agnew insisted, "Leave members of a liberal profession free to go as advocates of truth wherever called"—(including into consultation with homeopaths)—"and error will be less arrogant and dominant." It was partly in the name of liberalism that they successfully fought the move by Flint and his followers to reinstate the consultation clause (Agnew 1883b, 347). Looking with concern toward the forthcoming 1883 meeting of the state society, where the code issue would reemerge, one opponent of the AMA Code wrote to another affirming their shared commitment to "this movement for freedom" and stressing the importance of doing all that was possible "to prevent our profession in this state from abandoning the Free Republic of Letters" (Dimon 1883).

Among the leaders of the liberal movement were physicians who sought the abolition of *all* written codes of medical ethics, not merely the consultation clause. Advocating "a gentleman's code," Roosa, a particularly outspoken proponent of this stand, proclaimed that "we who argue for a simple declaration would allow even this to be unwritten" (Roosa 1883a, 422). "A physician," agreed Lewis S. Pilcher (1845–1934), a prominent Brooklyn surgeon, "is not a member of a guild or corporation, the rules of which he must comply with in order to retain his membership therein, and to enjoy its benefits, but a member of a liberal profession, the rules of which are the unwritten laws of humanity." Invoking the support of free trade and middle-class opposition to trade-unionism that typified liberalism during this period, he went on to assert that "the physician is a freeman; he has ceased to recognize paternal interference with his judgment; he wears the livery of no employer; he acknowledges the restrictions of no trades-union" (Pilcher 1883, 44, 45). The abolition of the consultation clause from the code of the New York society, while it did away with the most odious limitations on the individual physician's freedom of action, was, for these reformers, an expedient compromise with their more moderate colleagues. As a Rochester physician in 1883 explained the action that he and others who wanted only "the unwritten code of gentlemen" (Ely 1883, 12) had taken, they "voted for the new code, and accept it provisionally, as a step toward their more advanced position, and thus better than no change whatever" (Ely 1883, 10).

The coalition of New York physicians who dissented from the AMA Code consolidated their efforts by founding an organization with the unwieldy name, "The Association for Preventing the Re-Enactment in the State of New York of the Present Code of Ethics of the American Medical Association" (fig. 1). And in 1883 they compiled a volume to refute Flint's book that they titled *An Ethical Symposium: Being a Series of Papers concerning Medical Ethics and Etiquette from the Liberal Standpoint* (Post et al. 1883). At a meeting held at the Manhattan home (on W. 34th Street) of Drs. Abraham Jacobi and Mary Putnam Jacobi, members proclaimed that their objective was "to preserve to each physician perfect liberty to decide with whom he shall act in order to secure the best interests of the sick and the honor of his profession" (Report 1883, 2). "As far as is known," one activist explained, "no scientific body places prohibitory rules upon scientific men in matters of ethics" (Ely 1883, 21). It was for this reason that Abraham Jacobi, as president of the New York Academy of Medicine (which had several years earlier weathered a stormy battle during which the allegiance of fellows to the AMA Code was first affirmed then annulled), could reassure its members by 1886 that "the absence of ethical codes" from the academy was testimony to what he termed its new "scientific spirit" (Jacobi 1886, 608).

For these physicians, personal liberty warranted by scientific expertise provided a compelling sanction for doing away with the consultation clause. "Having been always regarded as 'high church' in all that relates to recognition

THE ASSOCIATION
—FOR—

PREVENTING THE RE-ENACTMENT IN THE STATE OF NEW YORK
—OF THE—

PRESENT CODE OF ETHICS OF THE AMERICAN MEDICAL ASSOCIATION.

ALFRED C. POST, M.D., President,
 291 MADISON AVENUE.
F. R. STURGIS, M.D., Secretary,
 16 WEST 32D STREET.
H. G. PIFFARD, M. D., *Chairman Com. on Correspondence*.
 10 WEST 35TH ST.

New York   May 3,   1883.

Figure 1. On letterhead stationary such as this, from the Cornelius Rea Agnew Papers, the liberal coalition of physicians in New York fought the efforts of conservatives to restore the AMA Code of Ethics in their state medical society. *(Courtesy of the History of Medicine Division, National Library of Medicine, Bethesda, Md.)*

of or association with 'irregulars' of all sorts," one physician wrote to Agnew, "I yet cannot but feel that the multiplication of 'thou shalts' and 'thou shalt nots' is an offense to the self-respect of a man who feels and knows that he no longer needs the aid or restraint of a leading string" (Andrew 1883). They saw their move, not as a sanction for homeopathy, but as a denial that sectarian distinctions were helpful any longer and as a declaration that the ideal of orthodoxy should be supplanted by an enlightened therapeutic egalitarianism. It was a necessary step in the creation of what another opponent of the AMA Code called a "pure, *scientific* democracy" (Hunt 1882).

Opponents of the AMA Code looked forward to a profession made up of doctors educated as experts in natural science—and, just as important, educated as well to accord that scientific expertise a new place in their identity as professionals. At the 1882 meeting of the Medical Society of the State of New York at which the consultation clause was voted out, Abraham Jacobi urged in his presidential address that "if we have reason to believe, not only that medical science is one and indivisible, and based on logic and experimentation, but that we, the profession of the State of New York, are sufficiently imbued with that spirit of logic and experimental science, characteristic of modern medicine," then the physicians who made up his audience should feel free to meet with homeopaths "with a spirit of reconciliation" (Jacobi 1882, 11). Those who had embraced a new conception of professional identity were asserting that with the advancement of science, exclusive medical creeds and the artificial rules that sustained them would disappear. "To-day the discussion is a heated one and full of perplexity," an Albany medical student noted in his M.D. thesis written in 1884, the very year the state society divided over the code. "Ten years from now the interests of humanity will influence and guide the profession and a code of ethics will be only known as a matter of history" (Craig 1884).

In the short run, the issue of consultation and the posture toward orthodoxy for which it stood split the leadership of the medical profession (see King 1983a, 1983b). American plans to host the Ninth International Medical Congress in 1887, a plan Flint had initially proposed in his 1884 presidential address to the AMA, were fundamentally disrupted when the AMA sought to exclude from the event physicians who had forsaken orthodoxy (Jacobi and Roosa, for example, originally on the planning committee, were expelled for their stand against the Code of Ethics). Embittered by Flint's "utter immobility" on the code issue, in 1885 the University of Pennsylvania medical professor William Pepper (1843–98) privately complained to Philadelphia ophthalmologist and medical editor Isaac M. Hays (1847–1925): "The truth is, he has arranged to use the Int. M. C. as a Club to finish off all the New Coders in N.Y.; and has sold himself to those who would prostrate this great scientific organization to that local petty purpose" (Pepper 1885). At the International Medical Congress 1887—held in Washington, D.C., with conservative Nathan Smith Davis (1817–1904), a founder of the AMA and first editor of its journal, as congress president—the sparse representation of American medicine's scientific leaders was striking. "Oh! my dear doctor what must they think of us abroad," an Ohio physician lamented to Agnew as plans for the congress were being finalized. "Our profession is in the dust and years will pass before our profession will recover from its present humiliation. They know as well as others, that no society of scientific character can succeed loaded to the muzzle with such missiles as codes of ethics" (Culbertson 1886).

Instead of giving in, however, those who most vigorously renounced the consultation clause made plans for an alternative Congress of American Physicians and Surgeons, conceived as a reaction against the AMA's policies, controlled by the recently founded and highly selective societies of medical specialists, and convened in 1888 as a forum for those practitioners most consecrated to the new experimental sciences. Among the constituent societies that backed this congress was the newly created Association of American Physicians, an exclusive society representing the most scientifically eminent among the nation's physicians (see Appel 1987; King 1983b). In this divisive climate, New York pathology professor Francis Delafield (1841–1915), as president of the Association of American Physicians, declared at its inaugural meeting in 1886: "We want an association in which there will be no medical politics, and no medical ethics" (Delafield 1886, 1). While the "Constitution and By-Laws" stated that a member could be expelled "for conduct unbecoming a physician and a gentleman" (Constitution 1886, xxiii), as medical historian Chester Burns (1985, 403) pointed out, this association, like most organizations of medical scientists and clinical specialists founded from the 1870s through the first quarter of the twentieth century, eschewed any written code of ethics.

During the 1890s the professional leaders of American medicine would gradually come to share a perception of the ideology of orthodoxy as cumbersome baggage inherited from an earlier age, a burden to be shed rather than a faith to be revered. At the University of Michigan, to cite one example, where the medical school had both regular and homeopathic departments, declining homeopathic enrollments in 1895 encouraged the regents to propose that the separate homeopathic department be abolished and that a professor of homeopathic materia medica and therapeutics—"the only distinctive feature of the system"—be appointed in the hitherto regular medical department. Victor C. Vaughan (1851–1929), dean of the school, circulated a letter to physicians across the country soliciting their judgments on the proposal, and the diversity in their replies made it abundantly clear that by the mid—1890s the orthodox consensus had been ruptured (Vaughan 1895).

Some regulars, though a small minority, wrote back to Vaughan protesting that the established boundaries should be maintained intact and that no homeopathic professor should be appointed to the same faculty as regular doctors. Others applauded the move as a measure calculated to subvert homeopathy and urged that "the past policy of ridicule and opposition" had been one source of homeopathic distinctiveness and thereby strength (Dodge 1895). Most regular physicians, however, counseled Vaughan that the touchstone of judging a good doctor was no longer orthodox practice but was, instead, scientific knowledge. "After all," William Osler (1849–1920) told Vaughan, "the differences which, in matters of treatment, separate members of the rational school are not greater than those which separate some of us from our homeopathic brethren" (Osler 1895). To establish a chair of homeopathic therapeutics in the medical school "would be one of the greatest strides onward toward the final solution of the pathy problem," one Michigan physician asserted. "All medical teachings must eventually come under one head, i.e., Science of Medicine so called." He noted that "to-day the best of both schools is constantly stepping over the proscribed boundary," and concluded that establishing a homeopathic chair in the otherwise regular medical school "is simply the foreshadowing of the future uniting" (Handy 1895).

In 1903 the AMA would delete the consultation prohibition as part of a larger revision of its Code of Ethics, which, in a document drafted chiefly by Johns Hopkins pathologist William H. Welch (1850–1934), was reconfigured as an advisory "statement of principles." New York's two state medical societies soon thereafter merged under the name and rules of the liberal organization that had spearheaded the 1880s revolt, and within the decade Abraham Jacobi, once denounced as a traitor, would be named AMA president (Burns 1985; Hamstra 1987, 177–200; King 1983b). By 1910 Abraham Flexner (1866–1959) was marching in step with other elite reformers by openly eschewing notions of orthodoxy and heresy in favor of a professional order that took science as its polestar. In his *Report* on medical education, Flexner dismissed homeopathy and allopathy alike as "medical sects," urging that both must give way to what he called "scientific medicine." Flexner looked for authority to the doyen of regular clinicians: "'A new school of practitioners has arisen,'" he quoted from Osler, "'which cares nothing for homeopathy and less for so-called allopathy.'" As Flexner insisted in his own voice, "Science, once embraced, will conquer the whole" (Flexner 1910, 156, 161, 162; and see Rogers 1998, 84–90).

In the rebellion of the 1880s, then, we see not a turning away from ethical principles, but a questioning of the idea that a fixed and punitive code of behavior could accommodate individual freedom of action by the modern physician. More than this, we see a concerted attempt to throw off the ideology of orthodoxy, an intellectual and political maneuver that marked the contested emergence of a new order of *scientific medicine*—a "scientific democracy"—in which trust in science was to be the best guarantee of technically and morally right conduct. The Code of Ethics rebellion thus displays in the medical profession an early harbinger of the Progressive Era faith and the progressive fallacy that an allegiance to science offers a value-free arbiter of social and moral issues.

Acknowledgment

Sections of this chapter that explore the link between late-nineteenth-century ideals of science and codes of medical ethics draw heavily on Warner 1991.

References

Agnew, C. R. 1883a. Letter to Austin Flint. New York (23 October). In Cornelius Rea Agnew Papers, History of Medicine Division, National Library of Medicine, Bethesda, Md.

———. 1883b. On Dr. Squibb's Resolution to Abolish the Code of Ethics of the Medical Society of the State of New York. *New York Medical Journal* 37:345–47.

Andrew, Geo. L. 1883. Letter to C. R. Agnew. La Porte, Ind. (3 April). In Agnew Papers.

Appel, Toby A. 1987. Biological and Medical Societies and the Founding of the American Physiological Society. In *Physiology in the American Context, 1850–1950*, ed. Gerald L. Geison, 155–75. Bethesda, Md.: American Physiological Society.

Bartholow, Roberts. 1872. Experimental Therapeutics. Introductory Address. Quoted in Medical College of Ohio, *Cincinnati Lancet and Observer* n.s. 15:635–36.

———. 1884. *A Practical Treatise on Materia Medica and Therapeutics*, 5th ed. New York: D. Appleton.

Bigelow, Horatio R. 1882. Letter to C. R. Agnew. Washington, D.C. (23 October). In Agnew Papers.

Burns, C. R. 1985. Science and Medical Ethics: The Dualism of William H. Welch (1850–1934). In *Proceedings* 2:403–8. Cairo: Twenty-ninth International Congress of the History of Medicine.

Clarke County Medical Society—February Meeting. 1875. *Cincinnati Lancet and Observer* n.s. 18:159–65.

Code of Ethics of the American Medical Association. Adopted May 1847. 1848. Philadelphia: T. K. and P. G. Collins.

Constitution and By-Laws. 1886. *Transactions of the Association of American Physicians* 1:xxi—xxiv.

C[oventry], C. B. 1847. Medical Convention, Utica, N.Y. (17 April). *New York Journal of Medicine and the Collateral Sciences* 8:371–74.

Craig, Joseph Davis. 1884. Modern Clinical Research. M.D. thesis, Albany Medical College. In Archives of Albany Medical Center, Albany, N.Y.

Culbertson, H. 1886. Letter to C. R. Agnew. Zanesville, Ohio (14 May). In Agnew Papers.

Delafield, Francis. 1886. Chronic Catarrhal Gastritis, with Opening Remarks by the President. *Transactions of the Association of American Physicians* 1:1–10.

Didama, Henry D. 1884. The President's Annual Address: Conservative Progress. *Transactions of the New York State Medical Association* 1:19–32.

Dimon, Theo. 1883. Letter to David Webster. Auburn, N.Y. (2 February). In Theodore Dimon Letters, Manuscripts and Special Collections, New York State Library, Albany.

Dodge, J[?illegible] T. 1895. Letter to Victor C. Vaughan. Big Rapids, Mich. (15 February). In folder marked Homeopathic Medical School, 1895, University of Michigan, School of Medicine Records, Box 135 (hereafter, Vaughan Letters), Bentley Historical Library, University of Michigan, Ann Arbor.

Ely, William S. 1883. The Questionable Features of Our Medical Codes. In *An Ethical Symposium: Being a Series of Papers concerning Medical Ethics and Etiquette from the Liberal Standpoint*, ed. Alfred C. Post et al., 8–25. New York: G. P. Putnam's Sons.

Flexner, Abraham. 1910. *Medical Education in the United States and Canada: A Report to the Carnegie Foundation for the Advancement of Teaching.* New York: Carnegie Foundation.

Flint, Austin. 1879. *Clinical Medicine: A Systematic Treatise on the Diagnosis and Treatment of Disease, Designed for the Use of Students and Practitioners of Medicine.* Philadelphia: Henry C. Lea.

———. 1883a. Letter to [C. R. Agnew]. New York (23 October). In Agnew Papers.

———. 1883b. *Medical Ethics and Etiquette: The Code of Ethics Adopted by the American Medical Association, with Commentaries.* New York: D. Appleton.

———. 1886. *Medicine of the Future: An Address Prepared for the Annual Meeting of the British Medical Association in 1886.* New York: D. Appleton.

F. R. S. 1883. Preface. In *An Ethical Symposium: Being a Series of Papers concerning Medical Ethics and Etiquette from the Liberal Standpoint*, ed. Alfred C. Post et al., iii–vii. New York: G. P. Putnam's Sons.

Hamstra, Kenneth Warren. 1987. The American Medical Association Code of Medical Ethics of 1847. Ph.D. diss., University of Texas at Austin.

Handy, Jno. H. 1895. Letter to [Victor C. Vaughan]. Flint, Mich. (14 February). In Vaughan Letters.

Hun, Thomas. 1883. A Plea for Toleration. In *An Ethical Symposium: Being a Series of Papers concerning Medical Ethics and Etiquette from the Liberal Standpoint*, ed. Alfred C. Post et al., 56–71. New York: G. P. Putnam's Sons.

Hunt, David. 1882. Letter to C. R. Agnew. Boston (22 November). In Agnew Papers.

Jacobi, Abraham. 1882. Inaugural Address, Delivered February 7th, 1882, at the Opening of the Seventy-sixth Annual Meeting. *Transactions of the Medical Society of the State of New York*, 8–16.

————. 1886. The Anniversary Discourse: New York Academy of Medicine. *Medical Record* 30:608.

Kaufman, Martin. 1971. *Homeopathy in America: The Rise and Fall of a Medical Heresy*. Baltimore: Johns Hopkins University Press.

King, Lester S. 1983a. The AMA Gets a New Code of Ethics. *Journal of the American Medical Association* 249:1338–42.

————. 1983b. The Changing Scene. *Journal of the American Medical Association* 249:1897–1900.

Nichols, H. W. 1882. Letter to C. R. Agnew. Canandaigua, N.Y. (14 July). H. W. Nichols Letters, Manuscripts, and Special Collections, New York State Library.

Osler, Wm. 1895. Letter to [Victor C.] Vaughan. Baltimore (16 February). In Vaughan Letters.

Pepper, Wm. 1885. Letter to Isaac M. Hays. Newport, R.I. (4 July). In Isaac Minis Hays Papers, Manuscript Department, American Philosophical Society Library, Philadelphia, Pa.

Pilcher, Lewis S. 1883. Codes of Medical Ethics. In *An Ethical Symposium: Being a Series of Papers concerning Medical Ethics and Etiquette from the Liberal Standpoint*, ed. Alfred C. Post et al., 42–55. New York: G. P. Putnam's Sons.

Post, Alfred C., et al., eds. 1883. *An Ethical Symposium: Being a Series of Papers concerning Medical Ethics and Etiquette from the Liberal Standpoint*. New York: G. P. Putnam's Sons.

Proceedings: First Annual Meeting of the New York State Medical Association, Held at the Murray Hill Hotel, in New York City, November 18, 19, and 20, 1884. 1884. *Transactions of the New York State Medical Association* 1:585–609.

Report of the Association for Preventing the Re-Enactment in the State of New York of the Present Code of Ethics of the American Medical Association. 1883. Meeting of the General Committee, 20 April 1883. New York: n.p.

Rice, John B. 1855. Notes on Lectures by Alonzo B. Palmer, Materia Medica and Therapeutics, University of Michigan College of Medicine and Surgery, Ann Arbor, lecture of 4 December. In John B. Rice Papers, Manuscript Collections, Rutherford B. Hayes Presidential Center, Fremont, Ohio.

Rogers, Naomi. 1998. *An Alternative Path: The Making and Remaking of Hahnemann Medical College and Hospital of Philadelphia*. New Brunswick, N.J.: Rutgers University Press.

Roosa, Daniel B. St. John. 1883a. The Necessity for a Code of Medical Ethics. *New York Medical Journal* 37:421–23.

———. 1883b. Objections to the Code of Ethics and to the Disciplinary Authority of the American Medical Association. In *An Ethical Symposium: Being a Series of Papers concerning Medical Ethics and Etiquette from the Liberal Standpoint*, ed. Alfred C. Post et al., 101–22. New York: G. P. Putnam's Sons.

Rosenkrantz, Barbara Gutmann. 1985. The Search for Professional Order in Nineteenth-Century American Medicine. In *Sickness and Health in America: Readings in the History of Medicine and Public Health*, ed. Judith Walzer Leavitt and Ronald L. Numbers, 219–32. Madison: University of Wisconsin Press.

Rothstein, William G. 1972. *American Physicians in the Nineteenth Century: From Sects to Science*. Baltimore: Johns Hopkins University Press.

Stillé, Alfred. 1874. *Therapeutics and Materia Medica: A Systematic Treatise on the Action and Uses of Medicinal Agents, Including Their Description and History*, 4th ed., vol. 1. Philadelphia: Henry C. Lea.

———. 1884. An Address Delivered to the Medical Class of the University of Pennsylvania, on Withdrawing from His Chair, April 10, 1884. *Medical News* 44:433–38.

"Truth." 1883. Letter to the Editor. Misstatements about the New York Code. *New York Medical Journal* 37:54.

Van der Warker, Ely. [1884]. Comments. In *Minutes of a Convention Held in the City of Albany, February 4th and 6th, 1884, at Which the New York State Medical Association Was Organized on a Permanent Basis*. n.p.

Vaughan, Victor C. 1895. Letter to Dear Doctor. University of Michigan, Ann Arbor (11 February). In Vaughan Letters.

Warner, John Harley. 1987. Medical Sectarianism, Therapeutic Conflict, and the Shaping of Orthodox Professional Identity in Antebellum American Medicine. In *Medical Fringe and Medical Orthodoxy, 1750–1850*, ed. W. F. Bynum and Roy Porter, 234–60. London: Croom Helm.

———. 1991. Ideals of Science and Their Discontents in Late Nineteenth-Century American Medicine. *Isis* 82:454–78.

———. 1992. The Fall and Rise of Professional Mystery: Epistemology, Authority, and the Emergence of Laboratory Medicine in Nineteenth-Century America. In *The Laboratory Revolution in Medicine*, ed. Andrew Cunningham and Perry Williams, 310–41. Cambridge: Cambridge University Press.

Wood, Geo. B. 1856. Annual Address before the American Medical Association, by the President. *American Medical Gazette and Journal of Health* 7:398–409.

Wood, Horatio C. 1880. *A Treatise on Therapeutics, Comprising Materia Medica and Toxicology, with Especial Reference to the Application of the Physiological Action of Drugs to Clinical Medicine*, 3rd ed. Philadelphia: J. B. Lippincott.

———. 1883–84. The Principles of Modern Therapeusis. *Philadelphia Medical Times* 14:633–35.

———. 1891–92. General Therapeutic Considerations. In *A System of Practical Therapeutics*, vol. 1, ed. Hobart Amory Hare, 17–52. Philadelphia: Lea Brothers.

4

The Challenge of Specialism in the 1900s

ROSEMARY A. STEVENS, PH.D.

The AMA's 1847 Code of Ethics set out professional duties, reciprocities, and rights for an honorable profession of fee-for-service generalists. In contrast, the dominant themes of medical professionalism in the twentieth century were specialization, institutionalization, and third-party payments. Through much of the century the code was to be pushed and pulled in different ways to express these very different conditions. It was not clear whether the code should act for the profession as a ruling body of doctrine, upheld by effective sanctions such as expulsion from the American Medical Association (AMA) or its constituent societies, or whether it should be regarded more flexibly as a set of guiding principles. In this chapter I explore specialization and the challenges it posed to the profession—to specialists, to general practitioners, and to the AMA—in the first two decades of the twentieth century. How were these challenges reconciled with the AMA's supposedly unifying Code of Ethics?

My first theme is that the instrumental role of the code changed between 1900 and 1920. If its nineteenth-century role was as a vehicle for defining and upgrading a responsible profession, the code was an unwieldy, even irrelevant instrument for rampant specialization in the twentieth century. By the 1920s, the code was to take on new roles in forging political unity through the socioeconomics and politics of medicine. Its present-day role is different yet again. Thus the first two decades of the twentieth century form a distinct period in the history of the code.

A second theme is versatility. In this period an attenuated code imposed few barriers to specialism: the AMA accepted professional segmentation based on specialist roles and skills without much comment and was quiet about the role of new specialty power structures. Once these had been accepted, notably through the establishment and success of the American College of Surgeons between 1913 and 1920, the code was once more available as a vehicle for a unified profession.

The rift in the fabric of the AMA in the late nineteenth century portrayed by John Harley Warner (see chap. 3, this volume), an instructive lesson on the symbolic power of the code to mobilize dissent, is one element in the AMA's largely quiescent position toward specialization in the early years of the twentieth century. But by the first decade of the new century, powerful new forces were in play. First and foremost, medicine was becoming fractionated into specialties at the same time that the AMA was reorganizing into a federation based on membership in county and state medical societies following constitutional changes in 1901. There was an acute sense of the need for compromise between the interests of university professors and those of grass-roots practitioners, and among differing agendas in the states. Membership in the medical societies rose from 35,000 in 1901 to more than 70,000 in 1908, ensuring the association increasing national visibility and prestige (Simmons 1933, 1). Dissent was to be avoided wherever it threatened harmonious professional relations.

Fortuitously, for a brief period between the late 1890s and the 1920s, the interests of general practitioners, big-city specialists, and medical school teachers in the leading schools were aligned around the AMA's agenda of national reform of medical education. In 1896 the AMA *Journal* issued its first report on medical colleges in the United States; in 1901 the journal added a compilation of medical practice laws; in 1904 the AMA formed its influential Council on Medical Education, whose members were professors from the leading schools; and in 1910, with the council's active cooperation, Abraham Flexner published his devastating critique of the schools, thus affirming and strengthening the AMA at a critical stage of its development (Flexner 1910; Stevens 1998, 58–74). Educational reform held the promise of upgrading scientific standards for practice, thus appealing to the adherents of the "pure scientific democracy" described by Warner. However, the reforms also demonstrated the effectiveness of organized medicine as a "political democracy," able to limit the future supply of physicians by pressing for the merger and elimination of medical schools. Not unnaturally, this was a matter of interest to the army of general practitioners and part-time specialists who were struggling financially in an overcrowded profession.

However, while the AMA's reform agenda for medical education was overtly directed to creating a better education for the general practitioner, it was actually a de facto endorsement of specialty departments (and thus specialists) in the schools. Specialty sections flourished as scientific entities within the AMA, providing a base for solidarity among specialists. The AMA was led by distinguished specialists and medical administrators, a major reason for its success in educational reform and national public health policy in the first two decades of the century. AMA presidents included, among other prominent physicians, surgeons William and Charles Mayo of the already well-known Mayo Clinic (who began their terms in 1906 and 1917, respectively); Surgeon General of the Army William C. Gorgas (1909); Rupert Blue of the U.S. Public Health Service (1916); William C. Braisted of the U.S. Navy (1920); distinguished pathologist William H. Welch (1910); and renowned pediatrician Abraham Jacobi (1912) (AMA 1958).

Obvious problems existed in the hurly-burly of unregulated specialist practice throughout the United States, both for quality of practice and for the development of a harmonious profession. Self-attribution as a specialist suggested superior knowledge and skill. Yet anyone could claim the title, from university professor to the six-week graduate of a proprietary postgraduate school or someone who had hung out in the cafes of Europe with minimal attendance at specialty clinics. Specialization made the ethics of consultation more complex. General practitioners were particularly concerned about losing patients for good, once they had been referred to a specialist. This was typically referred to as "stealing" patients. Kickbacks were common, particularly from surgeons to referring practitioners. The 1847 Code had also failed to produce desirable patient behavior. Patients seemed insensitive to the importance of adequate (and relevant) specialist education, crowding fashionable specialists' waiting rooms, predominantly those of surgeons, whatever their perceived complaint. One speaker to a county medical society in Illinois called the public's attitude toward surgeons "idiotic" (Reid 1908, 582). All of these concerns raised ethical issues.

How far could and should the AMA, champion of a homogenous profession, act as the parent of specialization? Let us turn first to contemporary views of specialization, next to what it meant to general practitioners, and then to organizational and ethical questions more specifically. I want to illustrate, in particular, the coalescence of interests between general practitioners and the specialist elite.

Specialism and Specialists

By 1900 specialism was an established fact, represented both by specialists in practice and by successful national associations, such as the American Surgical Association (1880) and the Association of American Physicians (1886), led by university teachers and based on professional distinction. The leading medical schools included, as a matter of course, specialized teaching and research departments in skin and venereal diseases, ophthalmology and otology, gynecology, laryngology, neurology, psychiatry, and pediatrics, together with the newer specialties of rhinology, orthopedic surgery, and genitourinary surgery. Some of the lesser schools included proctology, gastrology, and abdominal surgery. Meanwhile, outside of the schools, popular demand encouraged specialists in such fields as rheumatism, appendicitis, intubation, fever and catarrh, and hair and complexion (Zeisler 1901). It was not unusual, wrote an eminent Chicago physician, "to find an invalid whose suffering depends upon one principal thing, visiting an oculist, a stomach specialist, a dermatologist, a urinalyist and several other specialists, at one and the same time, acting independently of one another, while the family physician, the general man of the constellation stands by as umpire, occasionally throwing in an anti-constipation pill" (Billings 1898, 99). Specialization was proliferating to such an extent that the role of the general practitioner was being questioned in urban areas across the United States. A specialist in throat surgery from Philadelphia put the point nicely in a talk in Columbus, Ohio, in 1899: "Hitherto, the general practitioner has been regarding the specialist somewhat as the small boy regarded the arrival of his baby brother when he said, 'A little dog would have been better.'" His point was that the boy loved his brother in the end (Makuen 1899, 179). For organized medicine, the question was how this love—friendly cooperation between generalists and specialists—was to be defined, managed, and expressed.

Specialism was both a matter of pride and a source of concern in the medical circles of 1900. Science offered one justification; the proliferation of knowledge, another; the technology of surgery in burgeoning new hospitals, a potent third. "Old dividing lines are broken down," wrote one critic, who blamed the exigencies of the overcrowded medical marketplace. Specialties "have been so broadened as to disappear, and even the practice of surgery as distinguished from that of medicine seems unlikely much longer to be confined to a special class" (Kelsey 1900, 629). Drawing on evolutionary rhetoric made popular by Herbert Spencer and others, speaker after speaker described medical specialism as a necessary and desirable aspect of twentieth-century progress, an intrinsic element in society's larger "struggle for existence." "Is specialism a psychic advance or a retrogression?" asked one psychiatrist. The expected answer was of course that it was an advance (Alexander 1906, 438). Business, law, and other professions seemed to be thriving on subdivision, and the assumption was that medicine would too.

Nor was the enthusiasm for specialism confined to leading centers of medicine in the East and the Midwest: Boston, New York, Chicago, and Philadelphia. Participants in a discussion of medical specialism at the Utah State Medical Association in 1905 echoed the same general rhetoric. The "progressive division of labor" in all fields was a "stern necessity" (Snow 1905, 359). This was the "age of specialism," and every member of the profession should confine himself to a particular line of work (Ewing 1905, 361). One speaker was assigned as his topic the "unwarranted encroachments of the general practitioner upon the fields of the eye, ear, nose, and throat specialist from the latter's standpoint." He likened the person who would put back the clock to someone who rejected modern travel and invested his money in an old stagecoach line running through the United States. The "encroachments" were improper diagnosis and treatment by general practitioners for conditions that a specialist could handle easily, such as prescribing a simple spray or douche for nasal catarrh without making a rhinoscopic examination, missing adenoiditis, or ignoring the possibility that a patient with a headache might need her eyes tested (Stauffer 1905, 357).

The two most visible fields for specialization were ophthalmology and abdominal surgery. Since few general practitioners of the 1890s were able to use the ophthalmoscope, the eye specialists had a clear technological advantage. By 1908 there were some 2500 to 3000 practitioners in ophthalmology in the United States, together with thirty-five special hospitals and many more departments in general hospitals and medical schools; and there was substantial professional and public concern about the prevalence of eye diseases, notably in the newborn, and among workers as a result of eyestrain in the workplace. Vigorous competition was also alarming the best specialists on two fronts: from poorly trained doctors who held themselves out as experts, and from an army of well-organized (nonmedical) opticians who were seeking their own separate license in the states (Stevens 1998). In ophthalmology as well as in the related fields of ear, nose, and throat, ill-trained specialists posed problems of competition to general practitioners as well as to the better-trained, research-oriented specialists. But general practitioners were limiting their own fields too, for example by referring eye cases or surgery to specialists, and thus were no longer truly generalists. The chair of the AMA section on laryngology, otology, and rhinology claimed in 1912 that in some cities more doctors were limiting their work to these four special areas than were engaged in the whole field of general practice (Shambaugh 1912). Professional roles were becoming unclear.

Surgery in ill-trained hands posed potential dangers that twentieth-century Americans treated cavalierly. Surgery was glamorous and thrillingly modern. It could produce demonstrated cures (for example in acute appendicitis) and was regarded as relatively safe in the sterile operating environments of the new modern hospitals. "In these days," wrote an observer laconically, "operative intervention is so easy, that mistakes as a rule cost less" (Editorial 1900, 70). Surgeons were repairing gunshot wounds, draining abscesses in the brain, removing fluid accumulated in the chest during pleurisy, relieving the "running from the ear" that often accompanied scarlet fever and other infections, removing enlarged tonsils and adenoids, and cutting out tumors in all parts of the body. However, as AMA president and surgical professor W. W. Keen remarked in a nice damning phrase, the abdomen and pelvis were the particular "playground of the surgeon" (Keen 1901, 254). Abdominal and gynecological surgery became the focus of major efforts to reform surgery.

The vogue for surgery suggested agreement between doctor and patient that surgery was a risk worth taking. Indeed, public enthusiasm for surgery was to become a lasting trait of the American system. Yet unnecessary surgery—for example, exploratory laparotomies to settle a diagnosis rather than to benefit the patient or unnecessary hysterectomies and caesarian sections—was a serious, commonly recognized problem from the beginning of the century. Surgical professor Arthur Dean Bevan, then chair of the Council on Medical Education and later AMA president (1918), estimated in 1906 that 30 percent of gynecological operations were unnecessary (Bevan 1906).

One essential ethical question was whether it was professionally responsible to assume that all surgeons were of equal standing and skill. To the surgeons who pored over the new journal *Surgery, Gynecology, and Obstetrics* (established in 1905) and who thronged to the first Clinical Congress of Surgeons in 1910 to observe the latest in surgical techniques, common sense was likely to suggest that it was not.

A rather different, but related question was whether any ethical code in the twentieth century could impose duties on patients beyond the simple courtesies outlined in the 1847 Code of Ethics. Rationally, in a system fragmented into specialties, patients would be discouraged, in their own basic interests, from going straight to specialists, because direct access to specialists assumed members of the public were competent to make the initial diagnosis of which specialist they might need. Arguably, twentieth-century patients were much more knowledgeable about medicine than their predecessors—such as the longshoreman or housemaid described by a New York doctor in 1910 "who can tell with surprising accuracy all about the human appendix and discourse with glibness upon the germ theory" (Hillis 1910, 751). But unfortunately this knowledge was often partial and sometimes wrong. Direct access to specialists also weakened the position of the family practitioner, since patients were more ready to discount the advice of the practitioner who merely sent them on to a specialist or who counseled inaction and patience.

In Britain in this period, a formal system of referral was emerging that was to protect both the generalist's and the specialist's position. The general practitioner was the patient's primary physician (as we would now call it), and a limited cadre of specialists acted as consultants, monopolizing the staff of leading hospitals. Denial of direct access of patients to specialists was usually accomplished by the consultant's refusal to take such patients without a referral from the general practitioner. This basic generalist-specialist referral system, however, was doomed to fail as a pattern for practice in the egalitarian professional system of the United States. It assumed that general practitioners were competent as diagnosticians (a matter of some difference of opinion among specialists); it ignored the fact that middle-class patients liked going directly to specialists and talking about their experiences with friends; and it suggested limiting hospital appointments to an elite (a matter of continuing dissension in American medicine). In a profession trying to achieve unity, the power struggles between generalist and specialist were best ignored.

Between 1900 and 1920 basic ethical questions posed by specialism were thus either shunted aside or were displaced from the context of the code of ethics by being defined as practical problems for immediate attention. Two questions attracted the most attention. How could specialty practice be upgraded or "standardized" so that reputable specialists could be trained and identified by patients and practitioners? And how could one pernicious aspect of GP-specialist relations—the secret splitting of fees between a surgeon and a referring physician—be outlawed?

The case for defined specialist training was self-evident. As medicine became more complex, specialists needed not only adequate skills in their special field but also—of particular importance in a system where patients had direct access to specialists—the ability to put the patient's condition in proper context. For instance, kidney specialists needed to be able to treat heart diseases or diseases of the digestive system, the eye specialist should know about Bright's disease and syphilis, and the obstetrician should know about the impact of prolonged labor on the neurology of the infant. Instead, by 1900 there were two identifiable kinds of specialists—dubbed by contemporaries as the true and the pseudospecialist, or exclusivist—and pseudospecialists could be dangerous. "I will not say that all such specialists are bad or stupid men," said a professor from the Medical College of Virginia. "I would rather say that they are misguided men, that they are contracted men, that they are narrow men" (Johnston 1897, 289). Too often the specialist could "see no further than the organ he has selected as his special plum" (Billings 1898, 99).

The AMA had to balance out the demands of democratic reorganization, focusing on increased membership in county medical societies (and including the "pseudospecialists," many of whom were also general practitioners), with the logic of establishing a specialist elite. Professional leaders sent a mixed message about specialty skills in talks before their local medical societies. Frank Billings is a good early example. A key figure in both the Chicago Medical Society and the AMA (becoming AMA president in 1902) and reportedly a man who "radiated power," Billings was a laboratory-oriented physician who had studied bacteriology in Europe. He was a leading member of the Association of American Physicians, opponent of proprietary medical schools, specialist in the newly defined field of internal medicine, and professor at Rush Medical College (later merged with the University of Chicago). Billings addressed the Chicago Medical Society on the topic of specialism in 1898. The themes he raised were echoed by many other speakers in the first decade of the century: that the only sound way to become a specialist was through a rigorous general understanding of medicine; that since this was not then available in medical school, this meant a period in general practice before specialization; and that specialism was "disorganizing the medical profession" and "spoiling the patient," even though virtually everyone believed that specialists were necessary (Billings 1898, 99).

However, even well-trained specialists posed problems to an inclusive, egalitarian code of ethics, for they set up new hierarchies above general practice, suggesting a two-class system. This ethical issue was a far cry from the problem of ill-trained opportunists holding themselves out as specialists, to be sure, for they suggested unfair competitive cliques brandishing specialty status as a proscribed trademark. Nevertheless, the acceptance of a justifiable elite was also problematical. It says much about the difficult conditions of practice at the time that to the body of the profession, who were predominantly in family practice, the development of a well-trained elite seemed to be the lesser of two evils and the better approach for the care of patients. There were "too many specialists, but not enough good ones" (Zeisler 1901, 2).

General Practice and the Problem of Fee-Splitting

In theory, specialism widened the range of general practice by having experts standing by for consultation in cases such as major surgery, intubation, or a complicated obstetrical case. But there were vexing questions: Who should control the patient? How was specialist practice to be brought together for the full benefit of the patient? How should the specialties be regulated, and how should specialists be trained? And if every doctor was to be a specialist, then what was the general practitioner's field?

The traditional ideal of the family practitioner, someone serving all fields of medicine and acting as family counselor, chum, and intimate seemed largely to have disappeared. "Some of you might well ask if there is anything left for the general practitioner," a professor declared to freshmen at the year's opening exercises at Northwestern University Medical School in 1900. His answer was a resounding yes, citing the need for good management of acute diseases, normal deliveries, dealing with most eye diseases (but not cataracts or specialized diagnoses), and the perhaps mythical role of trusted family counselor (Zeisler 1901, 1). Others were not so sure. An obstetrics professor in Kansas City voiced a fairly common turn-of-the-century view: that "ere long the generalist would ebb out into the sea of oblivion, whilst astride the crest of the topmost incoming wave of public sentiment the different specialists ride triumphantly past the breakers into the harbor of ease, plenty and affluence" (Ritter 1898–99, 355; Konold 1962, 46). The long debates about the role and future of the generalist, lasting for more than one hundred years and still taking place, had begun.

Looking at the bright side, as did, for example, leading ophthalmologist Edward Jackson of Denver, one might claim general practice as an emerging specialty in its own right (Discussion 1899). But this was easy if one were a specialist. It was not so easy to find oneself a "residual legatee" to whatever was left after the surgeon, the neurologist, the gynecologist, and many other specialists had claimed their own expert jurisdictions (Reid 1908). There was no clear specification of the role and function of general practice in an age of specialization. Nothing came of a resolution to the AMA House of Delegates in 1919 to encourage the designation of general medicine or family physician as a "distinct and dignified specialty." Among the fifteen specialty committees organized by the AMA Council on Medical Education in 1920, family medicine was nowhere to be seen (Stevens 1998, 151, 155; Fishbein 1947, 314). It would take another half-century for family practice to achieve the formal accolade of specialty status: its own specialty certifying board in 1969.

Some science-oriented specialists were condescending to the general practitioner on occasion. Internist Heinrich Stern of New York, who was to found the American College of Physicians in 1915, described general practitioners as solvers of human, rather than scientific problems, serving an entirely different purpose from those in scientific fields. The practitioner, he said, was properly concerned with what worked, not why it did (Stern 1905). Thus general practice was branded as unscientific. This was a double blow since the proposed alternative, the role of human advisor, was discouraged by the public's (and much of the profession's) fascination with twentieth-century technology and the role of experts. Nor was family counseling encouraged by the culture of the reforming schools, by a sustaining system of medical ethics, by the marketplace, or by the geographical mobility of families and individuals. Patients were allegedly much more willing to pay the specialist's bill for specific techniques and treatments than the general practitioner's bill. A professor of surgery remarked in Saint Louis that most people would be insulted if the doctor charged for "mere advice," because Americans paid "for medicine not words" (Lanphear 1906, 24). Specialists, meanwhile, took to the high moral ground whenever it was suggested that they should share their fees with the referring practitioner, even though it was only the *secret* division of fees that was strictly unethical, not the division of fees in itself.

The generalist was caught on the horns of a dilemma. On one hand, the vastness of the special branches and the impossibility of mastering them acted as a "depressant," it was said, making the general practitioner less useful and less self-confident than in earlier days; making him someone who lacked the belief in himself that marked the successful practitioner (Bulkley 1899; Saint John 1904). On the other hand, those who did assert self-confidence—for example, declaring to a patient that she needed major surgery before the surgeon had made a separate diagnosis—were castigated in leading journals for their hubris (Editorial 1900). At the very least, the medical societies might have tried to insist more forcefully that specialists inform their patients that they should pay their family doctors for giving knowledge, comfort, and advice as well as for a procedure, a prescription, or a pill. The hard-working practitioner who went to pains to find the right specialists for his patients felt aggrieved that often the specialist, not himself, would receive a fee.

The fairly common practice of "fee-splitting" carried the weight of all these considerations. By fee-splitting was meant the practice whereby a specialist, typically a surgeon, gave an under-the-table kickback to a general practitioner for referring a patient—without informing the patient of this transaction. The practice reflected the worst of commercialism and underhanded dealing, but it also reflected a market that unfairly advantaged the specialist. There was no generally acceptable method in individual, fee-for-service practice, where all physicians were considered equal, for charging the patient a total fee for diagnosis and treatment of a particular condition with due account taken to the contribution of the patient's own practitioner. One alternative discussed in the contemporary press would be to have *open* division of fees, with the general practitioner and the surgeon presenting a joint bill for service, thus setting up what we might now call a practice network (Campbell 1903). The perceived problem was that this might advantage certain practitioners over others in the marketplace and raise new ethical issues about unfair competition. Instead, the AMA and leading surgeons organized parallel battles against secret fee-splitting.

In the absence of a formal general-practitioner-to-consultant referral system, and in the absence of a system of joint billing, what other options were there to regulate a medicine based on specialism? One approach would be to identify a relatively small cadre of full-time specialists who would limit their practices to consultation, perhaps through a second license or a university degree (both discussed at the time), leaving the general practitioner as the dominant agent in the care of patients. Not surprisingly, for general practitioners the idea of role differentiation and a limited role for specialists was appealing. Another approach would have been to organize multiple-specialty practice arrangements through hospitals or clinics. This approach, however, suggested unfair competition with respect to those who might be excluded and was to be opposed by the AMA for many years. The egalitarian principles that were built into the 1847 Code of Ethics, strengthened by the egalitarian assumptions of the AMA's reorganization as a professional democracy, ensured the outcome. This was not the time to create new distinctions within the association. Distinctions would have to come from other organizations.

In both cases—fee-splitting and defining specialty qualifications—the research-oriented, university-based specialists and the general practitioners had a common enemy: the ill-trained specialist who competed with both, to the detriment of each. Kickbacks from specialists to referring physicians provided incentives for those practitioners to refer to the highest bidder rather than to the most competent or best trained. The adoption of a reputable mark of specialist training, particularly for surgeons, would help eliminate the specialty diploma mills on which many of the "pseudospecialists" based their credentials. Moreover, if specialists were encouraged to abstain from general practice, they posed less danger of "stealing" patients, and all doctors might become more ethical practitioners. Prevailing practice patterns encouraged unethical behavior. An early commentator described the tensions in vivid terms: "It is useless to discuss ethics with the double-barreled specialist who is loaded for both special and general practice. It is equally useless to argue with the general practitioner whose deliberate purpose is to starve out the specialist" (Benedict 1899, 169). By the time of the Flexner report (1910), it seemed reasonable for specialists to establish a defining mark, so that both the public and the profession knew who was reputable and well trained. The most urgent need, then, for leading specialists and general practitioners alike, was to establish some form of education and credentialing for specialists—but not within the AMA.

Medical Ethics and the Challenge of Specialism

In this context—the proliferation of specialism, the problems for general practice, the dangers of surgical excess, and a movement to establish credentials for surgeons—the AMA grappled with the future of its code of ethics between 1900 and World War I. It was clear that the ideal of a homogeneous profession based on a well-educated general practitioner, the ideological core of the ethical code of 1847, was breaking down as a model for practice in the cities. On the organizational front, however, the AMA was committed to professional unity, not professional fragmentation, and the educational reform movement took as a given that all physicians should be educated as general practitioners, no matter what their career intentions. The AMA thus largely ignored the ethical issues of specialty practice, except where these appealed to a powerful bloc, as was the case for abolishing fee-splitting. With the AMA's reorganization, the primary responsibility for ethical issues devolved, in any event, to the local associations and the states.

The AMA meetings of 1902 set the stage both for an official position against fee-splitting and for the subsequent acceptance of specialist credentialing. Professor Arthur Dean Bevan introduced, on behalf of the AMA section on surgery and anatomy, the resolution that any member of a county medical society proven to engage in secret fee-splitting be "held guilty of misconduct, for which he may be expelled from the county medical society." The resolution carried, becoming AMA policy (AMA 1958, 265). However, this injunction was readily ignored at the county level, where the focus was on building membership and unity and where there were often mixed feelings about fee-splitting. In 1912, following a report from the Judicial Council on the continuing prevalence of fee-splitting, the AMA tried a more forceful move, agreeing to expel fee-splitters from the AMA itself. But the problem did not go away, for there was a third stage of action in 1924, when the AMA agreed to annul the charter of any "recalcitrant society" containing so many fee-splitters "as to make it impossible to enforce the ethical standards of the medical profession" (AMA 1958, 265–66). Behind these events lies some ambivalence about the relative roles of the AMA and the state and county associations in enforcing ethical behavior, leaving the door open for academic surgeons to act more effectively. At the first meeting of the new American College of Surgeons in 1913, each of the 1,059 founding fellows of the college took an oath to shun "dishonest money-seeking and commercialism," to refuse "all secret money trades with consultants and practitioners," and to teach the patient his "financial duty" to the physician (Davis 1960; Stevens 1998). Thus, an acknowledged ethical problem was built into the concurrent agenda for specialty standards and enforced through a specialty organization.

Other action at the AMA meeting of 1902 led to the attenuation of the AMA Code of Ethics in 1903, sparked by the New York State Medical Association, which worked for a year revising the code (see chap. 3 in this volume). The New York version followed the 1847 Code in structure and general principle but updated it to meet changing circumstances. For instance, it clarified the section on obligations by patients to their physicians by stating that the "first duty of a patient is to select as medical adviser one who has received a sound general and special education." This version also attempted to strengthen the role of the family physician and to encourage an orderly referral system, declaring that "the patient or relatives should never send for a consulting physician without the express consent of the medical attendant" (AMA 1902). Nevertheless, contemporary confusions were reflected in what should be done when two physicians disagreed. Under this version (as under the 1847 Code), a general practitioner might call in another physician on a case (who could well be a specialist in 1902), and if they disagreed, a third physician could then be called in. If the new consultant was a specialist and the two specialists agreed with each other, then under the terms of the code the general practitioner, in the minority, would be expected to withdraw quietly. The patient would then choose one of the specialists as her attendant, thus ignoring the general practitioner and encouraging direct patient access to specialists. The AMA's revision of the code in 1903 attempted to fix this by stating that the consultant should not take charge of the patient "merely on the solicitation of the patient or friends" (AMA 1903). However this solution too was unlikely to appeal to everyone, including the patient. Given the volatile state of medical practice, the code was a minefield of potential differences of opinion.

The New York Association offered its revision as a replacement to the AMA Code of Ethics in a resolution to the House of Delegates in 1902. The House agreed to publish the revision in the AMA *Journal* three times before the 1903 meetings, and deferred the question to a committee chaired by Dr. E. Eliot Harris of New York. This committee did its own careful revision, drawing on the existing code, the New York version, and its own judgment. Some problems were immediately avoided by omitting the sections on the obligations of patients and of the public to physicians. The committee made a stronger statement about pharmacy, praising pharmacy on the one hand but adding opposition to pharmacists' prescribing, as well as substituting or adulterating drugs, and selling quack or secret remedies. In the thick of AMA reorganization, the committee also added an explicit connection between professional duties and membership in county medical societies (made less specific in 1912). The ethical physician, as stated in chapter 2 of the 1903 version, should belong to the local society, help set up a local or county medical society if one did not exist, and support it for professional and public good. This too was a potentially divisive statement.

Perhaps the most brilliant political move, softening this and other potential threats, was the addition of a very brief disclaimer at the beginning of the document published in the AMA *Journal*, stating that "the American Medical Association promulgates as a suggestive and advisory document" a code now re-entitled "Principles." In this short phrase the overtones of legal force and moral weight that distinguish a "code" were jettisoned. As stated in the *Journal*, the overt reason for this move was that in the new AMA structure it was up to the state associations, not the AMA, to establish codes and penalties to regulate the practice of medicine in their domains, albeit within broad principles set out by the national association. The strategy was clearly also a means of deferring difficult decisions about how specialist practice should be managed and of deflecting disagreement.

Hard work and brilliant political maneuvering followed. Within the span of the 1903 meeting, an enlarged committee was established, including one delegate from every state—acknowledgment that the AMA was now a federal organization. This committee unanimously agreed to the 1903 document, which included some revisions of the 1847 Code and some of the New York suggestions, and lobbied delegates to approve the resolution in the interests of organizational success. The proposal to adopt the new Principles of Medical Ethics was moved by Dr. Harris and seconded by outgoing AMA president Charles A. L. Reid of Ohio. Reid, in a quiet warning to the delegates, noted the "absolute harmony" that had marked the 1903 meetings as a whole. He urged them to adopt the motion and "put an end to a confrontational question which has disturbed our councils for many years." The delegates adopted the proposal unanimously, "amid tumultuous and prolonged applause" (AMA 1903).

The AMA's stand-aside position on medical ethics lasted though the next few years, supported by reports of its Committee on the Elaboration of the Principles of Medical Ethics in 1908 and 1910 that it was "not expedient to take any action at present." The Principles were revised in 1912, still called

"Principles" but without the exculpatory "advisory" remark at the beginning (AMA 1958, 234; AMA 1912). By then the AMA was becoming a powerful national force, engaged in national policy making. By this time, too, the AMA's major concerns about professional behavior were centering on socioeconomic questions, such as fee-splitting and contract practice, rather than on the broader challenges of specialism. Economic relations between practitioners and the state were highlighted with the passage of workers' compensation laws: a federal law in 1908, and laws in thirty states between 1910 and 1915. The 1912 Principles included the sweeping statement that it was "unprofessional for a physician to dispose of his services under conditions that make it impossible to render adequate service to his patient or which interfere with reasonable competition among the physicians of a community" (chap. II, art. VI, sec. 2). It was on the basis of the 1912 Principles, extended over the years, that the AMA was to formulate its growing opposition to organized multiple-doctor practice, the "corporate practice of medicine," and state intervention into the practice of medicine.

The revised Principles of Medical Ethics of 1912 embodied contemporary dilemmas of generalism and specialism without focusing on them specifically. It specified honorable and gentlemanly conduct by all physicians, including avoidance of "insincerity, rivalry or envy," and set out ideal patterns for consultation. Where appropriate, the doctor in charge of the case was to send the patient's case history to a consultant, and in turn, the consultant was to advise the first doctor of his results, both reports being on a confidential basis. If they disagreed, another consultant would be called and the first was to withdraw; but this consultant was free to tell the patient his views, "since the consultant was employed by the patient in order that his opinion might be obtained." A physician attending a case as a consultant was not to become the patient's primary attendant for that illness without the permission of the referring doctor. However, the patient was still free to make choices, merely being expected to advise the family doctor whenever he or she wished someone else to take the case. Thus the situation was still far from clear.

Advertising continued to be forbidden. Fee-splitting was unprofessional unless the patient or his "next friend" was fully informed about the terms of the transaction. The patient was to "be made to realize that a proper fee should be paid to the family physician." The code said nothing specific about specialist identification except where it banned an "exclusive dogma or sectarian system," but this phrase clearly did not apply to reputable specialties. It did not hinder the establishment of the American College of Surgeons, which was organizing at the same time, and it allowed fellows to put the letters FACS after their names. The American College of Physicians followed shortly afterward, in 1915.

In direct contrast to reform of undergraduate education, the educational and certifying aspects of specialization—and to some extent the ethical issues faced in specialist practice—developed outside of the AMA. The specialties grew as self-regulating entities in a free-for-all professional environment of powerful national specialty groups whose members were aligned with specialty departments in medical schools, the major hospitals, and the AMA's specialty sections. The present Byzantine system of specialty boards and residency review committees is one result of this; there are now twenty-four certifying boards and seventy-eight distinct types of specialty and subspecialty training programs. Recognizing the levels of concern at the time, the first boards were the present American Board(s) of Ophthalmology (1917), and Otolaryngology (1924).

A second result of the accommodations made between 1900 and World War I was that the AMA approached many of the issues of modern specialized medicine on an ad hoc basis, rather than addressing broad philosophical or ethical themes. More attention was to be given, for example, to opposing the salaried employment of radiologists by hospitals or compulsory health insurance, than to how well patients were doing in a specialized system: clinical progress through enhanced science was a given.

A third result, arguably, was that in trying to advance the cause of all physicians, the AMA failed to protect the generalist. The official AMA view in the 1920s was that general practitioners ought to be able to handle 90 percent of all medical complaints. However, there were already 15,000 full-time specialists in 1923, numerous other practitioners were specializing on a part-time basis, and the trend was moving toward specialization (Stevens 1998, 154, 162).

The specialty groups grappled with their own role as guardians of ethical standards for the practice of medicine. In the contested ethical domain of fee-splitting, the American College of Surgeons, a new national elite organization, proved to be an effective regulator of ethics, for its fellows at least, while the AMA was attempting to unify a diverse profession. Yet at the same time, the 1912 Principles gave the AMA moral force and legitimacy in the national political arena and helped shape the profession's responses to the socioeconomics of specialized medicine. The power of the code as a body of doctrine was strengthened in 1914 by making the AMA Judicial Council an appellate jurisdiction in the case of ethical controversies at the state and local level. From the 1920s to the 1960s, the code became both less and more important: less necessary as an internal instrument of professionalization—a unifying symbol for the entire profession—but more important for regulating economic competition and more potent as an instrument of the AMA's national political positions.

The question remained: Was there a need, or a case, for inventing a new code of ethics for specialized medicine? In terms of specialist insignia, the answer was no. Change in ethical expectations became a *fait accompli* with the foundation of the American College of Surgeons, which was designed specifically to establish distinguishing marks on qualitative grounds. The provision of specialist marks was thus one change in ethical practice, even if not one clothed in traditional ethical discourse. The desirability of higher (specialist) degrees and mandatory specialist licensing for surgeons was also debated. An unsuccessful bill for mandatory licensing of surgeons was introduced into the Illinois legislature in 1913, the year the college was established. To leaders of the AMA, a private national specialty organization with high standards—the college—might have seemed a much better alternative than specialist licensing across the states. But the key to AMA acceptance of specialist insignia for surgeons lay in two factors: general practitioners were quiescent or in favor; and the leaders of the AMA and the college were often the same university professors, specialists such as John B. Murphy (AMA president, 1911) and Arthur Dean Bevan (1918).

The college's requirement that its fellows abstain from fee-splitting demonstrated a shifting organizational locus for enforcement rather than changes in overall ethical principles, for by 1913 the AMA had been formally against fee-splitting for over a decade. The primary difference was that, as a selective, prestigious organization, the college could enforce its requirements on new fellows; while the AMA, a democracy, depended on the practices and views of its county and state medical societies. After its first year, when there was a separate fee-splitting statement, new fellows of the American College of Surgeons had to make a broad fellowship pledge that included proscription of fee-splitting among other declarations. The goal of the college was clearly stated by its first president, John M. T. Finney of Johns Hopkins: to elevate professional, moral, and intellectual standards; to foster research; and to educate the public to distinguish between the "honest, conscientious, well-trained surgeon, and the purely commercial operator, the charlatan and the quack" (Davis 1960, 481–82). In short, specialty ethics implied appropriate training, honorable behavior, and a scientific caste of mind.

The foundation statements for the American College of Physicians included no statements about fee-splitting, which was largely irrelevant to the nonsurgical specialties. However, the statements reveal how far twentieth-century medical practice was already intertwined with national and state legislation and policy making. The college was designed to promote the advancement of science and the practice of medicine, develop biologically oriented physicians, improve medical education and licensing (including support of a national licensing board), establish a National Board of Health, promote good relations among physicians, enlighten public opinion, and recognize distinguished achievements in medicine. In the pledge, adopted in 1916, fellows promised "faithfully to obey all the rules and regulations of the College, and always to conduct myself as a member of a learned profession and as a gentleman" (Morgan 1940, 133–34).

For both colleges, as with the specialty certifying boards, ethical principles were an intrinsic but subsumed element of a broader agenda. The primary goals were high standards of clinical practice in the specialties based on science and designated training, with action taken to achieve this. Thus, as part of its agenda, the American College of Surgeons began to accredit hospitals and set up a cancer registry. These goals constituted, or substituted for, a separate code of ethics. They *were* the ethics. In the AMA too, contributions to ethical standards for medicine were achieved along similar lines: upgrading the standards of medical schools and licensing of physicians; unifying the profession and developing county medical societies; and pressing for passage of national food and drug legislation, a direct assault on quackery and secret nostrums. In the twentieth century, ethical issues and public policy were to become increasingly enmeshed, as is quite evident today.

The establishment of the American College of Surgeons elicited little comment in the AMA *Journal,* although there were rumblings in other journals and in some AMA constituencies. The Chicago Medical Society, for example, claimed that the college was un-American, undemocratic, unjust, and inequitable, and urged its members to oppose and to resist. Nevertheless, 103 members of the society were among the college's first fellows. Differences of opinion were nicely expressed in resolutions from the Illinois delegation at the AMA meetings in 1914. One deplored the college as "violating the fundamental democratic principles on which the American Medical Association is based," while the other hailed the college as "filling a long-felt want, which the American Medical Association has hitherto failed to meet" (Davis 1960, 131–32; Stevens 1998, 89).

What was *not* included in the debates on specialism and the parallel evolution of the AMA's ethical statements is also of interest. In the first two decades of the twentieth century, specialization was addressed in terms of advancing science, providing specialist insignia, and battling against fee-splitting, but not in terms of new organizational forms of practice that would link generalists and specialists together in an evidently "disorganized" medical care system (Davis Jr. 1916). The ethical stance was, rather, the reverse: to protect the individual fee-for-service practitioner, whether generalist or specialist, against "unreasonable competition," hewing to the message of the 1912 code. The specialist system that developed in the United States for much of the twentieth century was thus one of free-standing individual private practices, of direct access by patients to any specialist they chose, and of continuing ambivalence about family practice in terms of training, role, and function. The results of this legacy are evident in the present organization of practice in the United States. We are still working on an effective design for specialized medicine.

In the twentieth century, the code of ethics became a policy document whose role is negotiated and whose content depends on changing coalitions and on policy debates, as well as on emerging ethical questions. These processes can be seen in the history portrayed here. The coalition of interest between general practitioners and academics was both successful and contingent. Indeed, from time to time ritual warnings were issued against specialists going too far in presuming to speak for the entire profession, particularly in economic and political areas. Two striking examples are of former AMA presidents. In 1916 the Judicial Council took action against John B. Murphy, who had completed his term as AMA president only four years before, for grossly advertising in the public press. Five years later, former president Frank Billings, a major orchestrator of the 1903 Principles and chair of the Judicial Council in 1912, had to publicly deny his alleged support of compulsory health insurance and legislation for the protection of maternity (the Sheppard-Towner Act) in a statement of disavowal at the AMA meetings of 1921 (Fishbein 1947, 289–90, 324–25). The success of organized multiple-specialist practice in the military hospitals in Europe during World War I was insufficient to move the profession toward support of organized practice; in fact, quite the reverse was true. From the 1920s on, the academics were less visible in setting AMA policy as a whole. The egalitarian principles of the code had held. Each physician competed with the next.

The history of medical ethics in the early twentieth century is a story of organizational success. In the short period, 1900–20, the challenge of specialism was contained, the profession unified, the schools upgraded, and the ethical principles saved; the AMA became a national force. This was no mean feat, speaking to extraordinary leadership. The resilience, versatility, and multiple roles of the code were demonstrated. Given changing conditions that advanced the profession, such as the provision of specialty credentials, the code was moved aside as a barrier to change. Given the growing concerns of fee-for-service practitioners, the code could be brought forward again as a policy instrument. It carried the virtues of both constancy and change.

References

Alexander, Harriet C. B. 1906. Is Specialism a Psychic Advance or a Retrogression? *Alienist and Neurologist* 27:438–51.

American Medical Association. 1902. Code of Medical Ethics. 1902. *Journal of the American Medical Association* 38:1649–52.

———. 1903. Principles of Medical Ethics. *Journal of the American Medical Association* 40:1379–81.

———. 1912. Principles of Medical Ethics. *Journal of the American Medical Association* 58:1790–93.

———. 1958. *Digest of Official Actions, 1846–1958.* Chicago: American Medical Association.

Benedict, A. L. 1899. The Ethics of Specialism. *Bulletin of the American Academy of Medicine* 4:166–71.

Bevan, Arthur Dean. 1906. Unnecessary Operations on Women. *Surgery, Gynecology, and Obstetrics* 3:591–92.

Billings, Frank. 1898. The Relation of General Medicine to the Specialties. *Chicago Medical Recorder* 14:93–100.

Bulkley, L. Duncan. 1899. How Far Has Specialism Benefited the Ordinary Practice of Medicine? *Bulletin of the American Academy of Medicine* 4:174–78.

Campbell, Don M. 1903. Should the Specialist Divide His Fees? *Journal of the Michigan Medical Society* 2:74–80.

Davis, Loyal. 1960. *Fellowship of Surgeons: A History of the American College of Surgeons.* Springfield, Ill.: Charles C. Thomas Publishers.

Davis Jr., Michael M. 1916. Organization of Medical Service. *American Labor Legislation Review* 6:16–20.

Discussion on J. Cheston Morris, "On the Effects of Specialism on the Medical Profession." 1899. *Bulletin of the American Academy of Medicine* 4:183–86.

Editorial: The Physician and the Surgical Consultant. 1900. *Boston Medical and Surgical Journal* 142:70–71.

Ewing, A. C. 1905. Discussion of papers by Stauffer and Snow (cited below). *Northwestern Lancet* 25:361.

Fishbein, Morris. 1947. *A History of the American Medical Association, 1847 to 1947.* Philadelphia: W. B. Saunders.

Flexner, Abraham. 1910. *Medical Education in the United States and Canada: A Report to the Carnegie Foundation for the Advancement of Teaching.* New York: Carnegie Foundation.

Hillis, Thomas J. 1910. Specialism in Medicine: Is It Overdone? *Medical Record* 77:748–51.

Johnston, George Ben. 1897. The Prevalence of Specialism and Who Shall Be Specialists. *Medical Register* 1:285–91.

Keen, W. W. 1901. Surgery. In *The Progress of the Century*, ed. Alfred Russel Wallace et al. New York: Harper and Brothers.

Kelsey, Charles B. 1900. The Future of Specialties. *New York Medical Journal* 72: 629–31.

Konold, Donald E. 1962. *A History of American Medical Ethics, 1847–1912.* Madison: University of Wisconsin Press.

Lanphear, Emory. 1906. Should the Specialist Pay a "Commission" to or Divide a Fee with the General Practician*[sic]*? *American Journal of Clinical Medicine* 13: 22–26.

Makuen, G. Hudson. 1899. Some Obstructions to the Progress of Specialism. *Bulletin of the American Academy of Medicine* 4:179–82.

Morgan, William Gerry. 1940. *The American College of Physicians: Its First Quarter Century.* Philadelphia: American College of Physicians.

Reid, David W. 1908. Influence of Specialism on the General Practitioner. *Illinois Medical Journal* 14:580–86.

Ritter, C. A. 1898–99. The Specialty of the Generalist. *Kansas City Lancet* 4:355–59.

Saint John, S. B. 1904. President's Address: Specialism in Medicine. *Proceedings of the Connecticut Medical Society* (12th Annual Convention), 117–35.

Shambaugh, George E. The Specialist in Medicine. *Journal of the American Medical Association* 58:1827–29.

Simmons, George H. 1933. Some Fragments of the History of the AMA. Part 2, The Reorganization. *AMA Bulletin* 28:124.

Snow, L. W. 1905. What the General Practitioner Should Know About the Specialties. *Northwestern Lancet* 25:359–61.

Stauffer, Frederick. 1905. Unwarranted Encroachments of the General Practitioner upon the Fields of the Eye, Ear, Nose, and Throat Specialist from the Latter's Standpoint. *Northwestern Lancet* 25:357–59.

Stern, Heinrich. 1905. Led Astray. *Journal of the American Medical Association* 45:1535–40.

Stevens, Rosemary. 1998. *American Medicine and the Public Interest.* Berkeley: University of California Press. New edition with updated preface. (First published in 1971 by Yale University Press.)

Zeisler, Joseph. 1901. Specialties and Specialists. *Journal of the American Medical Association* 36:1–6.

5

Medical Ethics and the Media

Oaths, Codes, and Popular Culture

SUSAN E. LEDERER, PH.D.

In 1850 Dr. James Platt White (1811–81), professor of obstetrics at Buffalo Medical College, introduced a new method of obstetrical teaching that would have far-reaching repercussions not only for physicians in Buffalo but also for the newly formed American Medical Association. White's innovation was to allow his students, after obtaining the permission of his patient, Mary Watson, to observe while he attended her during childbirth. His students, aware of the historic importance of demonstrative obstetrics, publicly commended their professor in the local newspapers, as did a local newspaper editorialist in Buffalo (Drachman 1979).

The "exposure" of a woman patient to the "curious eyes" of male medical students prompted discussion both within the Buffalo medical community and in the lay public. White became embroiled in a public controversy over medical education and medical ethics that ended with a libel trial and a ruling from the fledgling AMA. The professional objection to White's pedagogical innovation was not so much over the entry of male medical students into the birthing room as it was over the public discussion of the method in newspapers. As the AMA Committee on Education commented in its 1851 report on demonstrative midwifery, "It is to be regretted that this subject has been brought at all upon the popular arena. It is wholly a professional question, and should be discussed by the profession in a calm, considerate and dignified manner. It is no subject for newspaper warfare, nor for warfare in medical journals in newspaper style" (Report 1851). Reflecting their sensitivity to popular opinion and the tenuous position of the orthodox medical profession at mid-

century, the AMA Committee on Education rejected demonstrative midwifery as both unnecessary and inappropriate.

Long before bioethics became a discipline and bioethicists became media
pundits, issues of medical ethics were debated by physicians and the lay public in popular newspapers, magazines, and other media—although, as in the
case of Dr. White, the organized medical profession seldom approved of the
practice. Some commentators credit popular media, especially the books of
medical journalist Paul de Kruif and novelist Sinclair Lewis, with opening
medicine and medical science to a wider public. For years following the publication of Lewis's *Arrowsmith* (1925), observed Joanne Trautmann, one of the
founders of the field of literature and medicine, "American doctors named this
novel as their chief literary inspiration" (Trautmann 1978, 1012). Paul de
Kruif's *Microbe Hunters* (1926), with its "stirring tales of discovery and heroism," according to molecular biologist John Coffin, "influenced the career
choices of many senior scientists practicing today" (Coffin 1997). But the extent to which popular culture played a role in shaping popular expectations
about the nature of medical responsibility and professional obligations in the
twentieth century has received little scholarly attention.

In the second half of the nineteenth century, prominent American novelists explored aspects of the American Medical Association's 1847 Code of
Ethics. Although not invoked explicitly by name, the AMA Code and some of
its specific clauses, particularly the restriction on consultations with such
nonorthodox practitioners as homeopaths, gained wider currency when featured in novels like William Dean Howells's *Dr. Breen's Practice* (1881) and
Elizabeth Stuart Phelps' 1882 novel *Doctor Zay* (Burns 1988). These novels
appeared in the same decade in which some members of the New York State
Medical Society revised the AMA Code to permit consultations with legally
qualified medical practitioners, orthodox or nonorthodox. The controversy
precipitated by this step received considerable newspaper coverage, and the
novelists could thus assume that their readers would be somewhat familiar
with the challenge to the code, the ethical issue of restricting consultations,
and its implications for patients.

Beginning in the 1920s and 1930s, the Hippocratic Oath, rather than the
AMA Code, received greater attention from novelists and playwrights. In part,
this reflected the resurgence of the Oath and a general revival of Hippocratic
holism in American medicine. Amid the challenges to medical practice in the
first half of the twentieth century, some physicians looked to the distant past
to locate enduring professional values (Smith 1996). In novels, plays, and short
stories, writers used features of the Hippocratic Oath to address such contro-

versial moral issues of the day as abortion and euthanasia. Indeed, it is worth recalling today that the Hippocratic Oath remains familiar to lay audiences from its continuing appearance in popular culture. In reviewing David Rabe's play *A Question of Mercy* in 1997, critic John Lahr quotes a line from the work in which one of the characters begs a physician to hasten the death of his lover, suffering with AIDS: "He's asking for help to lessen his pain. . . . Isn't that your task, your oath as a doctor?" (Lahr 1997).

Examining several twentieth-century cinematic and literary treatments of medical ethics offers a window onto the ways that popular culture has shaped the discussion of medical morality for both physicians and the public alike. Confining the history of professional ethics to exchanges in medical journals and at medical meetings assumes that physicians themselves are unaffected by popular attitudes and by the culture that produces them. If it is somewhat unorthodox to consider Hollywood and women's magazines like *Good Housekeeping* and *Ladies' Home Journal* as platforms for discussion of medical ethics and professional responsibility in medicine, it is nonetheless true that we ignore these outlets at the peril of diminished understanding of the ways in which issues of medical ethics reflect the complex interactions between physicians and laypeople.

That films could be a powerful force in shaping popular opinion and belief was an article of faith for many members of the American medical profession. In the 1930s, for example, those individuals who closely monitored cinematic portrayals of physicians and surgeons did so with an eye to averting what they considered to be damaging and erroneous depictions of medical activity and attitudes. Such leading medical researchers as physiologist Walter Bradford Cannon and Harvard surgeon Elliott Cutler, who chaired the AMA Committee on the Protection of Medical Research, actively tried to suppress several 1930s films featuring experimentation involving animals because they believed these movies played no small role in harming the prestige of medical research and in gaining public sympathy for the antivivisectionist cause (Lederer 1993).

Medicine attracted enormous attention in the popular culture of the thirties. A number of books with medical themes—both fiction and nonfiction— attracted American readers of the 1930s, a group "chastened, weary of strident rebellion, and more tolerant of bolder comment on sex and criticism of entrenched ideas" (Mott 1947, 253–54). Best-selling books of the decade included Lloyd C. Douglas's *Green Light* (1935), French surgeon Alexis Carrel's *Man the Unknown* (1936), Victor Heiser's *An American Doctor's Odyssey* (1936), *The Citadel* by British physician-writer A. J. Cronin (1937), Eve

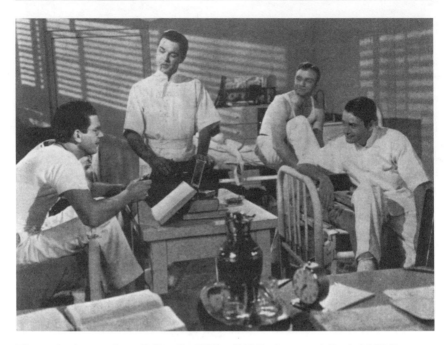

Figure 2. A scene from *Calling Dr. Kildare* (1939), the second film in MGM's popular Dr. Kildare series. (Courtesy of *Hygeia* (1939) 17:488.)

Curie's *Madame Curie* (1937), and Arthur Hertzler's autobiographical *The Horse and Buggy Doctor* (1938). The immensely popular Doctor Kildare character developed by novelist Max Brand also made his first appearance in 1936 (fig.2).

Given the intense popular interest in medical life, it is perhaps not surprising that playwrights and novelists would turn to issues of medical ethics, and especially to the Hippocratic Oath, in their work. To be sure, authors singled out some principles of the Oath for use as dramatic devices. Three ethical precepts in particular attracted both novelists and filmmakers in the 1930s: the imperative against abortion, the prohibition on euthanasia, and the injunction to keep secret those things that the physician might learn in connection with his professional practice.

The issue of abortion and the physician's responsibility received explicit attention in popular plays, novels, and films of the 1930s. In 1933 playwright Sidney Kingsley offered Broadway audiences a seldom-portrayed slice of medical life in his dramatic play *Men in White* (Raben 1993).[1] The production, which ran for 367 performances in New York City, garnered enthusiastic responses when it was performed in Chicago and also in London, Vienna, and Budapest. The play not only earned Kingsley the 1934 Pulitzer Prize for drama, but it was followed by a successful Metro-Goldwyn-Mayer Studios screen version, starring Clark Gable and Myrna Loy (Couch 1995).

Explicitly invoking the ideals of the Hippocratic Oath, the play prominently featured the issue of abortion (fig. 3). The young surgical intern at the center of the play has a sexual encounter with a student nurse, who becomes pregnant as a result. After an illegal abortion, she develops sepsis and is taken into the operating room for emergency surgery, performed by none other than the intern and his mentor. In what Morris Fishbein, editor of the *Journal of the American Medical Association,* described as the "most authentic and dramatic operating scene ever put into a play," the surgeons attempt to save her life without success (Fishbein 1934).

As part of his preparation for writing the play, Kingsley had witnessed in the Bellevue morgue an autopsy performed on a young girl who died as a result of septic abortion. The playwright recalled that he was "horrified to learn there were more than a million abortions being performed every year in this country—all illegal and mostly done by incompetents in septic, crude circumstances" (Couch 1995, 6). To be sure, most theater critics preferred to

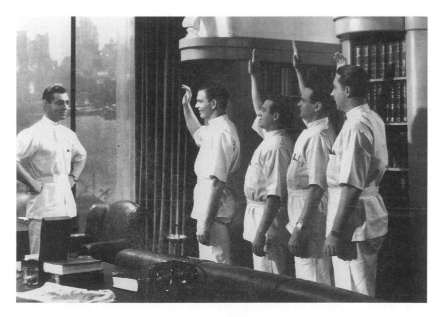

Figure 3. Dr. Ferguson (played by Clark Gable) watches as his fellow interns recite the Hippocratic Oath. (Courtesy of *Men in White* © 1934 Turner Entertainment.)

avoid mentioning Kingsley's use of the nurse's illegal operation; only *New York Times* critic Brooks Atkinson commented on the playwright's treatment of abortion (Atkinson 1933). In both the popular press and medical journals, discussions of the play suggest that many American physicians and surgeons were pleased with the depiction of medicine, despite the abortion issue. They liked Kingsley's portrayal of the demanding nature of a career in medicine and the moral gravity of the senior physicians he created on stage. The playwright was pleased that the Nazis banned the film version of *Men In White* because it was "not consistent with Nazi philosophy" (Couch 1995, 6).

The issue of abortion and the Hippocratic proscription against the practice also figured prominently in a novel entitled *The Hippocratic Oath*, published in 1938 by New York physician Edgar Dittler. The novel focused on the experiences of a young intern and his encounters with the medical system at Hippocrates General, a large urban hospital. The Oath of Hippocrates, the book jacket informs readers, was formulated more than two thousand years ago and remains the code of ethics followed by physicians: "Is it possible for a young man to remain true to this Oath when faced with the law of self-preservation, the lust for flesh, and the desire for success and prestige?" The novelist concludes that unfortunately it is not: "The need for money and the urge of unfilled desires bring about debauchery and evil practices that inevitably leave tell-tale scars on character and destroy honor" (Dittler 1938, jacket cover).

As in *Men In White*, the Hippocratic Oath is explicitly recalled in the context of abortion. In this case, the issue is money and what young physicians have to do in order to survive. As two interns discuss the framed copy of the Hippocratic Oath on the wall of the doctor's lounge, one recalls that "the dean of our medical school read it to us. Just in case we remembered to forget." After the lowly junior intern, the novel's main protagonist, reads the Oath's proscription on abortion ("in like manner I will not give to a woman a pessary to produce abortion"), his fellow intern informs him that "Hippocrates was very old-fashioned" (Dittler 1938, 179–80). Readers soon learn that the low salary the married intern receives has compelled him to accept money for referring "fair ladies of considerable means" to physicians who will perform the criminal abortions.

The book reviewer for the *New Yorker*, who described the book as "frank and lively," was right in predicting that "the doctors probably won't like it much" (Books 1938). The depictions of issues of medical competency, abortion, and questionable financial arrangements, together with the portrayal of the hospital as a hotbed of illicit sexual encounters between doctors and nurses, did not endear the book to physicians. Unlike *Men in White*, which had addressed the troubling issue of abortion in an environment ennobled by Hippocratic wisdom and idealism, Dittler's novel suggested how the high standards of the medical profession were corrupted by greed and arrogance. The Book Notices column of the *Journal of the American Medical Association* dismissed the novel's discussion of the "old question" about whether a physician or intern could resist the temptations of money while remaining true to the profession's ideals, concluding, "Obviously there are a few that cannot, but the vast majority can. All the old situations of life and love in the hospital are here reflected without much literary quality" (Hippocratic Oath 1939).

In these portrayals the Hippocratic Oath functioned as an emblem of the moral calling and professional responsibilities of American physicians. But the oath did not always receive respectful attention from writers. In his 1935 short story "The Hippocratic Oath," writer Sinclair Lewis, whose 1925 novel *Arrowsmith* is credited with inspiring many to enter the medical profession, dismissed the oath as a "solemn, churchly formula" that was "intended to make a youngster who has just disgraced himself by balling up the stylopharyngeus and salpingopharyngeus muscles, when any twelve-year-old boy knows the difference, feel that after all he has magically become a doc, and is now capable of treating boils, common colds and the bill-psychosis, or paymentia, of dead-beats—all three of which are incurable, though the happy medic hasn't yet learned it" (Lewis 1935, 24). Despite this less than favorable characterization, the physician at the center of Lewis's story nonetheless acknowledges that it was less the oath than what it stood for that influenced his conduct as a physician: "In itself an Oath is nothing, as in itself a Cross is only a trick of ebony and silver, and a Flag a streaky swatch of cotton or wool. It was the feeling behind the Oath: that a doctor must never betray anyone who depends upon him, no matter how vile" (Lewis 1935, 161). In Lewis's short story, the doctor's dilemma is his desire to reveal what he has learned in the course of caring for a patient. Despite the temptations (in the form of the patient's seductive wife), he resists in light of his Hippocratic commitment to refrain from breaking patient confidences.

This issue of confidentiality and the commitment to one's fellow physicians served as a focus of the best-selling novel of 1935, *Green Light*, by former minister Lloyd C. Douglas. In the 1930s and 1940s, Douglas's books, which often featured physicians and their moral problems, were extraordinarily popular. Douglas's first novel, *Magnificent Obsession* (1929), a tale of one man's redemption through his work as a surgeon, went through some fifty editions and three filmings (Dawson and Wilson 1952). Many of Douglas's novels, like *Green Light* and *Magnificent Obsession,* became Hollywood films.[2]

The hero of *Green Light* is a rising young surgeon, who takes the blame for a patient's death when his revered mentor, Dr. Endicott, frantic after learning about the collapse of his fortune in the stock market, makes a surgical mistake leading to the death of his patient. Endicott's decision to allow his protégé to take the blame creates a moral problem for the younger surgeon. Bound by his loyalty to his fellow physician and the Hippocratic Oath he has sworn to follow, he abandons his promising career and, after a series of adventures, eventually lands in western Montana, where he joins a bacteriologist conducting experiments with Rocky Mountain spotted fever (Douglas 1935). The older surgeon's failure to rise to the idealism embodied in the Hippocratic Oath provides the younger doctor the opportunity to lead a life of Christian self-sacrifice (he submits to self-experiment with infected ticks but survives his ordeal). Warner Brothers bought the film rights to the novel in 1936 and released a screen version the following year, starring Errol Flynn as the heroic young surgeon. Flynn, together with actress Olivia de Haviland, also starred in a radio version of the novel in 1938.

That these popular works in print, screen, and radio were seen as influential is evident from the attention they received from members of the medical profession in professional journals and in recollections of medical life from this period. Medical journals frequently reviewed both popular novels and films about the profession. In his 1944 *As I Remember Him: The Biography of R.S.*, microbiologist Hans Zinsser recalled that his own experiences of the Serbian typhus epidemic of 1915 were "on the whole rather prosaic and completely—try as I may—unconvincing of the heroism which the *Arrowsmith* type has made so familiar in prose and cinema, and which, despite de Kruif and others, I have never—Thank God!—observed in any of my numerous professional colleagues in action" (Zinsser 1944, 208). Zinsser was critical of medical bravado, but other physicians embraced portrayals in films and books that emphasized the high ethical standards of the medical profession.

In the 1930s some physicians cooperated with lay groups to develop educational materials to accompany the showing of such feature films as *Arrowsmith* and *The Story of Louis Pasteur*. The Progressive Education Association, with funding from the Rockefeller Foundation, created a discussion guide to accompany showings of *Men in White*. Among suggested questions for discussion—which did not include abortion—were: "Is there adequate medical care in the United States for everyone? How do we provide now for those who cannot afford private medical care? What objections are raised to state control of medicine? To group medical practice?" (Study Guide 1939). The Progressive Education Association's study guide for the films *The Story of Louis Pas-*

teur (1936) and *Arrowsmith* (1931) also featured explicitly medical ethical issues, including questions about the morality of experimenting with human beings.

The Motion Picture Production Code Administration, which after 1934 reviewed films from major Hollywood studios, worked closely with members of the organized medical profession to ensure that filmmakers depicted physicians with respect. In 1935, when Hollywood filmmakers, responsive to extensive newspaper discussions of voluntary euthanasia, proposed to make a film featuring a physician who ended the suffering of a dying patient, the Production Code Office required a number of changes in the script to ensure that the film presented the medical profession in a positive light (Lederer 1998).

In the 1930s mercy killing attracted considerable newspaper coverage amid efforts in the British Parliament to legalize voluntary euthanasia. As ethicist Ezekiel Emanuel has shown, newspapers on both sides of the Atlantic competed with each other to attract readers' interest in this issue (Emanuel 1994). In addition to publishing physician accounts of practicing euthanasia, magazines such as *Time* printed stories of "willing candidates" for mercy killing, together with vigorous denunciations of the practice from physicians and clergy (The Right to Kill 1935).

Joseph Breen (1890–1965), head of the Production Code Administration Office charged with ensuring the "decency" of Hollywood films, argued in 1936: "The worldwide interest that seems to have been revived concerning this question of 'mercy killing' so-called, has naturally resulted in a number of studios giving serious consideration to the possibility of producing a motion picture based upon this sensational theme" (Crime of Doctor Forbes 1993, 420). Among those studios was Twentieth-Century Fox, which began to develop *The Mercy Killer,* eventually released in a much modified form as *The Crime of Doctor Forbes* in 1936. The original screenplay closely followed the British debates and included a meeting in England in which seven distinguished men organize a "right to die" society to campaign for legalized euthanasia, dramatizing the actual origins of the Voluntary Euthanasia Society in December 1935. Although the studio was compelled by Breen's office to dilute the presentation such that no mercy killing actually occurred in the film, but only a confession of mercy killing, the film was nonetheless seen as a vehicle for dramatizing the arguments for voluntary euthanasia. The reviewer for the *New York Times,* for example, noted that the film laid an interesting groundwork for "consideration of the right or wrong in mercy killing" (Review 1936, 29). Other films that introduced mercy killing as a dramatic device in the 1930s and 1940s included *Moonlight Murder (1936)* and *Girl from God's Country* (1940), which featured a "brilliant surgeon" arrested for helping his terminally ill father to die. Newspapers, popular magazines, short fiction, and film thus provided a wider cultural context in which members of both the public and the profession responded to discussions about the morality of euthanasia.

The issue of mercy killing was not the only medical ethical question that generated considerable public discussion. Truth-telling and information disclosure to patients, especially when involving a diagnosis of cancer, prompted extensive reporting in popular journals and newspapers after the Second World War. Indeed, enlarging the focus to include popular media suggests that the recent history of information disclosure by physicians should be revised. For the most part, bioethicists have focused their attention on changes in professional attitudes toward truth-telling or information disclosure to patients since the 1960s and 1970s (Brown 1995). Routinely cited, for example, is Chicago psychiatrist Donald Oken's 1961 report of physician behavior after diagnosing cancer. In his survey of approximately two hundred physicians, he found that nearly 90 percent usually withheld the diagnosis from their patients. By 1977 a repetition of Oken's survey found physician behavior to have undergone a profound change; 98 percent of physicians reported being totally frank with patients diagnosed with cancer (Reiser 1980). Not included in such accounts is how popular discussions of disclosing a poor prognosis may have influenced professional behavior.

In the 1950s and 1960s, American popular magazines often reported on the question of what a patient should be told about his or her diagnosis. In April 1950, for example, the *Rotarian* magazine posed the question of what to tell a patient with prostatic cancer in its "What Would You Do" Series, which focused on practical problems in business and professional ethics. Six physicians and surgeons were asked to respond to the question "Do you tell the man the truth?" The only American physician participant, a general practitioner from Denver, Colorado, responded, "The truth, of course" (Symposium 1950). In 1956 President Eisenhower's bout of ileitis renewed public interest in the issue. In light of the survey conducted by the American Medical Association in 1956, which revealed a public desire for medical candor, incoming AMA President Dwight Murray told his fellow physicians that the experiences of World War II and the Korean conflict had forged a growing demand for frankness with patients: "The desire to know what's going on has become a part of the makeup of most Americans. In everything in which we participate we insist upon knowing the full story" (Should Doctors Tell All? 1956, 104). Given the changing character of Americans, Murray advised physicians to provide greater details about a patient's disease and treatment and specific answers to patient questions. He did concede that some patients would be better served by full disclosure than others, and that doctors reserved the discretion to act in a patient's best interests.

In the early 1960s, about the same time that Oken was conducting his often-cited survey documenting physician nondisclosure, a different picture emerges from the popular literature. The *Science News-Letter* in November 1961 reported a Science Survey poll of experts taken during the scientific sessions of the American Cancer Society meeting in which nearly all the participating physicians reported that doctors tell the patient the diagnosis of cancer (Davis 1961). One year later two popular women's magazines, the *Ladies' Home Journal* and *Good Housekeeping*, both addressed the "painful dilemma" of whether doctors should tell the truth to a cancer patient. Here too, readers of these magazines learned that American doctors differed about disclosing a diagnosis of cancer. In *Good Housekeeping*, physician Claude Forkner cited several surveys of lay attitudes about the issue, including a survey of 1200 adults in which 91 percent of the respondents insisted they would want to know the truth, a poll of cancer patients in which 89 percent favored being informed about their condition, and a survey of 560 "next of kin" in which the majority indicated that their family member should be told the truth (Should They Be Told the Truth? 1962).

These surveys of lay attitudes and how they influenced medical opinion seldom appear in discussions of the recent history of truth-telling or information disclosure. Yet they may be as salient as Oken's survey of physician behavior in understanding the changes in physician behavior and public expectation. Examining lay attitudes and popular discussions of this ethical issue calls into question the assumption that Oken's survey should automatically be regarded as representing mainstream American medical practice in 1961. Moreover, the examination of the broader social context challenges the interpretation that the changes in physician behavior occurred suddenly in the years between 1961 and 1977. The process may, in fact, have been more gradual, in response to growing patient and lay demand for being told the truth about a bad diagnosis.

The popular culture of the twentieth century—plays, novels, films, magazines, and newspapers—offers an important and under-utilized resource for understanding both the process and the context in which issues in medical ethics were shaped and reshaped for both professional and public needs. Most lay people today, it is fair to say, remain far more familiar with the Hippocratic Oath (if ignorant of its specific precepts) than with the AMA's Code of Ethics. This public awareness comes, not from reading articles in medical ethics or medical history journals, but from its continuing appearance in mass culture and the popular media. Broadening the scope of historical and ethical inquiry to include such unconventional sources as films and magazine articles will serve to enhance understanding of the complex history of medical ethics and its meanings for physicians and the public alike.

Notes

1. The only earlier play with a cast composed almost entirely of doctors was George Bernard Shaw's *The Doctor's Dilemma (1906)*.

2. It is more than a little surprising that Douglas has received virtually no critical attention, given his wide popularity.

References

Atkinson, Brooks. 1933. Men of Medicine. *New York Times,* 27 September.

Books: The Hippocratic Oath. 1938. *New Yorker,* 7 May, 94.

Brown, Kate H. 1995. Information Disclosure. In *Encyclopedia of Bioethics,* rev. ed., ed. Warren T. Reich, 3:1221–25. New York: Macmillan.

Burns, Chester R. 1988. Fictional Doctors and the Evolution of Medical Ethics in the United States, 1875–1900. *Literature and Medicine* 7:39–55.

Coffin, John M. 1997. Book Review: Microbe Hunters—Then and Now. *New England Journal of Medicine* 336:1264.

Couch, Nena, ed. 1995. *Sidney Kingsley: Five Prizewinning Plays.* Columbus: Ohio State University Press.

Crime of Doctor Forbes, The. 1993. *The American Film Institute Catalog of Motion Pictures Produced in the United States, Feature Films, 1931–1940,* ed. Patricia King Hanson. Berkeley: University of California Press.

Davis, Watson. 1961. Tell Cancer Victims Truth. *Science News-Letter* 80:299.

Dawson, Virginia Douglas, and Betty Douglas Wilson. 1952. *The Shape of Sunday: An Intimate Biography of Lloyd C. Douglas.* Boston: Houghton Mifflin.

Dittler, Edgar. 1938. *The Hippocratic Oath.* New York: Liveright Publishing Company.

Douglas, Lloyd C. 1935. *Green Light.* Boston: Houghton Mifflin.

Drachman, Virginia G. 1979. The Loomis Trial: Social Mores and Obstetrics in the Mid-Nineteenth Century. In *Health Care in America,* ed. Susan Reverby and David Rosner, 67–83. Philadelphia: Temple University Press.

Emanuel, Ezekiel J. 1994. The History of Euthanasia Debates in the United States and Britain. *Annals of Internal Medicine* 121:793–802.

Fishbein, Morris. 1934. New Books on Health: Men in White. *Hygeia* 12:58–60.

Hippocratic Oath, The. 1939. *JAMA* 113:1158.

Lahr, John. 1997. Death-Defying Acts. *New Yorker,* 24 March, 86.

Lederer, Susan E. 1993. Laboratory Life on the Silver Screen: Animal Experimenters and the Film Industry, 1930–1940. Paper presented at the History of Science Society, November 12, Santa Fe, New Mexico.

———. 1998. Repellent Subjects: Hollywood Censorship and Surgical Images in the 1930s. *Literature and Medicine* 17:91–113.

Lewis, Sinclair. 1935. The Hippocratic Oath. *Hearst's International-Cosmopolitan* (June).

Mott, Frank Luther. 1947. *Golden Multitudes.* New York: Macmillan.

Raben, Estelle Manette. 1993. *Men in White* and *Yellow Jack* as Mirrors of the Medical Profession. *Literature and Medicine* 12:19–41.

Reiser, Stanley Joel. 1980. Words as Scalpels: Transmitting Evidence in the Clinical Dialogue. *Annals of Internal Medicine* 92:837–42.

Report of the Committee on Education in Relation to "Demonstrative Midwifery." 1851. *Transactions of the American Medical Association* 4:436–37.

Review. Crime of Doctor Forbes. 1936. *New York Times,* 2 December, 29.

Right to Kill, The. 1935. *Time,* 25 November, 39–40.

Should Doctors Tell All? 1956. *U.S. News and World Report* 41:104.

Should They Be Told the Truth? 1962. *Good Housekeeping* 155:70–71, 200–206.

Smith, Dale. 1996. The Hippocratic Oath and Modern Medicine. *Journal of the History of Medicine* 51:484–500.

Study Guide to Men in White. 1939. Pamphlet, Progressive Education Association Commission on Human Relations.

Symposium. 1950. You Are the Doctor: What Would You Do in the Case of an Incurable Disease? *Rotarian* 76:24–26.

Trautmann, Joanne. 1978. Medical Ethics in Literature. In *Encyclopedia of Bioethics,* ed. Warren T. Reich, 3:1008–15. New York: Free Press.

Zinsser, Hans. 1944. *As I Remember Him: The Biography of R. S.* Boston: Little, Brown.

II

Professionalism and Professional Ethics

6

One Hundred Fifty Years Later

The Moral Status and Relevance
of the AMA Code of Ethics

EDMUND D. PELLEGRINO, M.D.

*Not for self, nor for the fulfillment of any earthly desire or gain, but
solely for the good of suffering humanity should you treat your patients
and so excel all.*

Charaka Samhita, D. C. Muthu

One hundred fifty years ago, when Isaac Hays, John Bell, and their colleagues
framed the first code of ethics for the then-nascent American Medical Association (AMA), the profession was in the midst of one of its recurrent identity crises. Standards of medical education were virtually nonexistent. Unorthodox practitioners and treatments flourished and enjoyed the favor of
public and press. "Orthodox" medicine, itself, was on shaky scientific
grounds. Venal physicians, charlatans, and internecine dissension discredited
the whole profession. American medicine seemed well on its way to becoming a trade like any other, its practitioners bent on the pursuit of untrammeled
self-interest.

Today, we face another, but far more complicated, moral crisis. The enormous power of medical technology, coupled with the legitimization of the
market ethos in health care, threatens to overshadow both physician and patient. What will our moral response be? What place in that response should
and will the moral guideposts of the Hippocratic Oath, and the AMA Code of
Ethics play? Should professional codes of ethics be abandoned entirely in an
autonomy-obsessed society? Should the traditional medical ethos be replaced
entirely by a new code, one modified to suit current economic and political re-

alities? Is a universal code even possible in our multicultural, morally plural-istic, democratic society?

The urgency, complexity, and problematic nature of these questions are justification enough for reconsidering the importance of the AMA Code of Ethics. I argue that the AMA Code is, indeed, still important, that it will re-main so because it embodies certain central moral truths about the universal human experiences of illness and the obligations that derive from that experi-ence, that the code translates these obligations into the language of daily med-ical practice, that commitment to that code is a promise of fidelity to trust that the profession owes those whom it treats, and that, despite the call for a "new" ethic, the moral heart of the 1847 Code remains viable even in the face of con-temporary deconstructionist trends in moral philosophy, in the profession, and in society.

I support these assertions in the following steps: first, I set out what I take to be the central moral precepts of the 1847 Code; then I examine the past and present criticisms of the AMA Code that give rise to the demand for a "new" ethic; following this I outline the social importance of the code today; and I close with a closer look at the grounding of the code in the internal morality of medicine and with a critique of the call for a "new" ethic. For purposes of this discussion, the moral "center" of the 1847 Code is located in article I and in the "Principles and Elements" of the current code. This is not to ignore or de-preciate the ethical significance of the other articles of the 1847 Code or the many issues developed in the "Reports" and "Current Opinions." Rather, it is to concentrate on what is unique to being a physician: the clinical relation-ship with patients. This is what is most at risk of deteriorating today and what gives meaning to the remaining parts of both codes.

At the outset, it is important to recognize that the AMA Code is a complex document in four parts, which have developed over the years since 1847: (1) the Principles; (2) the Fundamental Elements of the Physician–Patient Rela-tionship; (3) the Reports; and (4) the Current Opinions of the Council on Eth-ical and Judicial Affairs. The 1996–97 edition runs to 174 pages of text (Coun-cil 1996–97). The ethical compass points of the code are located in the "Principles" and "Elements," while the Current Opinions apply these prin-ciples to some 135 ethical issues for which the Reports provide the rationale. To express approbation for the Principles and Elements does not entail an ap-probation of everything in their detailed applications delineated in the Cur-rent Opinions and Reports.

The Moral Inspiration of the 1847 Code

In his introduction to the 1847 Code to the AMA convention of that year, Dr. John Bell said that it was framed on a tradition that went back to "the age of Hippocrates" (Appendix B, 317). Bell made no specific citation of any of the books of the Hippocratic corpus, nor does the code itself do so. Perhaps Bell did not elaborate because it might be presumed that the educated physicians of his time were familiar with the Hippocratic tradition to which, as far as ethics goes, those physicians had access through the writings of eighteenth-century English colleagues like Thomas Percival (Pellegrino 1985).

Most of the specifically moral content of the 1847 Code, as well as the etiquette of interprofessional relationships, was derived from the Hippocratic Oath and the other so-called deontological books—*Decorum, Precepts, The Physician* (Edelstein 1967, 328–29). To a lesser extent, the Hippocratic tradition also drew from the *obiter dicta* scattered throughout the other books of the corpus. The ethical content of the Hippocratic corpus was elaborated and commented upon over the centuries in many countries. A core of moral precepts gradually became identifiable as a tradition "Hippocratic" in spirit and content.

The central features of the oath are several. The preamble established the Hippocratic physicians as a moral community: a group of physicians bound together by a voluntary oath to observe a specified set of moral tenets. Next, there are a series of positive moral commitments to beneficence, nonmaleficence, obtaining consultation, leading a virtuous life, and maintaining fidelity to the oath itself. There is also a set of negative moral prescriptions: to avoid abortion, euthanasia, disclosure of confidences, and sexual relations with patients or their families. Finally, violation of the oath brought with it moral disgrace and alienation from those who remained faithful to its precepts.

In recent years objections have arisen to the idea of an integral Hippocratic tradition. The fact that many physicians in antiquity and later violated all or some of the precepts of that tradition is adduced as evidence. Specifically, reference is made to contradictions in the other books of the Hippocratic corpus that seem to counter the altruistic precepts of the oath and to cast doubt on its acceptance even by "Hippocratic" physicians.

One example is the treatment of incurable diseases (Prioreschi 1992). The Hippocratic text makes clear the physician's concern for reputation if the patient were to die (Hippocrates 1981, 4). But this could be simply a warning to prognosticate correctly. Elsewhere, the physician is urged to study incurable cases in order to prevent or ameliorate them (Hippocrates 1968, 339). At yet another point, there is emphasized the responsibility to recognize when patients are "overmastered" by their illnesses and medicine is "powerless" to aid them (Hippocrates 1981, 193). Here the intent seems to be to avoid futile treatment, not to refuse care to the patient.

Another example is the matter of fees. The physician may justly lay claim to them but should avoid pressing the patient and be willing to provide service without charge when the situation requires it. Strangers and recalcitrant patients should not be neglected (Hippocrates 1972, 317, 319).

With respect to patient participation, in one place the physician is counseled to "conceal most things" (Hippocrates 1981, 297), and in another the patient is advised to gain medical knowledge and learn how to choose a good physician (Hippocrates 1988, 7). The books of the Hippocratic corpus, other than the oath, thus had a more practical and prudential tone than the oath itself (Carrick 1985). Their variable and sometimes contradictory ethical precepts are the result of multiple authorship, different philosophical influences, and the different eras in which they were written. They do not, of themselves, vitiate the moral center of the Hippocratic tradition, which is its focus on the conduct of the physician-patient relationship. That is the focus of Bell's linkage of the 1847 Code with Hippocrates.

Bell defined the essence of the Hippocratic tradition to which he had referred as beneficence and benevolence, attendance to duty, and membership in a moral community, deduced from the conduct of centuries of eminent predecessors who from the time of Hippocrates had exhibited "their devotedness to the relief of their fellow creatures from pain and disease" (Appendix B, 317). Bell and his colleagues proposed to recapture by their code "a sense of ethical obligation rising superior . . . to considerations of personal advancement" (317). In a word, the central moral commitment in the code was its dedication to something other than the physician's self-interest, that something being the primacy of the welfare of the patient. This was a necessary reaffirmation, given the self-serving conduct of the physicians of this time from whom Bell wished to set the members of the AMA apart.

This same commitment to a certain degree of altruism was the moral heart of the 1847 Code, as it had been the moral heart of the Hippocratic Oath (Hippocrates 1972) and of the other ancient medical teachers like Charaka in India (Muthu 1930); the codes or acts of moral commitment of Jewish (Bar-Sela and Hoff 1962) and Arabic (Levey 1977) physicians in the Middle Ages; of the later Chinese physicians (Lee 1943); and of John Gregory (Gregory 1772), Thomas Percival (Percival 1803), and Thomas Gisborne (Gisborne 1794) in eighteenth-century England. Bell called this moral commitment a "devotedness" that was binding "regardless of the privation and danger and not seldom obloquy encountered in return." The physician's skill, Bell insisted, was "held in trust for the general good" (Appendix B, 318). To achieve this end, veracity and fidelity to trust, benevolence, and acting in common for the common good were necessary medical virtues.

This "devotedness" is further spelled out in article I of the 1847 Code entitled "The Duties of Physicians to Their Patients." It calls physicians to "obey the calls of the sick," to bind themselves in conscience to the responsibility they incur in discharging their duties, remembering that the "health and lives of those committed to their charge depend on their skill, attention and fidelity." "Every case . . . should be treated with attention, steadiness and humanity" (Appendix C, 324). The article goes on from the basis of this primacy of the patient's welfare to deduce confidentiality, nonabandonment of the incurable, and consultation. All must be done with a "sincere interest in the welfare of the person" (325). These are paraphrased and virtually verbatim repetitions of words Thomas Percival used in his ethics (Percival 1803).

The moral message of this first article is, as John Bell said, the continuation of an age-old tradition of what today we would call the principle of beneficence dedicated to the welfare of the sick. We might quarrel with the overemphasis of the 1847 Code on the use of the therapeutic privilege to withhold information from patients so as not to deprive them of hope, or with some of the specific details of the other articles like the obligations of patients to physicians or duties of physicians to each other and to society. But unless we wish to attribute bad faith to Bell, Hays, and the other drafters of the code, we understand that underlying the whole code was a tradition that characterized the moral focus of medicine from its beginnings: a primary dedication to the welfare of the sick person. This is the thrust also of the sections of the contemporary code labeled as the *Elements*.

In the 1990 version of the *Elements,* updated in 1994, the emphasis is clearly on a more collaborative effort between physician and patient than in earlier versions (Council 1996–97). No doubt this is a response to the emergence of the rights of patient self-determination in the preceding decades. But here too, the cooperative effort is justified by the "health and well-being of the patient" and by the "benefit to the patient" for whom the physician should be an advocate. The shift from the 1847 language of beneficence and mutual duties to the 1990 language of collaborative decision making, is significant sociologically and ethically. Respect for patient autonomy could also be considered part of the duty of beneficence since respect for persons fosters the welfare of the patient (Pellegrino 1994). Further admonitions to respect the dignity of the pa tient, to respond to his or her needs, to protect confidentiality, to cooperate with other providers, and to be the patient's advocate follow from the primary duty of beneficent regard for the welfare of the sick as the root moral imperative for physicians.

The 1847 elements in the 1990 version, enlarged by the insights of participatory democracy, are echoes of the first expression of beneficence together with nonmaleficence as the fundamental moral precepts in the Hippocratic Oath: "I will use treatment to help the sick according to my ability and judgment but never with a view to injury and wrong" (Hippocrates 1972). All the detailed provisions of subsequent codes derive from this first ordering principle.

The Moral Validity of the Code

In 1847 and in the years following, there have been objections to the whole idea of a code, summarized exceedingly well by Baker (1995). I have drawn on Baker's analysis for this section of this chapter.

A first objection is that there is no need for an explicit code of ethics. Ethics is a matter of character. Virtuous physicians do not need a code; vicious physicians will not observe it. The exercise of character will, in fact, be impeded by rules of behavior or so the argument runs. Would that this were true. Yes, ethics is a matter of character, but most humans are fallible and need some guidance in character formation by repeated, clear exhortations regarding principles as well as virtue. Surely no virtuous physician has been deterred from virtue by a code. Virtue is learned by practice and imitation of good models. The code provides a benchmark etched into the consciousness of all physicians by the conduct of exemplary physicians among their predecessors and their contemporaries. The majority need this kind of a moral center of gravity. A code is the lodestone that centers the moral needle. It points the way out of the moral confusion that has recurrently beset medicine in its long history.

A second objection is that the code is self-serving, generated by the profession to gain a monopoly of power and money (Berlant 1975). In this view, ethics is simply a device to exclude irregular practitioners and protect a dominant group and their philosophy of medicine. This is the error the New York branch of the Kappa Lambda Society committed when it mixed an effort at ethical reform with secret preferences among its members (Baker 1996). Such an argument might explain the motives of some physicians or even the consequences of an ethical code. But it is presumptuous indeed, at such an historical distance from the events, to claim to know the intentions of the framers of the code. The evidence is good or better that their aims were genuinely altruistic (Kett 1968). If they did intend to deceive, then they were guilty of collective malfeasance or conspiracy. But conspiracies are notoriously difficult to establish. As Baker contends, the Philadelphia branch of Kappa Lambda Society to which John Bell belonged acted from publicly declared motives of beneficence and justice.

RobertVeatch (see chap. 9 of this volume) has taken serious exception to any professional code arrived at unilaterally. Inasmuch as he sees medical relationships as essentially contractual and not convenantal, no statement of professional ethics made without patient and public participation would be valid. Moreover, given the pluralism of moral value in our society, no code could represent anything but the beliefs of limited communities that shared the same values. No universal ethical obligations or principles would be tenable if uni laterally elaborated by professionals (Veatch and Mason 1987). But the truth of a moral statement lies in its truth or falsity, in its internal credibility as a moral statement, not in who makes the statement. One may justifiably argue that the public and patients should participate in future code making, without conceding that without their participation valid conclusions cannot be reached. The same is true of the sharp criticism leveled at the 1847 Code, whose physician–drafters dared to define the mutual obligations of patients to physicians. Today we would argue that the patient surely should participate in such a discussion. But the crucial question that remains is whether there is, in fact, a moral basis for reciprocal duties on the part of patients. The process whereby the duties of patients were determined in 1847 is surely ill–advised, but the validity of those duties must be argued on their own merits. Ethics in general involves a reciprocity of obligations, and medical ethics is no exception. Indeed, unless the patient fulfills certain obligations, the physician cannot carry out his obligations to serve the patient's well-being (Pellegrino and Thomasma 1987, 99ff).

A third criticism asserts that the 1847 Code and the present code are statements of etiquette, not ethics. Leake (1927) made this assertion about Percival's ethics because he failed to detect any formal ethical theory or argumentation behind Percival's code. Lacking this, he said, Percival's work was all just a set of rules affecting the relationships between doctors and designed to protect the gentility of the profession.

It is true that Percival did not provide a formal treatise on medical moral philosophy. Neither did his English, Scottish, or American colleagues, whether they were philosophers or physicians. Even John Bell's introduction to the 1847 Code is more a statement of medical morality (presuppositions and duties about right conduct drawn from a long tradition) than a rigorously derived argument for the code. But Percival and his contemporaries did draw on a set of moral principles implicit in a shared educational tradition (Reiser 1995). For Percival that tradition combined the ethics of the Bible, the Roman and Greek classics—especially Stoicism—and the notion of condescension —the eighteenth-century English gentleman's perception of the beneficence owed by the more- to the less-fortunate members of society[1] (Pellegrino 1986).

A fourth criticism is that the code is thoroughly anachronistic and inconsistent with contemporary changes in the role of physicians (Reed and Evans 1987). Physicians, it is alleged, are too closely tied to the dyadic physician-patient relationships; they ought to focus instead on social and population ethics, on economics, and on medicine's new industrialized and institutionalized functions (Emanuel 1995). These new roles are frustrated, we are told, by too narrow a focus on the welfare of individual patients. Our ethics must shift from attention on the good of individuals to the good of society, from personalist to population ethics. This, along with moral skepticism, is the gravest challenge to traditional medical ethics today. The problems with an entirely new ethic based in postmodern philosophy, economics, or population-based morality will be developed below.

The Applicability of the Code Today

Thus far I have examined negative objections to the AMA Code of 1847 and its current transformation and attempted a rebuttal of each. I turn now to positive reasons why, from a societal perspective, a code of medical ethics is essential to assure that medical power will be used in morally defensible ways.

The 1847 Code was intended by its framers as an impetus to return the profession to the moral core that they believed had distinguished the best physicians from past times from their less noble colleagues. In a significant measure it did just that. To be sure, venal physicians were not deterred by the code. Nonetheless, the code in its later versions has served until very recently as a standard of behavior. It gave assurances, to the extent that any human organization can provide such assurances, that physicians as a whole could be expected to exhibit a degree of effacement of self-interest in their relationships with patients. The public and the profession took this to be a sign of the uniqueness of medicine and other helping professions like ministry, teaching, and the law.

In recent years, however, an increasing number of physicians and members of the public have come to feel that there is no longer anything ethically unique about the professions. It is important, therefore, to examine some of the reasons why, despite this trend, the AMA Code is a societal necessity.

First, the AMA Code serves as a vehicle for the translation of ethical knowledge and commitment from the realm of theory and promise into daily practice. Physicians have neither the time nor the requisite background to analyze every relevant debate on every important issue facing modern bioethics. They need some help to see how these debates bear upon, and shape, their day-by-day decision making. The ethical code provides an essential link between theory and practice that conscientious physicians need to make ethically sensitive decisions.

Second, the code fosters development of the profession as a moral community. It provides a moral vision of what it means to be a virtuous physician. It binds physicians to each other in a common commitment to the welfare of those they treat. The code becomes, in effect, a collective promise of fidelity, a true "pro-fession,"[2] a declaration of commitment and a standard by which to measure that commitment. In this way the code unites physicians in what Harvey Cushing called a "common devotion" (Cushing 1929).

Third, the code is a vehicle for the transmission of a tradition of dedicated service going back to antiquity, one that underscores the fundamental moral nature of medicine. That all physicians did not historically remain truthful to the tradition does not vitiate the tradition or make it socially worthless. Traditions are important in the ethical formation of young physicians and in sustaining the ethical commitments of older physicians. Those traditions connect us with the exemplary physicians of the past at a time in history when models of virtue are sorely needed. A tradition helps to locate the young physician temporally and morally. It recalls for the older physician the pristine ideals to which he has dedicated himself. It gives to both young and old a moral impetus when times and things become difficult.

Fourth, the code serves as a moral guide for physicians to negotiate the practical ethical dilemmas that grow thornier by the day. That guide is, as always, the primacy of patient welfare against which all professional acts and public policy are morally assessed. This guide tells us that in the end healing can never be primarily a business, nor health a commodity, nor the therapeutic relationship a contract. It also defines proscriptions—things that ought never be done, even for reasons of exigency, economics, or politics. In a world of relativist, subjectivist, and ever-changing mores, a stable moral nucleus is indispensable to resolve the conflicts of loyalty, moral complicity, and confidentiality inherent in today's metamorphoses from physician-as-healer to the physician-as-"provider," "businessperson," "gatekeeper," or "guardian" of societal resources.

Fifth, the moral truth the code embodies is an indispensable benchmark in the current effort to define the ends of medicine. It is surely a sign of these times of moral confusion that two and a half millennia after medicine became a definable practice we are still earnestly asking what the purposes of medicine should be (Callahan 1995, 95–117). But however we define these ends, they must ultimately be judged by their impact on patients. The fact that patients become ill and need help is the reason for medicine's existence. All the multitudinous purposes to which we can put medical knowledge must focus on this end that is rooted in the nature of medicine as a special kind of human activity (Pellegrino 1997).

Finally, a distinct code of ethics is essential because it defines the integrity of medicine as a moral entity with its foundations in something more than mere social convention. Medical ethics, as I show in the next section of this article, is grounded in a universal human experience of illness and healing. When that code is compromised, something important to the whole of society is lost. This was the case when the Soviets took power in 1917 and suspended the Hippocratic Oath. They revived it in 1971 and reshaped to fit the aims and ideologies of the Presidium (Presidium 1971). This was also the case when the Nazi physicians horribly distorted the beneficence provision of the Hippocratic Oath to justify experimentation and involuntary euthanasia for the "good" of the Reich. Their subversion of medical ethics to political ideology stands forever as a warning of the dire consequences of defection from the moral integrity of the profession.

What Grounds the Moral Validity of the Code?

Ultimately, the moral validity of the code does not depend on acceptance or promulgation by physicians, professional bodies like the AMA, ethicists, or the general public. Rather, medical ethical codes derive their moral force from what is self-evident about the nature of medicine as a special kind of human activity (Pellegrino 1983). Medicine is humanity's response to the universal human experience of illness, which none can escape. The sick person is a vulnerable, anxious, dependent, and exploitable human being who needs the skill of the physician to be healed. The physician offers his or her skill to help in healing. If the physician is to heal and not harm or take advantage of the vulnerability of the sick person, the physician must be trusted. Indeed, the physician invites trust and, in so doing, makes an implicit promise to be faithful to that trust. The physician promises to be skillful and to use his or her skill for the advantage of the patient and not primarily for his or her own gain or some-one else's. This is not a contract but a solemn promise, a covenant arising out of the phenomenon of the clinical encounter itself. In this sense, it is "inter-nal" to medicine and the other healing professions like nursing, dentistry, or clinical psychology (Ladd 1983).

The fundamental aspects of illness are the same across history, culture, and national boundaries. They were realities in ancient Greece, are realities today, and will be realities on any planet we colonize in the future. Being ill and be-ing healed are universal human phenomena. They may be expressed in differ-ent languages, in different customs, and in different behavior; but the core ex-periences of vulnerability, dependence, and need for help remain the same. Illness and disease are everywhere an assault on the sick person's humanity.

All medical codes have recognized these phenomena, explicitly or implic-itly, as the source for the doctor's duties. They shape the virtues of medicine: fidelity to trust, honesty, compassion, effacement of self-interest, and courage. Virtuous physicians can be trusted to be competent and to use their compe-tence primarily in the interests of their patients. These are the characteristics that distinguished the Hippocratic physician from the self-serving and in-competent practitioners of their day. These are the same moral precepts taught by the conscientious physicians of all eras (Bar-Sela and Hoff 1962; Levey 1977; Gregory 1772; Percival 1803; Hooker 1949). All of those physicians rec-ognized the source and ineradicability of their obligations. They were acutely aware of the presumptions inherent in offering to treat another human in the vulnerable state we call sickness and of the obligations these presumptions en-tailed.

Do We Need a New Ethic?

Increasingly, we are told we need a "new" ethic to replace the AMA Code and the Hippocratic Oath and to prepare us for the new roles the physician must play in the twenty-first century—as gatekeeper, social engineer, entrepreneur, case manager, functionary, or as an investor in a business, an industry, or a "sys-tem" of care. We are urged to turn from our focus on persons to a population-based ethic, to become micro-allocators, or shareholders, and to share in the risks and profits of the business of healthcare delivery. Only a new ethic, it is claimed, can integrate these multiple roles and give us the new identity soci-ety requires (Robin and McCauley 1995). This new ethic is also prescribed as the antidote to our moral identity crisis. All we need do is become the managers, investors, and rationers of managed care and the healthcare business, and the decisions we make will ipso facto be both profitable and in the interests of patients (Engelhardt and Rie 1988; Hall 1994). Attractive as this may sound to contemporary ears, it is an illusion. Physicians who become investors or managers cannot escape the moment of truth: when cost containment and profits are threatened, ethics inevitably becomes the victim of exigency (Woolhandler and Himmelstein 1995).

But the challenges to the AMA Code and what it embodies are even more fundamental than the conflicts of interest generated by capitulation to a market or corporate ethos. The most serious threats arise from the corrosion of the foundations of moral philosophy itself. Here we confront contemporary radical attacks on any attempt to derive a stable morality of any kind. This threat arises in the complex, variously defined mode of thinking called *postmodernism*. Distant and esoteric as this movement may seem from the bedside, its influence is being felt there through the writing and thinking of contemporary philosophical bioethicists.

Postmodernism is characterized in many ways—philosophical, political, literary, esthetic, and moral (Cornell 1992; Norris 1993; Rockmore 1992). But all versions share an antipathy to stable moral truth that makes all philosophical systems—and even rationality itself—suspect. Postmodernism opposes overarching standards of conduct and denies the possibility of any objective morality. Postmodernism deals with a world of moral pluralism by giving equal credibility to all, since without a stable morality there is no way to decide among conflicting moral beliefs.

The implications of this worldview for the future of medical ethics in general, and for the code in particular, are profound. Postmodernism would oppose any such thing as a "foundation" for the code in the phenomena of medicine or in the 1847 Code or in the Hippocratic ethic. But postmodernist thought goes further: it denies the very possibility of rational discourse about medical ethics, and in this way it even attacks contemporary bioethics, which, at the moment, claims to be a rational enterprise.

Contemporary bioethics, as it has developed over the past twenty-five years, is a continuation of the post-Enlightenment search for morality free of religion and metaphysics—a morality based in an autonomous rationality. Since postmodernism specifically undermines all rationality, it robs contemporary bioethics of any claim it might make to arrive at a new ethic. In this postmodern view, if there is to be a new ethic, it will have to be a product of either social construction or pragmatic accommodation, each of which, in its own way, also results in an ethic of medicine that eschews traditional foundations in medicine or any other stable reality. Certainly, a code like that of 1847, or the present AMA code, would, on this view, have little claim to anyone's allegiance.

Ethical or social constructivism makes truth and value dependent on social relations, on those societal practices that endure but that are true only as long as they endure. Moral truth is constructed out of our beliefs and values and depends on our approval or disapproval as judged by their coherence with some appropriate system of beliefs. A pluralist society would "construct" a multiplicity of moral truths and therefore a plurality of moral codes. Given the breadth of beliefs and values in contemporary society, this is tantamount to the abolition of all ethics except what individual patients and physicians "construct" for their particular relationship. Communication between constructions of a moral code would become difficult or impossible since the values defining each construction would be so different.

Ethical accommodationism is even more pliable. It accepts the impossibility of any stable moral truth and therefore of a stable core for any code. Instead, the aim is to bring ethics into conformity, for reasons of exigency, with external forces like economics, politics, law, or managed care. This approach is irenic in aim. Its hope is that physicians can salvage something of the traditional physician-patient relationship by a suitable compromise with economics or politics. This is the view of those who urge us to abandon traditional medical ethics and move from individual patient to population ethics, to acceptance of gatekeeper, managerial, and institutional roles. In this view, the virtues of medicine should be adapted to the virtues of the competitive marketplace and self-interest. This makes the physician as much an instrument of social purpose as of patient welfare. It gives any code a degree of plasticity that robs it of normative power.

What all this makes clear is that the future of the AMA code is uncertain. With erosion of the traditional inviolability of a covenant of trust and the primacy of the welfare of the patient, the profession becomes ethically divided and fragmented. On one side will be those who remain faithful to the patient-centered ethic of tradition; and on the other, those who reject that ethic for the new moral plasticity. The traditionalists will most likely come from the ranks of those who hold to some principle-based or transcendental foundation for ethics in religion and metaphysics. On the other side, there will be a group of physicians following a variety of codes or no code at all—those who will adopt the ethics of business or the marketplace, or individually negotiated contracts for care. This, ironically, was the state of medicine when the Hippocratic Oath was formulated (Edelstein 1967).

Conclusion and Challenge

One hundred fifty years ago the AMA took two bold steps when it sought to unite all physicians in a profession held together by a common commitment. The first step was to seek reform in medical education; the other step was to reaffirm the ethical nature of medical practice. Though there has been dissonance and controversy, these efforts have made American medicine a profession—a group most of whose members are still committed publicly to stand for something other than the pursuit of self-interest.

Today we need to reaffirm that commitment. But we now must do so in cooperation with our fellow health professionals. It is now clear that we must talk less of "medical ethics" and more of "patient care ethics." The challenge for the AMA today is to take leadership in reasserting the primacy of the patient's welfare, and to join other health professionals in recommitting ourselves to the welfare of those we serve. Together we must insist that no public policy, no practice arrangement, no professional prerogative, no definition of roles that weakens our primary loyalty to the patient can be allowed to dilute that commitment. We are called to use our collective moral power as advocates for the sick even though there will be powerful forces urging us to yield to a more pliable accommodation to contemporary mores.

Critical and cynical as some may be about the motives behind the Hippocratic ethic, the 1847 Code, and its subsequent modifications, their central moral content is still as valid in 1997 and as it will be in 2047. Fidelity to the moral center of medicine is the only antidote to the moral malaise that afflicts our profession today. We do not need a "new" ethic of accommodation to economics, commerce, or the idolatry of the marketplace. Even less do our patients need such an ethic. The morally viable response to present and future crises rests in the daunting nature of our promise to help our fellow humans who come to us in the complex predicament of illness and seek our help—a predicament that transcends time, place, and culture because it is a universal mark of our common humanity. Recognition of this ineradicable fact gave the AMA code its relevance one hundred and fifty years ago, and by whatever name we call it, will give it relevance in the future.

Notes

1. See the definition of *condescension* in Samuel Johnson's *Dictionary of the English Language* (London: W. Stahan, 1755).

2. Pro-fession, etymologically, is "a solemn declaration, promise, or vow" according to the Oxford Dictionary (Oxford: Clarendon Press, 1961).

References

Baker, Robert. 1995. Introduction. In *The Codification of Medical Morality: Historical and Philosophical Studies of the Formalization of Western Medical Morality in the Eighteenth and Nineteenth Centuries.* Vol. 2, *Anglo-American Medical Ethics and Medical Jurisprudence in the Nineteenth Century,* ed. Robert Baker, 2–14. Dordrecht: Kluwer.

———. 1996. The Kappa Lambda Society of Hippocrates: The Secret Origins of the American Medical Society. *Fugitive Leaves from the Historical Collections,* Library of the College of Physicians of Philadelphia 11(2):1–7.

Bar-Sela, A., and Hoff, Hebbel. 1962. Isaac Israeli's Fifty Admonitions to Physicians. *Journal of the History of Medicine and Allied Health Sciences* 17:245–57.

Berlant, John. 1975. *Profession and Monopoly: A Study of Medicine in the United States and Britain.* Berkeley: University of California.

Callahan, Daniel. 1995. The Ends of Medicine: Shaping New Goals. *Bulletin of the New York Academy of Medicine* 72(1):95–117.

Carrick, Paul. 1985. *Medical Ethics in Antiquity.* Boston: D. Reidel.

Cornell, Drucilla. 1992. *The Philosophy of the Limit.* New York: Rutledge.

Council on Ethical and Judicial Affairs, AMA. 1997. *Code of Medical Ethics. Current Opinions with Annotations.* Chicago: American Medical Association.

Cushing, Harvey. 1929. *Consecratio Medici, and Other Papers.* Boston: Little, Brown & Co.

Edelstein, Ludwig. 1967. The Hippocratic Oath. In *Ancient Medicine: Selected Papers of Ludwig Edelstein,* ed. O. Temkin and C. L. Temkin. Baltimore: Johns Hopkins University Press.

Emanuel, Ezekiel J. 1995. Medical Ethics in an Era of Managed Care: The Need for Institutional Structures Instead of Principles for Individual Cases. *Journal of Clinical Ethics* 6(4):335–38.

Engelhardt Jr., H. Tristram, and Rie, Michael A. 1988. Morality for the Medical-Industrial Complex: A Code of Ethics for the Mass Marketing of Health Care. *New England Journal of Medicine* 319:1086–89.

Gisborne, Thomas. 1974. *An Enquiry into the Duties of Men in the Higher and Middle Classes of Society in Great Britain.* London: B. and J. White.

Gregory, John. 1772. *Lectures on the Duties and Offices of Physicians.* London: W. Straham and T. Cadckk.

Hall, Mark A. 1994. The Ethics of Health Care Rationing. *Public Affairs* 8:33–50.

Hippocrates. 1968. Hippocrates, Vol. 3. With an English translation by E. T. Whitington. Loeb Classical Library 149. Cambridge: Harvard University Press.

———1972. Hippocrates, Vol. 1. With an English translation by W. H. S. Jones. Loeb Classical Library 147. Cambridge: Harvard University Press.

———1979. Hippocrates, Vol. 4. With an English translation by W. H. S. Jones. Loeb Classical Library 150. Cambridge: Harvard University Press.

———1981. Hippocrates, Vol. 2. With an English translation by W. H. S. Jones. Loeb Classical Library 148. Cambridge: Harvard University Press.

————1988. Hippocrates, Vol. 5. With an English translation by Paul Potter. Loeb Classical Library 472. Cambridge: Harvard University Press.

Hooker, Worthington. 1949. *Physician and Patient.* New York: Baker and Scribner.

Kett, Joseph. 1968. *The Formation of the American Medical Association: The Role of Institutions, 1760–1860.* New Haven: Yale University Press.

Ladd, John. 1983. The Internal Morality of Medicine: An Essential Dimension of the Physician-Patient Relationship. In *The Clinical Encounter: The Moral Fabric of the Physician-Patient Relationship,* ed. Earl E. Shelp, 209–32. Boston: D. Reidel.

Leake, Chauncey. 1927. *Percival's Medical Ethics.* Baltimore: William & Wilkins.

Lee, Tao. 1943. Five Commandments and Ten Requirements (trans.). *Bulletin of the History of Medicine* 13:271–72.

Levey, Martin. 1977. Medical Deontology in Ninth Century Islam. In *Legacies in Ethics and Medicine,* ed. Chester Burns, 129–44. New York: Science History Publications.

McKinney, Loren C. 1952. Medical Ethics and Etiquette in the Early Middle Ages: The Persistence of Hippocratic Ideals. *Bulletin of the History of Medicine* 26:1–31.

Muthu, D. C. 1930. *The Antiquity of Hindu Medicine and Civilization.* Cited by Will Durant in *Our Oriental Heritage,* 530. New York: Simon and Schuster, 1994.

Norris, Christopher. 1993. *The Truth About Postmodernism.* Oxford: Basil Blackwell.

Pellegrino, Edmund D. 1983. The Healing Relationship: The Architectonics of Clinical Medicine, The Clinical Encounter, The Moral Fabric of the Patient-Physician Relationship. *Philosophy and Medicine* 4:153–72. Ed. Earl Shelp.

————. 1985. Foreword: Thomas Percival: The Ethics Beneath the Etiquette. In Thomas Percival, *Medical Ethics, or a Code of Institutions and Precepts Adapted to the Professional Conduct of Physicians and Surgeons* [Reprinted from the 1803 version]. Classics of Medicine Library, Birmingham, Ala.

————. 1986. Percival's Medical Ethics: The Moral Philosophy of an 18th Century English Gentleman. *Archives of Internal Medicine* 146:2265–69.

————. 1994. Patient and Physician Autonomy: Conflicting Rights and Obligations in the Physician Patient Relationship. *Journal of Contemporary Health, Law and Policy* 10:47–68.

————. 1997. *The Goals and Ends of Medicine: How Are They to Be Defined?* New York: Hastings Center.

Pellegrino, Edmund D., and Thomasma, David C. 1987. *For the Patient's Good: The Restoration of Beneficence in Health Care.* Oxford: Oxford University Press.

Percival, Thomas. 1803. *Medical Ethics or a Code of Institutes and Precepts Adapted to the Professional Conduct of Physicians and Surgeons.* London: J. Johnson.

Presidium of the Highest Soviet of the U.S.S.R. 1971. The Oath of Soviet Physicians, 26 March.

Prioreschi, Plinio. 1992. Did the Hippocratic Physicians Treat Hopeless Cases? *Gesnerus* 49:341–50.

Reed, Ralph R., and Evans, Daryl. 1987. The Deprofessionalization of Medicine. *Journal of the American Medical Association* 258:3279–82.

Reiser, Stanley. 1995. Creating a Medical Profession in the United States: The First Code of Ethics of the American Medical Association. In *The Codification of Medical Morality: Historical and Philosophical Studies of the Formalization of Western Medical Morality in the Eighteenth and Nineteenth Centuries.* Vol. 2, *Anglo-American Medical Ethics and Medical Jurisprudence in the Nineteenth Century,* ed. Robert Baker, 89–103. Dordrecht: Kluwer.

Robin, Eugene D., and McCauley, Robert F. 1995. Cultural Lag and the Hippocratic Oath. *Lancet* 345:1422–24.

Rockmore, Tom. 1992. *Anti-Foundationalism Old and New.* Philadelphia: Temple University Press.

Veatch, Robert, and Mason, Carol. 1987. Hippocratic Versus Judeo-Christian Ethics in Conflict. *Journal of Religious Ethics* 15:86–105.

Woolhandler, Steffie, and Himmelstein, David U. 1995. Extreme Risk: The New Corporate Proposition for Physicians. *New England Journal of Medicine* 333(35): 1684–87.

7

Professionalism and Institutional Ethics

ELIOT FREIDSON, PH.D.

Consider what has happened to American medicine over the past thirty years. The physician's relationship to patients has been drastically altered. Medicine's traditional methods of controlling economic competition and making a living have largely been destroyed. Independent, solo, fee-for-service practice is rapidly disappearing. The clinical freedom of the physician has been seriously weakened. Divisions within the profession have intensified. Taken together, these changes have the potential to destroy professionalism in medicine and reduce physicians to the position of technicians. What role can ethics play in saving professionalism?

Brennan observed that "medical ethics in the liberal state must address not only interpersonal relations, but also institutional relations" (Brennan 1991, 94). But most discussions of medical ethics have been concerned with the ethical problems that have been created by remarkable advances in medical technology, genetics, drugs, and clinical technique rather than with institutional relations. The focus is on the ethical conduct of individual physicians in their interaction with patients—what I shall call *practice ethics*. Certainly that focus is necessary, for when all is said and done, the clinical encounter is at the foundation of health care. But important as practice ethics are, they are not enough to guide the future of medicine. Equally important are the policies of professional institutions that shape the social and economic circumstances within which the clinical encounter takes place—what I shall call *institutional ethics*. In the absence of circumstances that encourage and support ethical conduct, I suggest, all but the most heroic physicians will be prevented or at least discouraged from acting ethically toward their patients.

In this chapter I argue that a new set of institutional, but not practice, ethics is needed by the medical profession in order to deal effectively with the transformation of its practice environment. I do so first by analyzing the 1847 Code of Ethics of the American Medical Association and showing that the bulk of its articles concern establishing a set of norms that were characterized by such critics as Leake (1927, 1–2) as "etiquette," but that might better be recognized as institutional ethics. I will show how those norms attempt to create circumstances fitted to the time and place of the 1847 Code that would allow physicians to establish a solidary professional community within which ethical relations with patients are facilitated. I go on to note that while most of the ethical principles of the 1847 Code addressed to the doctor-patient relationship are, with minor exceptions, still relevant today and may in fact be timeless, its *institutional* ethics are largely irrelevant to today's circumstances of practice. After elaborating the changes that have taken place in the circumstances of practice that I characterized so briefly at the start of this paper, I discuss a number of issues that have profound bearing on practice ethics and suggest the positions that the profession as a whole should take in order to maintain a milieu in which the practice ethics of individual physicians can flourish.

The Ethics of the 1847 Code

The traditional ethical principles of American medicine are clearly and simply presented in the sesquicentennial 1847 Code (Appendix C). Of course, it is only the first of a series of codes (see Three Ethical Codes 1888; those in Leake 1927; and most recently, Council 1997). It is not very complex, but it is sufficiently clear and concrete to allow us to visualize the ethical problems of medical practice in general, the particular circumstances of practice that the 1847 Code took for granted, and the policies it recommended for supporting ethical practice under those circumstances.

Since modern professionalism had not yet been fully established, the code paid more attention to establishing its jurisdictional boundaries than need be the case today. Aside from that,

- it established the ethics of the clinical encounter, specifying how physicians should deal with patients at the bedside or in the consulting room, both clinically, in conscientiously attending to their complaints and treating them, and socially, in protecting the confidentiality of the information their patients provide them;
- it asserted norms to govern professional relations between colleagues and with members of other occupations;

- it asserted norms governing the economic relations between colleagues and with members of other occupations;
- it asserted norms governing the economic relations between physicians and patients and the public in general.

The core of the Code is designed to protect the well-being of patients and establish the profession's practice ethics. Its very first article (Appendix C, 324) deals with the "Duties of Physicians to Their Patients," urging that "Every case submitted to the charge of a physician should be treated with attention, steadiness and humanity." It establishes the obligation of confidentiality, asserting that "secrecy and delicacy, when required by peculiar circumstances, should be strictly observed." It also discusses how often to visit a patient, the use of consultation in difficult cases, the avoidance of discouraging prognoses, and the like.

Significantly, however, the largest part of the 1847 Code does not deal with relations with patients at all. Some of it aims at avoiding conflict between colleagues. Thus, it deals at some length with avoiding the criticism of colleagues in public, collaborating with or referring patients to nonphysicians, and advertising in a self-aggrandizing fashion. In addition, it forbids patenting "any surgical instrument or medicine" or dispensing any nostrum whose composition is secret, asserting that to monopolize or keep secret remedies or techniques that cannot be freely evaluated or employed by all members of the profession "is inconsistent with beneficence and professional liberality."

The code also discusses at some length the norms that should govern instances of professional rivalry, or disagreement over diagnosis or proper therapy, specifying that when there is disagreement, either the majority opinion or that of the attending physician should prevail. In disagreements taking place beyond the bedside, it suggests adjudication by a committee of physicians, a "court medical," but cautions that the proceedings be kept secret so as to avoid discredit to the profession.

In addition, the code is concerned with tempering economic competition between physicians. It asserts the desirability of establishing minimum fees, thereby regulating but not preventing competition. It urges physicians to provide free care to colleagues and their families as an act of "professional brotherhood" and, more importantly, urges that as an act of professional beneficence, physicians provide care without charge "cheerfully and freely" to those who cannot afford to pay. Finally, it declares that it is the duty of physicians to give advice to the public on matters of public health and to provide their services during epidemics "even at the jeopardy of their own lives."

But the public owes something to physicians in return. The code concludes with a unilateral assertion of a contract between the profession and society: due to "the benefits accruing to the public directly and indirectly from the active and unwearied beneficence of the profession . . . physicians are justly entitled to the utmost consideration and respect from the community" (Appendix C, 334).

The Historic Circumstances of the 1847 Code

To understand some of its principles, it is important to understand how the code reflects the particular historic circumstances of medicine at that time. Physicians then formed a relatively small group of community practitioners, each in his own home or in the home of his patients, trying to make a living from patients' fees. They had lost a legally sanctioned monopoly over surgery and the prescribing of dangerous drugs. Their public esteem was problematic. Under circumstances of almost entirely free competition, academically trained physicians represented only one of a number of different kinds of practitioners. The competitive pressure of "irregulars" and "empirics" who claimed equal and cheaper skills must surely have tempted average "regulars" to adopt their rivals' techniques for generating paying patients and to share their patients by establishing referral relations with them. Some must also have been tempted to accept ruinously low fees in the hope of making a living by the volume of cases, to attract patients by making exaggerated claims about their special skills or exclusive remedies, to treat without charge some of those who could afford to pay in the hope of their future patronage or referrals, and to deprecate the competence of both their "regular" and "irregular" competitors.[1]

Abbott (1988) has shown in great detail how the establishment of firm jurisdictional boundaries is essential to the process of professionalization. However, the embattled position of American physicians in the middle of the nineteenth century encouraged them to respond to competition in ways that blurred any differences between them and their competitors. But if there were no distinct criteria by which to distinguish a "regular" from a "quack," how could clear jurisdictional boundaries be established as the basis for a license for exclusive practice? Furthermore, apart from competition with irregulars, no-holds-barred competition among academically trained physicians themselves discouraged the development of a sense of community or "brotherhood," of mutual respect, of common purpose through commitment to the same distinctive training and therapeutic approach.

The 1847 Code may be interpreted as an effort to establish both a distinctive jurisdictional identity and a cohesive occupational community. It defined its members by their academic training. It attempted to forge a cohesive professional community by excluding cooperation with those lacking such training, preventing ruinous (and bitter) economic competition between colleagues, banning the use of techniques or remedies that could not be shared by all, controlling forms of advertising and other public behavior that demeaned the competence of colleagues and reflected badly on the character of the profession as a whole, and establishing rules to prevent or adjudicate disputes between colleagues.

Etiquette and Ethics in the Code

The norms of the code that I analyzed as having established jurisdictional boundaries and nurtured a professional community have been scornfully termed mere etiquette by such writers as Leake (1927) and Berlant (1975). In his introduction to Percival's *Ethics*, which all writers agree was the major source for the articles of the 1847 Code (e.g., Baker 1993), Leake (1927, 2) writes that such codes are "designed to promote the dignity and pecuniary advancement of the individual physician and of the profession as a whole," and that they represent etiquette rather than ethics. He goes on to say that medical etiquette is "concerned with the conduct of physicians toward each other, and embodies the tenets of professional courtesy. Medical ethics should be concerned with the ultimate consequences of the conduct of physicians toward their individual patients and toward society as a whole" (Leake 1927, 2). However, Burns (1977) appears to argue in his commentary on Percival that those norms of etiquette are ethical in that they establish the circumstances that facilitate ethical relations with patients. There is, indeed, something to be said for that interpretation. If market conditions are so extreme that in order to make a living average practitioners are driven to cut their fees, increase the number of patients they see, and reduce the time and attention they give to each, perfunctory and even inadequate care can result. The sheer temporal and physical possibility of providing "attention, steadiness and humanity" may be destroyed. Thus, pressures from unregulated competition (or, in the present day, for example, from an inordinately high case-load and inadequate assistance) may influence what even the most virtuous physician can do for patients.

Of course, institutional ethics providing protection against circumstances that can discourage ethical practice are at least as likely to advance the practitioner's pecuniary interest as to advance the good of the patient. Professions can be, in George Bernard Shaw's famous phrase, "conspiracies against the laity." This is what many critics of medicine and other professions have charged with some justice. But without denying that self-interest can thrive with such protection, a strong argument can be made that ethical practice is even *less* likely to thrive without it. The 1847 Code can be interpreted as laying down two sets of norms, one constituting a *practice ethic,* and another constituting a supportive *institutional ethic.* Together they provided the rationale in the former case, and the circumstances in the latter, for the eventual licensing and growth of the American medical profession.

The Golden Age of American Medicine

American medicine did not succeed in becoming professionalized until some time after the adoption of the 1847 Code, and even after it gained exclusive licensing (Shryock 1967) there would be many economic ups and downs. In the late nineteenth century and during the Great Depression, many physicians lived in genteel poverty. For some, contract practice in mining communities in the West and in large cities in the East was an unpleasant necessity (see, e.g., Starr 1982, 200–209). The Golden Age of the solo, fee-for-service form of practice that the 1847 Code took as its model did not really begin until a full century later.

By 1947 medicine's competitors had either been effectively excluded from the marketplace or contained in limited practices, and attending physicians dominated the hospitals, which had grown into institutions of great importance.[2] The profession was at least nominally unified, though its unity was threatened by the continuous growth of specialties and the professional societies representing them. Despite the great changes that had taken place between 1847 and 1947, many of the ethical dictates of the 1847 Code of Ethics could still be practiced by individuals in their own offices or at the bedside of their hospital patients. Individual physicians were free to make their own decisions without much interference from patients or colleagues. Medicine was largely organized on a local, community basis, and it regulated the behavior of its members by norms that had close kinship to the institutional ethics espoused by the 1847 Code:

- it supported fee bills,[3] restrictions on advertising, and the boycotting of offending physicians;
- differences of clinical opinion were settled primarily by consensus among local practitioners or by seniority;

- criticism of colleagues, even within medical circles, was scrupulously avoided;
- the provision of free care to the poor was a matter of personal conscience and sometimes a quid pro quo requirement of the nonprofit hospital in which physicians had attending privileges;
- local community medical standards were taken to be authoritative in the courts, and physicians maintained what more than one critic has called a "conspiracy of silence," avoiding expert testimony against colleagues in malpractice cases;
- information provided by patients during the course of the clinical encounter reposed primarily in the records of individual consultants, which were virtually private property, not even available to the patient;
- financial, clinical, and "ethical" disputes between physicians were carefully shielded from public knowledge;
- state licensing boards were largely passive and secretive.

Most of these characteristics were attacked with increasing frequency and strength by critics who perceived more self-interest than dedication in the profession's performance.[4]

The Crippling of Traditional Practice

The events of the past three decades have resulted in radical changes in the circumstances of medical practice. This chapter began with a general statement of those changes. Now they may be elaborated.

First, the physician's relationship to patients has been drastically altered:

- Public and private health insurance has destroyed the direct economic relationship between physician and patient. Patients and physicians now rely primarily on insurers to pay for care.
- The proliferation of elaborate technologies and specializations has diffused the responsibility for providing care through a host of personnel. Responsibility has become embedded in a *system* rather than concentrated in the hands of one physician.
- The patient's record is no longer the virtual private property of the individual physician. It now circulates among a number of therapeutic and clerical personnel as well as to central insuring agencies and is theoretically available for the patient's scrutiny. The record's comprehensiveness,

permanence, and broad accessibility have been enhanced by computerization.

- Decisions to provide free care to the poor are no longer likely to be made by individual physicians but are made by the institutions in which they work.
- Medicine has lost much of its control over the information available to consumers and faces a more suspicious public. Public interest organizations seek the disclosure of previously restricted information about the care provided by both physicians and health care organizations; massive amounts of information about illnesses and their treatment are being disseminated to the public by private and public organizations and by the media; many previously controlled drugs may now be bought over the counter, and prescription drugs are being aggressively advertised directly to the public.
- Both in the courts and in ethical discourse, patients have gained a position of relative autonomy, with rights to information and decision making that discourage physicians from making unilateral decisions, however benevolently intended, concerning their care.

Second, traditional methods of controlling economic competition and making a living have largely been destroyed:

- Court decisions have swept away the practice of establishing minimum fees.
- Other decisions have swept away some (though not all) of the strictures on advertising, which, rightly or wrongly, has gained First Amendment status.
- Physicians now depend for their income on government agencies, large corporate employers, and health insurance companies, and must usually accept the economic terms offered by those organizations.
- An increasing number of physicians work for a salary or on a capitation basis in circumstances organized and financed by large for-profit organizations.
- Physicians are becoming divided into clinical practitioners, on the one hand, and managers or owners of practice organizations, on the other.

Third, the traditional freedom of the physician to make clinical decisions insulated from close examination and criticism by members of the medical community has been seriously weakened and divisions within the profession have intensified:

- Differences of clinical opinion are no longer adjudicated primarily by collegial opinion at the site of practice. In civil litigation, local "community standards" of care have lost privileged status in the courts, as has the absolute authority of expert medical testimony, by use of the doctrine of *res ipsa loquitur.* When "the fact speaks for itself," lay juries are no longer dependent on experts to provide authoritative testimony in the case of, for example, malpractice suits (see Freidson 1986, 106–7).
- Both public and private financing organizations employ authoritative protocols to decide whether or not medical services rendered are necessary or appropriate. Those protocols are created and administered by a new class of academic, research, and managerial medical specialists who establish clinical standards and supervise and administer their use in practice.[5]
- The technical specializations and subspecializations that have been growing steadily since the beginning of the century are multiplying and deepening divisions within the profession due to their sometimes conflicting therapeutic and economic interests.[6]

Finally, the economic foundation of medical practice has changed for many physicians:

- In traditional circumstances, the economic requirement of practice was solely that it provide a living (over-generous or not) to those who performed it. The growth of for-profit healthcare organizations adds the requirement that practice also yield an attractive return to investors. As Gray (1991) and others have noted, the expansion of the role of profit in health care can threaten the fiduciary obligation that is at the very center of medical ethics.

Taken together, I believe that these changes have the potential to destroy professionalism in medicine and to reduce physicians to technicians. It is true that, like professionals, some technicians perform extremely complex and skilled tasks that require considerable discretion. But unlike professionals, technicians have little voice in choosing the goals of their work, selecting the actual tasks they are to perform, or establishing the criteria by which their work is evaluated. It is different for professionals, who are committed to taking responsibility for their own work, preserving both its technical and moral integrity, and employing it to serve the good of their clients as well as the public. They do not serve passively, however, as a mere reflex of their clients' desires. Rather, they claim ultimate allegiance to some ideal goal—like health, justice, truth, or salvation—that transcends the interests of their immediate patron and even of the state.[7] By definition, technicians, on the other hand, serve their patrons literally as "freelancers" or "hired guns," doing whatever work is asked of them within their realm of competence. While a profession's members patently need to gain a living and must therefore seek economic reward, their more important reward is the recognition and respect that good work receives from colleagues, clients, and the public, and the intrinsic pleasure of doing interesting and challenging work of value to others.[8]

The basic ethical principle of devotion to the well-being of the patient that is expressed in the 1847 Code is central to professionalism. It is certainly as important today as it was then and, for that matter, as it has been throughout the history of medicine (e.g., Wear et al. 1993). But the policies of the 1847 Code that I have labeled institutional ethics are no longer adequate for the task of coping with the political and economic environment in which medicine finds itself today. While the ethical choices of individuals remain a fundamental component of practice, individual physicians have considerably less control over their immediate environment than was the case in the past. Nor can they as individuals alter the organization and financing of practice by third parties or the new economy that has been created. Now more than in the past, organized and coordinated activity of professional groups and associations assumes critical importance. Only they have the authority and leverage to press for policies that encourage and protect ethical practice by defending and creating the social and economic circumstances that support individual practitioners who are primarily concerned with the good of their patients.

Institutional Ethics for Our Time

The basic obligations of a profession truly concerned with the good of both its clients and the public can be advanced in part by the activities of individual members, but that is not enough. It must also take organized political action to gain an institutional environment that at least facilitates, but optimally supports and stimulates, the practice ethics of its members. It should do everything it can by political, legal, and other means to ensure that all who need its services receive them irrespective of their ability to pay. It should take active measures to ensure that the services its members provide are both competent and respectful of the needs of their clients. It should take active steps to ensure that its members are sufficiently insulated from unregulated economic pressure to minimize the influence of economic need on their practice. Finally, it must use every means possible to require working conditions that provide its members with the resources necessary for both competent and beneficent service. Let me discuss some of the policy positions implied by those statements.

One of the most important of the traditional ethical positions of medicine is the obligation to provide free care to the poor, whose needs are no less pressing now than they were a hundred and fifty years ago. It is widely recognized that tens of millions of Americans are not receiving adequate health care today. The voluntary activity of individual physicians may provide some care, but hardly enough; legislation is needed to finance and organize care for all. I believe that professional groups and associations have an ethical obligation to give forceful political support to programs that assure decent health care for all citizens, and to join with others who are concerned with providing care on some other basis than the present system of rationing by income (Reinhardt 1996).

The obligation to provide medical care regardless of ability to pay brings up an even broader ethical principle of professionalism, namely that the role of profit, of self-interest, must be limited. Health care is a public good, which is why it is regulated by the state and professional monopolies over service are permitted. There is no really free play of market forces in health care, fashionable rhetoric notwithstanding: what competition there is takes place within a regulated market. Therefore, the realistic policy questions are: How *much* of a living should be provided to health care professionals and executives of health-related organizations? And what *degree* of profit should go to investors? At present, efforts to lower the cost of care are reducing only the incomes of physicians and other professionals who provide direct services to the public. By contrast, the emphasis is on maximizing profits to the shareholders and executives of successful pharmaceutical and medical technology companies as well as insurance companies and managed-care organizations. Since health care is, and should remain, a *regulated* commodity, a kind of public utility, the industries connected with it should be treated as public contractors whose profits and operating costs require close public scrutiny and control. It is consonant with the profession's ethical obligation to provide care to all that it should spend less effort fighting modest reductions in the income of its members and considerably more effort fighting the huge contribution to the cost of care made by unconscionable profits for the manufacturers and purveyors of health-related products and the private organizers and insurers of health care.

On a related theme, recall that the 1847 Code attacked the patenting of remedies and procedures on the grounds that if they had any value they should be available for all physicians to use freely for the benefit of all their patients. This sounds quaint in a time when property rights that restrict free access to knowledge have been expanding far beyond what could have been conceived of then. This trend has received far less attention than its importance warrants. The public domain of knowledge and technique is shrinking. Many newly discovered therapeutic resources and techniques, even human cells, may become private property, available for the benefit of the public only at a price, and often a very high price, which contributes further to rationing by income. The flow of new scientific information has already been slowed and restricted (e.g., Blumenthal et al. 1997). It is consonant with the ethics expressed in the 1847 Code for the profession to strongly support the free use of new knowledge and technique by all its members for the benefit of all patients regardless of their ability to pay. This position is not, as it may have been in 1847, merely a device to forge a professional community; it is absolutely essential for providing all possible health benefits to the public.

While the profession should be ethically committed to limiting commercial property rights over therapeutic knowledge and technique, it should vigorously defend and enforce *patients'* property rights over personal information. The legal expansion of property rights has not been nearly as well secured for patients as it has been for commercial interests. The 1847 Code asserted an ethical obligation to protect the confidentiality of information provided by patients during the course of consultation. Today, this includes the findings of clinical examination, laboratory analysis, and other increasingly elaborate and sophisticated diagnostic methods. It is no longer possible for individual physicians to control the circulation and use of such information, because patient records cannot be secured unilaterally; consequently, the possibility of violating confidentiality and privacy by their exploitative use has increased markedly. The indiscriminate circulation of patient records for commercial, research, and law enforcement purposes can at the very least injure patients by violating their privacy, but it can also injure them in more concrete ways. If the profession takes its fiduciary relationship with patients seriously, it should be an active and publicly conspicuous advocate of patients' rights to privacy; and it should support all legal and administrative efforts that limit the distribution, use, and storage of clinical and personal information for any but the narrowest of purposes and by the fewest possible agencies. While justification for violating confidentiality was established early in this century in the case of patients with serious communicable diseases, all claims to do so should be closely scrutinized and honored as little as possible.[9]

Recall that the 1847 Code attempted to control advertising. The reasons for that effort may very well have been self-interested. Certainly efforts to prevent the advertising of competitive fees give that appearance, and that was at the center of the Supreme Court ruling striking down bans on professional advertising. But advertising can also injure patients by disseminating false, misleading, or inadequate information about healthcare products, procedures, and practice organizations, and by persuading them that they need some product that they can very well do without. The aim of commercial advertising is not to provide full and complete information to consumers so they can make choices in their best interest; rather, it is to exaggerate positive information and minimize, if not conceal, the negative in order to persuade the consumer to buy something.[10] The consequences of poor information for consumers may not be serious in the case of ordinary products or services about which they can easily learn from experience, but health care is a rather different commodity. I believe that commercial advertising of health-related goods and services should be much more strictly controlled than it is at present. Often such advertising (particularly by hospitals, insurers, and healthcare organizations) does not provide enough information for informed choice: it provides only superlatives and attractive symbols that convey no significant amount of information. More importantly, when information is provided, it is, as often as not, misleading, even if not false. Where "complete" information is required by law, it is too often in the traditionally illegible fine print, and written in technical language that is well beyond the capacity of most people (including the educated middle class) to understand and evaluate. The stakes are too high to condone laissez-faire in health-related advertising. Ethical concern for the public good demands that the profession organize action both to narrow the boundaries of what the Supreme Court chose to call "commercial speech" and to pursue legislation that requires advertisers to provide full information in accessible form.[11] Moves to this effect for HMOs are already being made in some states. The profession should not only strongly support them but also urge their extension and strengthening.

Finally, I turn to medical practice itself. There is an urgent need to undertake aggressive but responsible action to protect the right of physicians to exercise discretion in their treatment decisions. Without the right to exercise discretionary judgment, physicians become technicians. Note that the epidemiologically derived standards employed by those who finance and administer medical work apply to *populations* rather than individuals, and that patients must be respected as individuals. The mechanical imposition of such standards on treatment in the therapeutic encounter acknowledges neither the individuality of patients nor the professional judgment required to evaluate their cases. This is likely to seriously damage the well-being of many. Without returning to the rightly discredited easy collegial tolerance of the past, the profession must find some way to reinforce the physician's right to exercise responsible discretion.

Practitioners must also be in a position to maintain their fiduciary relationship with patients, which requires that the good of the patient come before all else. That prime practice ethic is threatened when physicians are either employed by, or under contract with, organizations whose obligation is above all to maximize financial yield to investors. Physicians today are losing control over their incomes, but that is less important for professionalism than the fact that they are losing control over the allocation of resources like time, case-load, equipment, and support personnel, which permit them to do good work. As Gray (1991, 339) notes, *organizational* resources, not merely individual dedication, are needed for good work. Often physicians appear unable to negotiate contracts that protect their economic and clinical rights, and in many cases HMOs can "terminate" physicians arbitrarily without cause. The bargaining position of physicians in their work settings must be strengthened so that their practice ethics can flourish even in managed-care organizations. But those who are employed are, like professors in private universities, seriously handicapped in exercising collective bargaining rights by the *Yeshiva* decision of the U.S. Supreme Court.[12]

Neither present-day American labor law nor traditional bread-and-butter trade unionism recognizes that professionals are neither managers nor conventional workers. But since professionals are classified as managers or supervisors by the *Yeshiva* decision, they do not have legal protection for negotiating collectively with employers about the work they perform and the resources they need to perform it for the benefit of their clients. If they were classified as employees, on the other hand, they would also lack protection for negotiating on those issues; for traditional trade unionism is concerned with compensation, safety, work loads, and fringe benefits, with employers retaining the right to determine the tasks workers are to perform and the equipment and time with which to perform them. But the position of professionals is considerably different from that of traditional industrial and clerical workers; for they or their colleagues are the authoritative source of the knowledge and skill employed in the work they do, the tasks they are to perform, and the criteria for evaluating them. And insofar as enough of their work is so unpredictable as to require discretionary judgment, they must be free of the mechanical constraints of mandatory routines so as to be able to serve the needs of individual patients. Today, when physicians are no longer independent practitioners, it is essential that they be able to negotiate collectively with employers, should they wish to do so, and most particularly negotiate about the resources they need for the benefit of their patients. As part of its primary ethical obligation to serve the good of its patients, the profession should fight for revisions in American labor law that would grant its employed members the right to negotiate collectively.

When considering new rights to bargain collectively under the protection of labor law, it is essential to avoid stereotyping the issue by invoking the specter of traditional trade unionism and its ultimate source of power, the strike. It is possible to imagine a new or revised labor law that recognizes a specifically professional form of unionization, one focused on negotiating working conditions bearing on the *capacity* to provide ethical care—on adequate staffing and support, on space and equipment, on case-load, on mechanical constraints on the exercise of discretionary judgment—without any necessary concern with compensation as such. Given the essential nature of health services, it is possible to imagine that such a law could withhold protection for strikes, though that is a matter for debate. Whatever that law may be in its details, however, it should protect the right to form a union or association for physicians within a practice organization and, if its negotiations with management prove fruitless, protect the right of that collective bargaining unit to engage in public demonstrations, issue statements to the press, and otherwise attempt to bring the force of public and legislative opinion to bear on the employer's policies. A highly publicized opinion by official representatives of the medical staff that management is failing to provide its physicians with the resources they need to provide good health care to their patients could have powerful consequences, especially if it is separated from self-interested issues of compensation. And if protected by labor law, those expressing their considered, critical judgment need have no fear of dismissal or blacklisting.

The Proof of Ethical Codes

Finally, it is essential to observe that it is not enough for a profession to create ethical codes, for its ethics committee to issue opinions and commentaries attempting to apply particular ethical principles to newly risen issues, and for its distinguished leaders to give thoughtful lectures on ethics. These do have some value, for they can provide guidance to ethical action. But if there is no significant action on the part of the profession as a whole to institutionalize those ethical principles and to create or preserve the circumstances that encourage ethical behavior, the profession has little defense against those who charge that its code is mere window dressing. In today's political and cultural climate, when the public has lost much (though by no means all) of its confidence in the primacy of professional ethics over self-interest, such vulnerability can prove fatal to the status of medicine. Because of its increasingly scientific and technical character, medicine is considerably more vulnerable than law, for example, or the professorate, to being reduced to technician status. Should its ethical commitment be questionable and the art underlying its adequate practice ignored or deprecated, it will truly be at risk. That is all the more reason why professional associations and groups need to undertake vigorous legal and political action to enforce the code of ethics and defend or create the institutional circumstances which encourage ethical practice.

An unambiguous case in point of an unenforced violation of medicine's ethics is the participation of physicians in the execution of capital offenders by lethal injection, which has been explicitly declared unethical by the AMA (Council 1997, 11–14) and other medical associations. This clear violation of medical ethics by individual physicians has been going on for some years, yet state licensing boards have chosen to ignore it despite their stated obligation to apply sanctions to those who violate ethical as well as legal and technical norms. If the medical profession's code is to be seen as more than empty posturing, its representatives must undertake vigorous legal action to force licensing boards to discipline such behavior even if that may conflict with legislation that requires physician participation. It is true that disciplining state executioners will raise difficult Fourteenth Amendment questions, but taking ethics seriously requires facing them. Professional ethics are similar to those of religious institutions in that they go beyond the state and its law.[13] To condemn the behavior of Nazi doctors and Soviet psychiatrists, whose behavior was technically lawful, without also condemning American doctors who act as state executioners is hypocritical.[14] As Pellegrino and Thomasma (1993, 51) put it, "Medicine should not be subject to the whims of the society in which it is found, and to its mores."

Physician participation in state executions is an unusually dramatic instance of the unethical practice of medicine that the profession has not yet been able to confront officially, and that damages the perception of its commitment to its code. Another example is the code's condemnation of patenting medical procedures, which does not sit well beside its approval of patenting surgical or diagnostic instruments (Council 1997, 150). Indeed, most of the issues discussed in this chapter are touched upon in today's code of ethics, but in only the most general terms, without any concrete recommendations for legal or political action to discipline individual offenders and create mechanisms to protect virtuous practitioners from a hostile environment.

When practice decisions must be made in today's complex social and economic environment, organized professional action to create circumstances that discourage or prevent violation of some ethical principles and encourage and permit others becomes indispensable. The practice ethics guiding the way individual professionals deal with their clients and the institutional ethics guiding the way professions as organizations create the milieu for practice are inseparable. As Brennan (1991, 88) put it, "Medical ethics in the future must have two not entirely separable aspects. One retains a focus on relations between doctors and patients. The other moves beyond that focus to address economic and political issues in health care. Traditional ethics allowed physicians to ignore the overall social repercussions of medical ethics. This is no longer possible." The fate of the professional status of medicine in the future will hinge in no small measure on its recognition of the truth of that statement.

Acknowledgments

An earlier version of this paper benefited greatly from the suggestions of Helen Giambruni and Robert Baker. Whatever virtues this expanded version has are owed to Helen Giambruni's critical editing.

Notes

1. The precarious economic and social position of physicians at that time is clearly presented in the histories of Rothstein 1972, Shryock 1947, and Starr 1982.

2. For excellent histories of the rise of the hospital in America, see Rosenberg 1987 and Stevens 1989.

3. See Rosen 1946.

4. For my contribution to this literature, see Freidson 1988, originally published in 1970. See the afterword to the 1988 edition, which reconsiders earlier criticism in light of political and economic change.

5. Should this new class continue to grow, it is possible that the medical profession will, like schoolteaching, split into two major segments with seriously conflicting interests—researchers and administrators on the one hand, and practitioners on the other.

6. In spite of centrifugal economic and jurisdictional forces, it is improbable that medicine will, like engineering, split up into virtually separate professions. Unlike en-

gineers, who are divided by serving such entirely independent industries as chemical, electronics, and nuclear energy, the vast majority of medical specialties are part of the single interdependent division of labor practiced within the health services.

7. These distinctions are developed at some length in Eliot Freidson, *Professionalism: The Third Logic* (Cambridge, UK: Polity Press), in preparation.

8. It is a reflection of a time ideologically dominated by the dogma of neoclassical economics that I must remind readers that even now, remarkable technical and intellectual achievements are produced by scholars, scientists, and other professionals who are motivated less by their modest economic rewards than by public and collegial respect and honor.

9. It should never be forgotten that patients are virtually coerced by insurers and providers to provide consent to the release of their records. If they do not consent, they may not receive their financial benefits or even treatment.

10. Little attention has been paid to what is surely one important source of the cost of health care—the deliberate and sophisticated stimulation of consumer demand.

11. Thus, *truly* informed consumers shopping for health insurance should not only know what disorders and services are excluded from coverage or provided limited or restricted coverage, but also, in light of their own medical histories and that of their immediate kin, what their actuarial risk is of needing services that are not covered. A *truly* informed consumer should have access to the same information as those who write their policies. In this case, as in others, there is a transparent double standard that favors producers rather than consumers and that belies the assumption of a truly free market with fully informed consumers.

12. For an introduction to the Yeshiva decision of the Supreme Court and the basic issues it involves for employed professionals, see Freidson 1986, 134–84. See Rabban 1991 and Rabban 1994 for more extended discussion.

13. The Council on Ethical and Judicial Affairs of the AMA observes that "ethical and legal principles are usually closely related, but ethical obligations typically exceed legal duties. In some cases, the law mandates unethical conduct. . . . In exceptional circumstances of unjust laws, ethical responsibilities should supersede legal obligations" (Council 1997, 1).

14. It should be emphasized that the question of physician participation in executions must be kept quite separate from a personal opinion supporting the execution of capital offenders. Participation in executions is as a physician rather than as a private citizen.

References

Abbott, Andrew. 1988. *The System of Professions: An Essay on the Division of Expert Labor.* Chicago: University of Chicago Press.

Baker, Robert. 1993. Deciphering Percival's code. In *The Codification of Medical Morality: Historical and Philosophical Studies of the Formalization of Western Medical Morality in the Eighteenth and Nineteenth Centuries.* Vol. 1, *Medical Ethics and*

Etiquette in the Eighteenth Century. ed. Robert Baker, Dorothy Porter, and Roy Porter, 179–211. Dordrecht: Kluwer.

Berlant, J. 1975. *Profession and Monopoly: A Study of Medicine in the United States and Great Britain*. Berkeley: University of California Press.

Blumenthal, D.; Campbell, E. G.; Anderson, M. S.; Causino, M.; and Louis, K. S. 1997. Withholding Research Results in Academic Life Science: Evidence from a National Survey of Faculty. *Journal of the American Medical Association* 277:1224–28.

Brennan, T. 1991. *Just Doctoring: Medical Ethics in the Liberal State*. Berkeley: University of California Press.

Burns, C. R. 1977. Historical Introduction to 1975 Reprint of Thomas Percival: Medical Ethics or Medical Jurisprudence? In *Legacies in Ethics and Medicine*, ed. C. R. Burns, 284–99. New York: Science History Publications.

Council on Ethical and Judicial Affairs, AMA. 1997. *Code of Medical Ethics. Current Opinions with Annotations*. Chicago: American Medical Association.

Freidson, E. 1986. *Professional Powers: A Study of the Institutionalization of Formal Knowledge*. Chicago: University of Chicago Press.

———. 1988 (1970). *Profession of Medicine: A Study of the Sociology of Applied Knowledge*. Chicago: University of Chicago Press.

———. Forthcoming. *Professionalism: The Third Logic*. Cambridge, UK: Polity Press.

Gray, B. H. 1991. *The Profit Motive and Patient Care: The Changing Accountability of Doctors and Hospitals*. Cambridge: Harvard University Press.

Leake, C. D. 1927. *Percival's Medical Ethics*. Baltimore: Williams and Wilkins Co.

Pellegrino, E. D., and Thomasma, D. C. 1993. *The Virtues in Medical Practice*. New York: Oxford University Press.

Rabban, D. M. 1991. Is Unionization Compatible with Professionalism? *Industrial and Labor Relations Review* 45:97–112.

———. 1994. Arbitration of Disputes over Professional Standards. In *Arbitration 1994: Controversy and Continuity*, ed. G. W. Gruenberg, 194–213. Washington: Bureau of National Affairs.

Reinhardt, U. E. 1996. Economics. *Journal of the American Medical Association* 275(23), 19 June, 1802–4.

Rosen, G. 1946. *Fees and Fee Bills: Some Economic Aspects of Medical Practice in 19th-Century America*. Baltimore: Johns Hopkins University Press.

Rosenberg, C. E. 1987. *The Care of Strangers: The Rise of America's Hospital System*. New York: Basic Books.

Rothstein, W. 1972. *American Physicians in the Nineteenth Century: From Sects to Science*. Baltimore: John Hopkins University Press.

Shryock, R. H. 1947. *The Development of Modern Medicine*. New York: Knopf.

———. 1967. *Medical Licensing in America, 1650–1965*. Baltimore: Johns Hopkins University Press.

Starr, P. 1982. *The Social Transformation of American Medicine: The Rise of a Sovereign Profession and the Making of a Vast Industry*. New York: Basic Books.

Stevens, R. 1989. *In Sickness and in Wealth: American Hospitals in the Twentieth Century.* New York: Basic Books.

The Three Ethical Codes. 1888. *The Code of Ethics of the American Medical Association, Its Constitution and By-Laws. The Code of Ethics of the American Institute of Homeopathy. The Code of Ethics of the National Eclectic Medical Society.* Detroit: Illustrated Medical Journal Co.

Wear, A., et al., eds. 1993. *Doctors and Ethics: The Earlier Historical Setting of Professional Ethics.* Amsterdam: Editions Rodopi B.V.

8

Doctor, Schmoctor

Practice Positivism and Its Complications

ARTHUR ISAK APPLBAUM, PH.D.

For it is, after all, with men and not with parchment that I quarrel.
—Henry David Thoreau, "Resistance to Civil Government"

The standard role of doctor as a learned professional devoted to the care and healing of the sick currently is under challenge by practices that require medical expertise, but that partially conflict with a commitment to serve the medical needs of each individual patient. Managed care has made some doctors into gatekeepers; clinical trials deny some patients treatment that the doctor-researcher has reason to believe is beneficial; consumer demand has turned some doctors into cosmetic and genetic technicians. The job of expert witness, company doc, public health official, and, many would say euthanist, all conflict in some way with the role obligations of standard doctoring.

On what grounds can these conflicting pursuits be criticized? One might say that the practice of medicine is a *natural role,* by analogy to natural law. On this view, the standard role obligations of doctoring follow from some truths about the kind of creatures we are. Doctors who pursue ends that conflict with the end of caring for each patient are making a conceptual mistake, for one cannot occupy the role of doctor and coherently pursue ends incompatible with what doctoring must be. In this paper, I explore this claim about the role of doctor and propose a different, more plausible, but more troubling way to think about professional roles and their connection to morality.

Role is not a well-defined and well-developed moral idea, and we will have to make do with some sloppiness around the edges. The term has theatrical origins, referring to the roll of parchment on which an actor's part was written and so, metonymously, to the part itself. It was pressed into service by anthropologists and sociologists to describe positions in society that come along with expected patterns of conduct related to the social function of those positions.[1] Moral philosophers ask normative questions about the social scientists' descriptive category: When, how, and for what reason are the social prescriptions attached to roles also moral prescriptions? When, how, and for what reason is the evaluation that a person is good at one's role also a moral evaluation that one is a good person? The theatrical metaphor is inspired, because it vividly calls to mind a determinate script that must be read by anyone who plays that role. But the image may assume too much at the start: perhaps the role player ought to be a Method actor, or an improvisationist. Provenance of the term *role* aside, the concept of distinctive positions in social practices and in stitutions that have distinctive duties, values, and virtues is very old, of course. Indeed, the conventional view of the ancient world, not unchallenged, supposes that what we would now call one's social role comprehensively governed moral life in heroic societies. On this view, Homeric characters and their author thought that different virtues attached to different social roles, the fifth-century dramatists began to recognize conflicts between overlapping social roles but saw no resolution, and the Socratics first asked about the virtues of a good man simply.[2]

Schmoctoring

I begin this exploration of professional roles with an old chestnut of a law case that is widely used in the teaching of legal ethics, *Spaulding v Zimmerman*. It is also a medical ethics case of first importance—and one with direct implications for some of the pressing challenges that confront the practice of medicine today. In 1956 John Zimmerman had a serious automobile accident. David Spaulding, a teenaged passenger in the car, sustained a severe crushing injury of the chest with multiple rib fractures, fractures of the clavicles, and severe cerebral concussion. Spaulding sought damages from Zimmerman. Zimmerman's auto insurance company sent the young Spaulding to a doctor in its employ for examination. The insurance company's doctor discovered a life-threatening aortic aneurysm that Spaulding's own doctors had missed and that Spaulding knew nothing about.

What do you suppose the doctor did with such information? He picked up the phone and placed an emergency call to . . . Zimmerman's lawyer. Lawyer, doctor, and insurance company decided to conceal the youth's condition, and Spaulding settled for $6,500.

Some time after settlement, the aneurysm was detected in the course of a routine medical checkup by Spaulding's own doctor, and Spaulding was rushed into surgery. He survived, and he successfully petitioned the trial court to set aside the settlement with Zimmerman, arguing that Zimmerman's lawyer improperly withheld information. The Minnesota Supreme Court upheld vacating the settlement but took pains to proclaim that "no canon of ethics or legal obligation" required the lawyer to inform Spaulding that without treatment he could drop dead at any moment (*Spaulding* 1962, 710). "There is no doubt that during the course of the negotiations, when the parties were in an adversary relationship, no rule required or duty rested upon defendants or their representatives to disclose this knowledge" (*Spaulding* 1962, 709).[3] It is this defense of the lawyer's actions that makes *Spaulding v Zimmerman* a notable case in legal ethics.

Our interest, however, is in the actions of the doctor, not the lawyer. Is there no canon of *medical* ethics that requires doctors—even doctors hired by insurance companies or lawyers—to tell Spaulding that his life is in danger? Now, this condemnation of the doctor might be overdetermined in that, quite apart from any role obligation the doctor has as a doctor, he (and we) have a common, preprofessional moral duty to warn others of grave danger when we are in circumstances where we can do so at little risk or cost to ourselves. But added to any responsibility he might have simply as a person, doesn't he have a professional responsibility, in his role as doctor, to care for his patient?

There are a number of arguments the doctor can make in his defense. He might claim that he did not take Spaulding on as his patient—that no doctor-patient relationship had been formed. You might imagine the doctor warning Spaulding before the examination: "Don't be fooled by the stethoscope. Yes, I am a doctor, but not yours. I have not taken you on as my patient." But the standard role of doctoring doesn't let doctors off so easily. In emergencies and in Good Samaritan cases, it is widely believed that doctors have a professional obligation to treat, whether they wish to take on new patients or not. More generally, the rules of the role of doctoring do not permit just any contractual relationship between a doctor employing her medical expertise and a consenting adult, and doctors are morally obligated to follow the rules of their role.

It has been claimed that it is not mere convention that the existing role obligations of doctors require that doctors attend to illness and suffering in a certain way and prohibit them from employing their medical expertise in other ways. Rather, on this view, the fact that we are the sort of creatures that fall ill and suffer creates a set of natural moral obligations that bind those who have the skills to cure and relieve suffering. On this view, one says in response to the insurance company doctor that he cannot coherently claim to be a doctor and then fail to attend in the right way to Spaulding's condition. No agreement with the insurance company or Zimmerman, and no agreement with Spaulding, can release the doctor from the obligations of his natural role.

Suppose the fellow in the employ of the insurance company responds like this: If doctoring indeed is a practice governed by such stringent rules and exclusive ends, then call what I do *schmoctoring*—a different practice with different ends and different role obligations.[4] It's not merely that Spaulding isn't my patient, but that I am not (at least not in this capacity) a doctor. Why am I not free to fashion some other way of employing my science and skill, as long as I do not violate the law or any preprofessional moral obligations that apply to all occupations? I may not lie, cheat, steal, or coerce, just as plumbers and sales clerks may not. But as long as Spaulding is properly informed that, as a schmoctor, my role obligations commit me to serve the insurance company, not Spaulding, what is wrong with occupying the role of insurance company schmoctor?

Similarly, as long as the customer is properly informed that managed-care schmoctors are under contract not to mention the word "transplant" in front of patients, what is wrong with the role of managed-care schmoctor? For a chance to get an experimental drug, consent to be the subject of a research schmoctor. Overweight? Try a pill-mill schmoctor. If you want a traditional patient-doctor relationship, stick with that other profession, the Doctor®.

Indeed, the insurance company schmoctor might go further and claim exemption from some preprofessional moral obligations that bind plumbers and sales clerks. Perhaps insurance company schmoctoring, like lawyering, is a morally justified adversary role. Lawyers claim permission to advance unjust ends, conceal wrongdoing, and persuade others of matters of fact and law that they themselves do not believe to be true on the grounds that, in equilibrium, good and just ends are served by the adversary system. Perhaps the schmoctor is exempt from the common moral duty to inform Spaulding because he has a fiduciary obligation to advance the interests of his employer in an adversary system where others are advancing the interests of Spaulding.[5]

Let me be clear about schmoctoring: I am not suggesting that the vast majority of physicians in the managed-care setting and the vast majority of clinical researchers are not deeply committed to the standard role of doctoring, and I am not suggesting that they are failing to put the needs of their patients first. Rather, I am imagining practices of schmoctoring that might someday come about as contractual and institutional arrangements such as cost containment, capitation, and for-profit ownership continue to press against the standard role. In the practice of schmoctoring that might someday come about, schmoctors will not enter into a fiduciary relationship with patients; rather, they will be contract employees of for-profit health-care providers who, in turn, have contractual relationships with consenting adult customers.

In contrast with the natural role view, call the view that admits the possibility of schmoctoring *practice positivism,* by analogy to legal positivism. On this view, the concept of a practice does not impose any general content requirements or restrictions on the rules of all practices. The rules of a practice simply are what they are, not what they ought to be or what we want them to be. If this view is correct, we cannot criticize the schmoctor on grounds that are internal to the concept of a professional practice or role. We can criticize an entire role or practice from the outside and ask if it is a morally permissible or worthy pursuit. But if practice positivism is the correct view of roles, then medical expertise can be put in service of a wide range of purposes without internal contradiction. I think practice positivism is the correct view of roles. To see why, we need to trace out some connections between roles and morality.[6]

Ways of Moralizing Roles

Suppose that a social or professional role has some moral force, by which I mean that the fact that a person occupies the role affects what he is morally required, permitted, or forbidden to do, and affects how his character and actions are to be morally evaluated. What is the route by which such roles connect to morality? Consider two ways: call them *direct moralization* and *mediated moralization.* In direct moralization, role prescriptions are themselves moral prescriptions for persons who occupy the corresponding role. So, the professional rule that requires doctors to maintain patient confidences is itself a moral rule for one who is a doctor, and the professional rule that requires lawyers to be the zealous advocates of clients is itself a moral rule for one who is a lawyer. This seems to be an unobjectionable way to account for the moral force of role prescriptions when they have such force, until we look at the implication of direct moralization for evaluation, where the view appears to require that role evaluations be themselves moral evaluations. So, if seeking to maximize shareholder value is a criterion for being a good business manager, then for a person occupying the role of business manager, seeking to maximize shareholder value is a criterion for being a good person. Direct moralization, one might think, is too direct.

In mediated moralization, the prescriptions that a role generates are not in themselves moral prescriptions, and standards for evaluating good role occupants are not in themselves moral evaluations. Rather, if one occupies a role that has moral force, one has one great moral reason to follow the role's non-moral prescriptions. So, the requirement of patient confidentiality is a professional rule of the role of doctoring, but is not in itself a moral rule. Morality enters because, by hypothesis, doctors have a moral obligation to obey the nonmoral rules that apply to doctors. Similarly, maximizing shareholder value makes one a good manager, but not, at least not directly, a good person. Under mediated moralization, "good doctor" and "good manager" are not in themselves moral evaluations any more than are "good hammer" or "good spy." Rather, if one's role has moral force of a certain sort, part of being a morally good person is to be good at one's role.

Neither scheme of moralization supposes that every role has moral force, or that every prescription and evaluation within a moralized role is morally dispositive. Each scheme still is in need of an account of which roles are moralized, and why; and each is in need of an account of how to act and evaluate action when practical reasons, both within and without the role, conflict. The two ways of moralizing roles amount to much the same thing when both conclude that the role occupant morally ought to follow the prescriptions of the role; but they may not always reach the same conclusion.

Direct moralization seems highly implausible if the role prescriptions that are said to be in themselves moral prescriptions include all the actual commands, rules, and customs of the role—the positive law of the role, so to speak. Many explicit rules and implicit customs of roles clearly are devoid of direct, substantive moral content—doctors are expected to complete lots of paperwork for insurance companies, and lawyers are expected to wear suits in court, but it seems odd to say that billing patients and dressing up are among the direct moral obligations of doctors and lawyers. If morality has something to say about those activities, it is by a more circuitous route. More important, the rule makers and exemplary practitioners in a role are not infallible—even the AMA's Council on Ethical and Judicial Affairs can err—so the content of actual practices, even in otherwise good roles, can be morally and professionally mistaken. If a doctor ought to comply with monopolistic rules prohibiting advertising, and if an army officer ought to comply with policies to suppress homosexuality in the military, the reason is not that these features of the role have acquired substantive moral correctness by virtue of their enactment. That would turn the governing mechanisms of various role-generating institutions—the AMA House of Delegates, the Joint Chiefs of Staff—into legislatures of morality. But beyond the borders of Kant's Kingdom of Ends, morality is not so enacted. We can recognize roles to have moral force without adopting a pure proceduralist view about the moral and professional correctness of actual practices.

There is an apt analogy here to political obligation and the moral force of the laws of the state. We distinguish between what the law of the state is and what the law should be. If, by hypothesis, there is a general obligation to obey the law, it is not because all laws are good laws (that is simply false) or because the law prescribes that the law be obeyed (that is circular) but because there are extralegal moral reasons to obey laws—even, generally, the bad ones. Similarly, we distinguish between what the role *is* and what the role *should be.* There may be moral reasons to comply with roles as they are, but that is not to be confused with the claim that all of the reasons for action given by a role, even a good role, are already moral reasons.

On the other hand, mediated moralization, the view that role prescriptions are nonmoral prescriptions that role occupants generally are morally obligated to obey, seems to put too much distance between the substantive content of a role and the sources of moral obligation. Mediated moralization might explain an obligation to defer to authority when the actual demands of the institutional role are in error, and might explain obligations to comply with conventions of practice that have no substantive content themselves but are useful in coordinating behavior in roles. But many role prescriptions and evaluations do have substantive moral content of their own, and not because the role prescription accidentally coincides with an ordinary, nonrole obligation, but because the role shapes or gives moral force to a reason or value. Something important is missed if a physician's commitment to heal the sick or a journalist's commitment to inform the public is accounted for by saying that role occupants are morally obligated to perform the nonmoral commands of their roles. That may be true, but it is not the only moral reason physicians and journalists have for pursuing the goods valued by their roles. A physician reproaching a colleague who does not care for patients properly or a journalist reproaching a colleague who handles the truth carelessly does not simply argue that the wayward colleague is obligated to perform her role. Such an argument would appeal to possible sources of a generic moral obligation to obey role prescriptions: that one ought to do well whatever one does, that one ought to do what one has agreed to do, that one ought to fulfill the reasonable expectations of others, or that one ought to be fair to other role occupants, to mention a few candidates. But a physician will also appeal to the substantive goods particular to medicine and remind the colleague that she once believed that healing the sick was a valuable pursuit; the journalist will recall shared commitments to supporting a free and educated citizenry.

Perhaps it is like this. All roles put forward actual, nonmoral, substantive prescriptions of the institution—what the role is: "Submit forms in triplicate," "Wear a tie in court," "Don't ask, don't tell," "Be home by ten o'clock, dear." Then there are reasonable constructions of substantive role prescriptions—what the role *should* be: heal the sick, pursue justice, defend the nation, love your parents. Here, then, is the truth in direct moralization: though actual role prescriptions are not in themselves moral prescriptions, reasonable role prescriptions may be. To the extent that what the role is tracks what the role morally should be, the role is, in this sense, directly moralized.

Similarly, roles put forward, with varying degrees of formality, actual structures of authority, ways of determining what person, group, text, or process gets to say what the actual substantive prescriptions of the role are. The umpire behind the plate gets to call balls and strikes, and the first-base umpire gets to call the runner out; there are rules of precedence for making other calls, and the commissioner of baseball gets to decide what these rules are and how large the strike zone is. The actual authority structures of some roles, such as doctors and lawyers, are by and large collectively self-governing. Others, such as the roles of artist and intellectual, are by and large individually self-governing. Still others, like the role of child or the traditional role of nurse, are governed by those who occupy other roles: parent and physician. A description of what the role is includes both the substantive prescriptions of the role and the procedures and structures of authority that generate those substantive prescriptions. This formulation poses many descriptive puzzles: what if authority to generate prescriptions is contested, or if the criteria for who occupies a role are contested, or if the prescriptions of a role are largely violated by role occupants? But descriptive puzzles are not conceptual puzzles. Just as actual substantive role prescriptions (what the role is) can be distinguished from reasonable role prescriptions (what the role should be), actual structures and procedures of authority in a role (who or what in fact says what the role is and who is in it) can be distinguished from reasonable structures and procedures of authority (who or what *should* say what the role is and who is in it). Just as there are reasonable constructions of the substance of role prescriptions, there are reasonable constructions of the authority of role prescriptions. Here, then, is the truth in mediated moralization: there can be moral reasons that obligate a role occupant to comply with the actual substantive prescriptions of roles even when the content of what the role is does not track the content of what the role should be. So if one is in a role, one can have two different sorts of moral reasons to obey the actual prescriptions of role authorities: direct reasons, when the actual substantive prescriptions track the reasonable construction of the role's substance, and mediated reasons, when the actual structure of authority in the role tracks the reasonable construction of authority in the role.

This account of the connections between morality and roles is not quite adequate, for in distinguishing between what the role is and what the role should be, it leaves room for ambiguity about the senses of "should." There can be reasonable criteria for evaluating a role and its prescriptions that are still nonmoral. Architects should design beautiful spaces that work. When the actual practice of architecture strays from that ideal, as it did, for example, when Brutalism was in fashion, architects are not doing what architects ought to do, they are not being good architects. But "should," "ought," and "good" are here aesthetic prescriptions and evaluations, not moral ones. Excellence in architecture may have nothing to do with morality, and appeals to what the role of architect should be need not be moral appeals. Similarly, reasonable constructions of authority in roles need not be moral constructions. Excellence in teaching English usage to schoolchildren requires having and transmitting a view about what is and is not standard grammar. It is perfectly intelligible to distinguish between what the rules of grammar are and what they ought to be, and it is perfectly intelligible to hold a view about whether, to be a good teacher or writer of English, one should follow the rules that are or the rules that ought to be, all the while using *ought, should,* and *good* in nonmoral senses. William Safire's linguistic prescriptivism is a view about good English, not good ethics, and a position on whether to obediently follow Safire on split infinitives is a position about linguistic authority, not moral authority.

We might stipulate that criteria of excellence in roles must operate within the morally permissible range, so that, though reasonable role prescriptions and evaluations can be nonmoral, they cannot be immoral. But such a stipulation is not conceptually required. Excellence in an executioner is not conceptually constrained by the bounds of what is morally permissible. Though perhaps mistaken, it is not incoherent to say that Charles-Henri Sanson, headsman for both Louis XVI and the Terror, was an excellent executioner but an evil man (see Applbaum 1995, 1999). The notion of a reasonable construction of a role neither captures all the connections between roles and morality nor reconciles roles with morality.

I have, in a somewhat roundabout way, noted distinctions that are worth emphasizing. A role is not simply whatever role occupants happen to do. Since many actual doctors commit malpractice and many actual parents are negligent and abusive, it would be quite odd to think that prescriptive and evaluative force flows directly from what occupants of the role of doctor and parent

actually do. The very notion of a good role occupant who does what is prescribed creates the possibility of a bad role occupant who does not do what is
prescribed. Indeed, the concepts of malpractice, negligence, and abusiveness
assume both a standard and a failure to meet it. If this seems too obvious to
mention, recall how common is the notion that art simply is what artists do.
This could be a deep insight about the practice of a role if the emphasis is on
the plural, what artists do. Practices are collective enterprises that connect
practitioners over time and across space, so standards of excellence are likely
to have some relationship to what actual practitioners, if only the best of them,
actually do. In contrast, the claim that art is whatever an artist does is fatuous.
This is not to exclude the possibility of iconoclastic artistic excellence, but to
include the possibility of art criticism.

Nor are the actual prescriptions and evaluations of a role necessarily what
the role should be. I likened the actual role to the positive law to emphasize
that, though an actual role prescription is presented as a practical reason for a
role occupant, it is not by itself a practical reason: the role occupant still needs
a reason to treat actual prescriptions as action-guiding. The reason might be
that the actual prescription adequately realizes substantive practical reasons,
moral or nonmoral, that the role occupant already has. A doctor who faces actual role prescriptions on patient confidentiality may find that following them
satisfies moral reasons to respect and dignify her patients. Or a cellist may find
that the conductor's interpretations accord well with his own aesthetic and historical sensibilities. Or a lawyer who faces the actual role prescriptions on zealous advocacy may find that following them satisfies her prudential reasons to
seek out challenge, gratification, and financial reward. Alternatively, some attribute of the actual role prescription unrelated to its substance might provide
the practical reason. This can be so if the role occupant has a moral reason to
follow actual role prescriptions regardless of their content—for example, a
judge may have acquired a moral obligation to follow the role prescriptions of
the court by swearing to do so. Or the role occupant can have a nonmoral, practical reason to follow role prescriptions regardless of content—for example, a
soldier may have a desire or interest in being good at his role in a role where
compliance with actual role prescriptions, ordinarily without regard to their
content, is part of being good at it.

An actual role prescription, however, can fail to generate moral reasons for
action. Not every role has or claims to have moral force, and there is no conceptual requirement that the actual demands of roles be compatible with the
reasonable demands of morality. Less obviously, actual role prescriptions can
fail to generate even nonmoral practical reasons. This may be so for unchosen

roles. Someone who is conscripted into an army against his will occupies the role of soldier but may lack any reason to be a good soldier (though threat of punishment gives him a reason to appear to be a good soldier). Or this may be so when an actual rule or custom of the role prescribes an action that is inconsistent with being good at the reasonable construction of the role, and the role occupant has a practical reason to be good at that.

To show the plausibility of practice positivism, let me offer an example where, unlike schmoctoring, we are likely to applaud, rather than condemn, a professional's refusal to take the rules of a role as his own. Suppose a librarian holds the outmoded notion that excellence in his role involves collecting books. For years, his professional colleagues have been computerizing their holdings and linking their users to the information superhighway, while he assembled carefully chosen collections on carefully chosen subjects. He is considered by virtually all professional librarians to be an antique, though he takes great pride in and gets much satisfaction out of what he does. Though he clearly is out of step with what the role has become, this does not yet provide him with a practical reason to give up his notion of excellence, for his commitment is to what he believes the role should be, not to what it is. He has a practical reason to be a good librarian on his criteria of good librarianship, not on the dominant view of the role.

One might say about him that if he is unmoved by the evaluative criteria of the role as it is he is not a good librarian (though he might be a good something else—book collector, perhaps); or one might even say that he is not a librarian at all, that he no longer occupies the role (though, again, he may occupy some other role). But these seem to be purely verbal distinctions, and not much rides on them. The important point to observe is that, if he is defined to be a bad librarian or not a librarian at all, that does not obviously give him a practical reason to become a good librarian. It might be that, if confronted with the prospect of having to concede that he is not a good librarian, he would discover that he does have a reason to be good at the role as it is: he may become convinced that the world of learning and the needs of library patrons have changed, or that he cares about the approval of his peers. But he may instead revise his account of himself, and rename his commitment "excellence in book collecting," rather than in librarianship. In response to the reproach, "Good librarians don't browse the stacks, they surf the net," he might respond, "If so, then I am not a librarian, so I have no reason to be a good one." Similarly, the schmoctor has no reason to be a good doctor.

But our antiquated book lover need not give up his claim to be a good librarian or a librarian at all so quickly: he might have good grounds to argue that his criteria of excellence, because they fit the traditional purposes, functions, and values of librarianship, are authoritative, and the database searchers are usurpers. If he is mistaken about the criteria for good librarianship, it is not simply because he is vastly outnumbered. The doctrine of *role realism,* on the model of legal realism, is wrong: a practice is not simply whatever role occupants in fact do. Recall that malpractice is possible. But if the book collector is going to put up an honest fight for the soul of the practice, his claim must be about what librarianship in fact is and how that in fact is decided, not about what librarianship ought to be and how that ought to be decided. Though role realism is wrong, the doctrine of practice positivism, on the model of legal positivism, is right: a role simply is what it is, and not what it ought to be.

Doctoring

If the content of the role of doctoring is largely conventional, not natural, what difference does it make? It is of course as important as ever that professional groups such as the American Medical Association continue to deliberate about and render collective judgments about what the rules of the role of doctoring are. But if I am right about the limitations of the claims about natural roles and right about the expansiveness of the claims about positive roles, it is not enough to render judgments. It is not enough because, over time, under various market and institutional pressures, those with medical training may come to question whether they are bound by the rules of doctoring, which they did not shape and did not choose. Instead, they may come to see themselves as schmoctors of various stripes. And if enough of them think so, *it will become so:* a new set of social meanings surrounding a new actual role, the role of schmoctor, will have emerged. For the role of doctoring is not discovered in the natural order of things. It is stitched together from the shared social meanings of those who profess to be doctors and those who call upon their services. To be clear: moral obligations are not legislated by social practice. Morality is a construction of reason, not a convention of society. But positive role obligations *are* conventional, and depend only on what the practice in fact *is.* Insofar as we are morally obligated to comply with positive role obligations simply because they are positive role obligations, it is only when the role that in fact is applies to us.

One way a role applies to us is if we agree to it; another is if we accept the benefits of the role generated by those who have accepted upon themselves the role's burdens (see Applebaum 1996). And this may be enough to obligate most current practicing physicians to the standard role of doctoring. But conventions and shared understandings are changing, and if enough doctors act like schmoctors, the time will soon come when it cannot be supposed that most of those with medical training have agreed to the role of doctor, not schmoctor. Once this happens—once medical practitioners fail to identify with and endorse the goods and virtues and commitments internal to the standard practice of doctoring—they indeed are morally free from the collective judgments of a social practice that is not their own and that does not apply to them.

What can the profession of doctoring do to prevent the emergence of schmoctoring? There always is denial. An organized profession can, wittingly or unwittingly, make claims about the source of its moral authority that are not true and hope that most practitioners believe them. Just as false claims about the divine right of kings served to keep subjects in line for a time, false claims about what the role of a medical practitioner must naturally be might hold sway for a time. But the march of transparency and reflection in our social relations will catch up to the myth of natural roles just as surely as it did to the myth of natural monarchy. The task, then, is to inspire medical students and practicing doctors to choose, upon reflection, to commit or recommit themselves to the standard role of doctoring, though they are free, and know that they are free, to do otherwise—though there are other institutional arrangements for the delivery of medical care that satisfy the constraints of common morality. Schmoctoring can meet the logical requirements of coherence and the minimal moral requirements of justice. The profession of doctoring must therefore understand itself as a calling that could have been otherwise, but argue why it still is a calling worthy of being answered by a reflective practitioner. Insofar as doctors continue to identify with their profession and look to their colleagues for guidance and support on what counts as good professional practice—that is, insofar as those with medical training wish to subject themselves to the judgment and approval of their peers—they will reject the label of schmoctor. The challenge, of course, is to continue to articulate in a clear and reasoned voice to both doctors and patients what would be lost if the practice of doctoring gave way, in substantial measure, to the various forms of schmoctoring that I have described.

Acknowledgments

This chapter was presented at a conference celebrating the 150th anniversary of the AMA Code of Medical Ethics in March 1997. A modified version of it appears in Applbaum 1999.

Notes

1. Montaigne may well be the first to have used the theatrical term in connection with vocations (Montaigne 1992, 3:1, 3:10). Nietzsche made good use of the metaphor (Nietzsche 1974; and see Kaufmann's introduction, 24). David Luban attributes the social scientific coinage to the anthropologist Ralph Linton in his 1936 book, *The Study of Man* (Luban 1988, 105). Dorothy Emmet says that G. H. Mead may have used the term in lectures given from 1904 onwards (Emmet 1966). See also Goffman 1961.

2. For more nuanced views, see Nussbaum 1985; Williams 1993. Cf. Nietzsche 1974, sec. 356 on role acting in Periclean democracy.

3. Why then uphold the trial judge's order to vacate? Using tortured logic, the justices faulted the lawyer for withholding information from the *court* when, acting as an officer of the court rather than as an adversary, he proposed approval of the settlement.

4. The schmoctor gambit is borrowed from Nozick (1974, 235n.).

5. For an elaboration of how such obligations are acquired, see Applbaum 1996 or Applbaum 1999, chap. 6.

6. For an elaboration of practice positivism see Applbaum 1998 or Applbaum 1999, chap. 5.

References

Applbaum, A. I. 1995. Professional Detachment: The Executioner of Paris. *Harvard Law Review* 109(2):458–86.

————. 1996. Rules of the Game, Permissible Harms, and the Principle of Fair Play. In *Wise Choices: Decisions, Games, and Negotiations*, ed. Richard J. Zeckhauser, Ralph L. Keeney, and James K. Sebenius. Boston: Harvard Business School Press.

————. 1998. Are Lawyers Liars? The Argument of Redescription. *Legal Theory* 4 (March):1.

————. 1999. *Ethics for Adversaries: The Morality of Roles in Public and Professional Life*. Princeton: Princeton University Press.

Emmet, D. 1966. *Rules, Roles, and Relations*. London: Macmillan.

Goffman, E. 1961. Role Distance. In *Encounters: Two Studies in the Sociology of Interaction*. New York: Bobbs-Merrill.

Luban, D. 1988. *Lawyers and Justice*. Princeton: Princeton University Press.

Montaigne, Michel de. 1992. *Les Essais* (1588). Ed. Pierre Villey. Paris: Quadrige/Presses Universitaires de France.

Nietzsche, F. 1974. *The Gay Science* (1887). Translated with introduction by Walter Kaufmann. New York: Viking.

Nozick, R. 1974. *Anarchy, State, and Utopia*. New York: Basic Books.

Nussbaum, M. 1985. *The Fragility of Goodness*. Cambridge, UK: Cambridge University Press.

Spaulding v Zimmerman, 116 NW2d 704 (1962).

Williams, B. A. O. 1993. *Shame and Necessity*. Berkeley: University of California Press.

9

Who Should Control the Scope and Nature of Medical Ethics?

ROBERT M. VEATCH, PH.D.

During the Interim Meeting of the American Medical Association (AMA) in 1979, a newly emerging leader, James S. Todd, M.D., offered the final report and recommendations of the Ad Hoc Committee on the Principles of Medical Ethics. That report contained the text of the soon-to-be-adopted revised Principles, which were to revolutionize professionally written medical ethics. The introduction to that report contained an insight even more revolutionary than the text itself. It stated that "the profession does not exist for itself; it exists for a purpose, and increasingly that purpose will be defined by society."

Whether the committee was endorsing the wisdom of relying on society to define the scope and nature of medical ethics or merely reporting the inevitable, this statement marks the beginning of a new era in professionally generated medical ethics. Stated more precisely, it marks the return to an earlier wisdom in which medical professionals saw themselves as an integral part of an ethic of the broader society and generated the ethic for professional conduct by close and spirited exchange with the intelligentsia of the day—the theologians, philosophers, lawyers, and literary elite who were the custodians of the morality of the culture.

By contrast, for a period between 1800 and the late 1970s, it was widely held that a profession was the source of its own ethic. One version of that claim was that the profession produced and enforced its own ethic (Durkheim 1958; Barber 1963; Hughes 1963). Sometimes this has been expressed with the claim that among professions there are goods or moral norms internal to, or inherent in, the concept of the practice (MacIntyre 1981). Thus for medicine, physicians have claimed that there is a morality internal to medicine (Brody 1994; Jecker and Schneiderman 1995; Pellegrino and Thomasma 1988). The claim that there is a morality internal to a profession has turned out to be hard—indeed, I would argue impossible—to sustain.

The Eighteenth-Century Grounding of Professional Ethics

The code ethics of the Anglo-American medical profession has its grounding in the Scottish Enlightenment of the late eighteenth century (Baker, Porter, and Porter 1993). The single most important figure was the philosopher-physician John Gregory (1724–73). He presented the lectures to the University of Edinburgh medical students that gave rise to the most important volume of the day: *Lectures on the Duties and Qualifications of a Physician* (Gregory 1772).[1] He influenced decisively the work of Thomas Percival (1740–1804), whose *Medical Ethics* (Percival 1803) became the model for the early American professional codifications including the 1847 Code of Ethics of the AMA. He also shaped the thinking of Benjamin Rush (1745–1813), who is acknowledged by the authors of the AMA Code as another major influence on their work.[2]

Gregory was from a family of physicians, but he was equally at home with humanists. He began his career in Aberdeen as a regent (from 1746–49), sometimes referred to as a professor of philosophy. He had the remarkable responsibility of taking a group of King's College, Aberdeen, students through the entire curriculum of the college education (Wood 1993). He was introduced to this environment by his cousin, Thomas Reid (1710–96), one of the leading philosophers of the day. Together they founded the Wise Club, a philosophical debating society common among the intelligentsia of the period. It was before that club that he gave a series of six lectures on faculty psychology that were eventually published as *A Comparative View of the State and Faculties of Man with Those of the Animal World* ([Gregory] 1765), a philosophically sophisticated discussion of some of the key philosophical issues of the day. After moving to Edinburgh in the 1760s, Gregory traveled in an inner circle of some of the most illustrious philosophers in Western history, including David Hume and Adam Smith.

Gregory was always a staunch defender of Christianity against the skepticism of Hume (Gregory [1774] 1821).[3] If pressed for an account of where his ethics were grounded, Gregory would most certainly have identified Christian theological sources. But he was also a man of the Scottish Enlightenment. His philosophical precursors were Francis Hutcheson (1694–1746), David Hume, Adam Smith (1723–90), and Gregory's cousin, Thomas Reid. The issues he pursued were those of the Enlightenment. His way of knowing was the common sense, an epistemological convention common to the branch of the Enlightenment critical of religious skepticism.[4]

This is not the moral epistemology of professional ethics of the Hippocratic tradition or of any other professional morality that grounds knowledge of the duty of the physician in the profession. Gregory was remarkably uninterested in the Hippocratic ethic. In a thorough search of Gregory's writings, I have yet to find a single reference to the Oath. He does occasionally express a mild interest in other Hippocratic writings. He believes that physicians should know good Greek, and he considers Hippocrates a writer of great skill (Gregory 1772, 96). He also has good things to say about Hippocrates' empirical method (43, 130), but he never mentions him as a source of ethics. The Hippocratic view that knowledge is reserved for those within the profession is not a position Gregory held. For Gregory the ethics of medicine is deeply embedded in the ethics of the culture, which had its grounding in Christianity and Scottish empiricist philosophy. Medical professionals conversed intimately with theologians and philosophers and derived their ethics from their foundations.

The same can be said of Thomas Percival, who was strongly influenced by Gregory and who acknowledges his indebtedness to him in the opening of his *Medical Ethics*, published in 1803 but having its origins in the previous decade. Percival's *Ethics* eventually provided the most decisive text for the drafters of the AMA's Code of 1847. Like Gregory, Percival was not inclined to turn to professional medical sources to develop his ethic for physicians and had little interest in the Hippocratic ethical tradition.[5] In addition to the important influence of Gregory, Percival acknowledges the influence of the cleric Thomas Gisborne (1758–1846), who had written a volume on the ethics of various professions including a chapter on medicine (Gisborne 1794). Gisborne's understanding of ethics is grounded in Christian religious doctrine. He holds that there are "duties of station," duties that attach to specific roles, including professional roles such as that of physician. What is critical, however, is that Gisborne and Percival would never attempt to rely on a professional group as the foundation of the ethical norms for their members. They would not even view the professional group as standing in any privileged position when it comes to knowing the duties of the physician. Rather, in terms of ethics, physicians are lay people. Knowledge of ethics might come through reason, revelation, the moral sense, or the teaching authority of theologians; it would never come through the medium of professional consensus. Great physicians such as Percival or Gregory may be pretty good at philosophy or theology. As such, they may have wisdom about the morality of their professional role. They would not claim, however, that merely by being wise in medicine, one was also wise in the ethics of the practice.

Attempts to Ground Ethics in the Profession

Soon after the beginning of the nineteenth century, the relationship of professional physicians to the theologians, philosophers, and literary leaders of the culture began to change. It seems to me quite clear that physicians, for the most part, simply quit talking with humanists. They became modern medical scientists (see chaps. 3 and 4, this volume). With the proliferation of knowledge from the Enlightenment, the concentration of medical education on medical science became overpowering. Especially in Britain, students entered their medical education directly from secondary school. At hearings in Edinburgh before the Commission for Visiting the Universities and College in Scotland beginning in 1826, the members of the faculty repeatedly referred to the young ages of the students. The dean of the faculty of medicine pointed out that they had a requirement that no one could be awarded a degree of Doctor of Medicine under the age of 21 (Commission for Visiting 1837, 195). While the cultural elite of the eighteenth century (including Gregory and Percival) would have started their classical education at home, the social class of the medical student was shifting so that such broadening could not be relied upon by the early nineteenth century. The typical physician, indeed even the elite physician, simply no longer had the exposure to the humanities that the previous generation had received.

The Isolation of the Medical Profession

My research suggests that it was at this point that the ethics for the profession of medicine became isolated from the broader religious and secular ethical sources of the surrounding culture. Not until at some point after this isolation did the Hippocratic Oath reemerge as a decisive moral text. I am still uncertain exactly when this rediscovery of the rather simplistic ethics of the pagan Greek mystery cult began to dominate Anglo-American medical ethics once again. It is clear that it was not critical in the late eighteenth century. The medical students at Edinburgh took an oath, but it had its origins in the same oath taken by all other graduates. It was a pledge of loyalty to the king, to the Scottish National Covenant, and to the university—not to any Hippocratic ethical tradition.

By the time of the emergence of interest in professionally generated medical ethics of the nineteenth century in Boston (1808), then in New York (1823), Baltimore (1832), and Philadelphia (1846), and finally in the founding meeting of the AMA in 1847, the members of the drafting committees had available to them only distant memories of the physician as philosopher. They were able to draw on Percival and Rush, but it seems unlikely that any of the key players—John Bell and Isaac Hays, for example—really understood the ethical bases of the sources they used. Certainly, they were out of their league in metaphysics, moral epistemology, and moral theology. There appears to be no evidence of interaction between the theologians of the mid-nineteenth century and the drafters of the AMA Code (Veatch 1995). The communication between organized medicine and secular humanists was a little more open. To be sure, occasional physicians cultivated their knowledge of secular moral philosophy. Worthington Hooker (1849) was an example in the nineteenth century, as is Edmund Pellegrino in the twentieth. But they were increasingly isolated from organized medicine, certainly not decisive figures in the articulation of professionally generated codifications.

The Ontological Claim to a Professionally Generated Code

Professionally generated codes of medical ethics carried with them two rather bold and strange claims. The most radical was that the scope and nature of medical ethics was controlled by an organized profession because it was the source of the moral norms for practitioners. It was as if the role of medical professional was the property of the profession. The claim was something akin to that of a college fraternity that could claim it was the ultimate source of norms for the brothers because it invented the rules. It was the origin of the handshake, the password, and the norms for behavior among members.

In the nineteenth and early twentieth centuries, some physicians claimed that they literally created the norms for the profession (Veatch 1972). Russell Roth, a speaker of the AMA's House of Delegates in the 1970s, entered the debate of the day over physician advertising with such a claim. Troubled by the fact that the lay population was challenging the authority of organized medicine to prohibit physician advertising, Roth (1971) claimed that the profession "has imposed upon itself certain proscriptions which are often poorly understood by the public." Little wonder that the public understood so poorly if the profession had imposed these proscriptions on itself. This is the boldest form of the claim that the profession might make regarding the control of the scope and nature of medical ethics. The claim is ontological—that the ethical norms come, not from God or from reason or from the moral laws of nature, but from organized medicine.

This view seems akin to the position taken by Mark Siegler in chapter 10 of this volume. He claims that medical ethics, or at least clinical ethics, is part of the discipline of medicine and that the goal of medical ethics is to improve medicine in practice by furthering patient care and improving patient outcomes. This shows considerable confusion even for one who has not studied the discipline of ethics in any formal, systematic way. First Siegler confuses the goals of the broad field of medicine with the goals of physicians. He seems to think that all of medicine is defined by what physicians do, and that the goals of medicine are set by the goals of physician practices. Sociologically speaking, however, medicine is a much broader sphere. It is the sphere of life having to do with organic well-being. As such, most medical decisions people make do not involve physicians at all. Medical decisions are made whenever one chooses to take a drug (or refrain from taking one), whenever one chooses to seek professional counsel about a bodily problem (or refrains from seeking such counsel), or whenever dietary and lifestyle choices are made. Medical decisions are made regularly, not only by ordinary citizens, but also by judges, legislatures, educators, and others in many other roles. Even among medical professionals most decisions are not made by physicians; they include the other health professions such as nursing, pharmacy, dentistry, or the allied health professions, all of which are commonly professions existing within a medical center. Medicine is no more the exclusive domain of the physician than education is the exclusive domain of teachers.

Thus, even if the purpose of medicine (even when restricted to the clinical setting) were to further the goals of medicine, it would be a serious error to assume that these goals were defined by, or generated by, physicians. Normative moral choices in the medical sphere are no more the province of the professional physician group than the morality of corporal punishment by means of electrocution is the province of electrical engineers or war is the province of the professional military.

It is a serious confusion to assume that the purpose of medical ethics, even at the clinical level, is to further any goals—let alone goals defined by a particular professional group. The very act of deciding what counts as a good outcome in a sphere of life such as medicine requires religious and philosophical evaluation that necessarily takes one outside the domain of the professional activities of physicians. Whether preserving a permanently vegetative life with aggressive life-support is a good or a horrible outcome requires theological or philosophical judgment. It may be morally right for an orthodox Jew, morally tolerable for Roman Catholic, and morally outrageous for someone of another religious or philosophical worldview. Asking what counts as the "medical good," independent of these normative enterprises, is a meaningless activity. Claiming that deciding the moral goals of life is the province of a professional cadre called physicians is hubris of the worst form.

If each profession invents its own norms, then the physician is logically in an exposed position when he or she is playing the role of layperson. When the physician is the client of the lawyer or the accountant, it would appear that these other professions would be in control of the ethical norms for their roles just as physicians are in control of theirs. Moreover, when physicians interact with other health professionals—nurses, pharmacists, or occupational therapists—they might also expect that these professionals would claim authority to control the norms for their roles. When the two groups must interact in a way that is governed by each profession's norms in a way that conflicts, chaos would reign.

Most critically, when members of the health professions interact with lay people, are they claiming, as Roth seems to imply, that the profession invents the norms not only for the professional actor but also for the layperson as well? That would seem to have been the model for the group gathering in Philadelphia in 1847. They articulated not only the "duties of physicians to their patients," but also the "obligations of the public to physicians" (AMA 1848, 1–14; see Appendix C). What right had they, a group of physicians, to obligate others? Imagine, for example, a physician in moral dispute with the Pope or some other prominent theologian, in which the issue is who is the authority for determining what is the right conduct for a physician with regard to some medical-moral issue such as euthanasia or abortion or autopsy. Is it really plausible that some nineteenth-century participant in the Philadelphia meeting of the AMA could say to the Pope, "We have imposed upon ourselves certain duties"?

To this day, there are interesting cases in which the profession and some secular or religious groups differ on the proper role of the physician. For example, until 1994 the AMA's Council on Ethical and Judicial Affairs took a more conservative position than the pope on the issue of forgoing life support for patients who are critically ill and suffering but not terminally ill (AMA 1986, 13; cf. Council 1994, 37). To this day, the AMA seems more open to Hippocratic deception in the informed consent process than is secular liberal political philosophy or the American courts (AMA 1996, 120).

The Epistemological Claim to a Professionally Generated Code

Sometimes medical and other professional groups that generate codes of ethics make a more modest claim, which can be called the epistemological claim. Those who make this claim hold that the norms of morality—including the morality in professional roles—have their foundation in more ultimate sources—in the deity, in reason, or in the moral laws of nature—but that only the professional group can understand and articulate the norms for the professional role. Perhaps this is the claim that Siegler is really making. That view, which may have its roots in the Hippocratic cult's view of esoteric knowledge, seems to come down to a belief that only by being socialized into the professional role can one know the duties of being a member of that profession. Lord Brock (1970, 661–63), a British physician participating in the House of Lords' debate on euthanasia, captured the notion when he said, "As an ordinary citizen I must accept that the killing of the unwanted could be legalized by an act of Parliament, but as a doctor I must know that there are certain things which are part of the ethics of our profession that an Act of Parliament cannot justify or make acceptable."

He claims that by being a member of the professional group he knows things that others do not know: something about the role of the physician. A similar claim is being made by some physicians in the current physician-assisted suicide debate and perhaps also by Siegler when he suggests that clinical ethics must be clinically relevant in improving medicine.

Is there any reason, however, to accept the claim that only those in a role can have knowledge of the duties that attach to that role? That certainly was not Thomas Gisborne's view when he wrote chapter after chapter on the duties of station of various roles, to none of which he belonged except the clergy.

The controversy is similar to the one over whether only military generals can determine the role of generals. Especially in the case of professionals, who by their very nature must be in constant interaction with lay people, there is no reason to hold that only members of the professional side of the lay-professional relation can know the duties of the lay and professional roles. Certainly, there is no reason to assume that knowing the technical aspects of doctoring will necessarily give one expertise on the moral norms of that role. In fact, there is good reason to believe that lay people are typically just as authoritative in articulating the norms for these roles. In a real sense, these roles are in the public nexus. The health professions (and many others) are licensed publicly. The public gives special privileges in exchange for requiring that licensed professionals accept certain publicly articulated norms.

Of course, if these norms are moral norms, they are not properly seen as grounded in mere public consensus. For the theologically inclined, they derive from the will of the deity. For the secular, they are grounded in reason or moral principle. Is there any reason to believe that being a member of a professional group should give one special expertise in knowing the deity's will or what moral reason requires for their professional role (but not for other professional or lay roles)? It is hard to imagine why.

The case for a broad public responsibility for articulating the moral norms of professional roles stems from a belief in human fallibility and human equality. Humans are fallible in their capacity to have moral knowledge, including knowledge of the norms for professional roles. They are more or less equally fallible; no individuals or groups are definitively authoritative in moral knowledge. As such, members of professional groups cannot claim to be the only ones who can define the norms for either professional or lay roles. The acknowledgment of James Todd's committee in 1979 of the role of the public in defining the purpose of medicine began reversing the professional elitism of over a century and a half beginning in the years building up to the AMA's code in 1847. The fact that patients are not playing a significant role in the ongoing revision of the principles and interpretations or in the adjudication of disputes about alleged unethical practices of professionals suggests that there is yet a long way to go.

Grounding Professional Ethics
Beyond the Profession

It is in the nature of ethics that they must be grounded in our most fundamental beliefs and values, not in personal opinions or tastes or the views of a social or professional group. They must be rooted in our most fundamental authority. For religious people, that is the deity; for secular people, it is reason, natural law, or truths held to be self-evident. They come not merely from the profession but from a more basic source.

Many systems of belief and value (religions or philosophies) claim to articulate ethical principles. The proper norms for medicine depend on these values, so there will be as many ethics for medicine as there are ethical systems. Each system includes an epistemology—a theory of who is authoritative in knowing the proper norms of conduct. For religious systems, that may be priests, church councils, scholars, or prophets. For the secular world, it may be reason or a group that possesses wisdom. For a democratic society, there is no generally recognized authority. All are potentially equally authoritative. In fact, that equality of moral authority could be considered a defining characteristic of a democracy.

For our most general societal norms, society will be the authority that controls and shapes medical ethics. But within that society, there will be many different groups that will attempt to articulate special ethics for various types of medical practice. Medical ethics is appropriately seen as derived from these broader religious and philosophical ethics, not from sources in the various professions.

For example, recently feminist bioethics has emerged as a theory of considerable interest, especially to those who identify with feminist thought. It is not a stretch to imagine feminists who conceptualize a type of medical practice with goals, modes of interaction between lay and professional, and moral norms derived from feminist theory (see Holmes and Purdy 1992; Sherwin 1992; Farley 1985; Little 1996). Understandings of the moral norms for the roles of physician or nurse as well as that of the layperson will be radically different, from this perspective, than from the perspective of, say, Talmudic medical ethics. The idea that there can be one all-purpose, generic perspective from something called the profession of medicine makes no sense.[6]

Since the AMA adopted its revisions of 1980, it has begun the process of reintegration into the mainstream of our culture, recognizing, at least in theory, the legitimate role that the broader public will play in articulating the moral norms for professional and lay roles. Recognizing the 150th anniversary of the original code of the AMA with this meeting, with its broad interdisciplinary sponsorship and participation, is a recognition that we are moving back to the reintegration of the profession of medicine into the broad intellectual conversation of our culture.

Notes

1. An early unauthorized version from student notes appeared as [Gregory] 1770.

2. See, for example, Benjamin Rush's *Lectures on the Mind* (1981). The influence of the Scottish Enlightenment figures on Rush is immediately apparent in this and other works of Rush: "I know the doctrine I am defending is considered by Dr. Read *[sic]*, Dr. Beattie, and Dr. Gregory as unfriendly to morality and religion; but I am happy in being able to oppose to those authors, the names of Hartley, Crombie, Priestley, and above all of them our illustrious countryman the Revd. Mr. Edwards" (Rush 1981, 525). It would be a rare nineteenth-century American physician who could write such a sentence.

3. This was best seen in his posthumously published advice to his daughters (Gregory 1774).

4. For appeals to *common sense,* see Gregory 1772, 62, 141, 185, 215, 234, 193; Gregory 1765, 47.

5. He makes brief mention of Hippocrates as a great physician (Percival 1807, ii; 1803, 95–96).

6. I cite feminist bioethics and Talmudic ethics as two examples of substantive ethics that will have direct implications for lay and professional medical roles. Others include the various other religious ethical traditions as well as secular systems such as liberal political philosophy or Marxist ethics. Viewed in this light, the Hippocratic tradition would be one among competing belief systems. All of these could be contrasted to empiricobioethics, which is descriptive ethics rather than normative ethics. Attitudinal surveys and other social science techniques may be used to measure the particular ethical positions of the various traditions but cannot, in themselves, determine what ethical stance is morally right or wrong any more than can consensus of professional opinion.

References

American Medical Association. 1848. *Code of Medical Ethics: Adopted by the American Medical Association at Philadelphia, May 1847, and by the New York Academy of Medicine in October, 1847.* New York: H. Ludwig and Company.

———. 1986. *Current Opinions of the Council on Ethical and Judicial Affairs of the American Medical Association, 1986: Including the Principles of Medical Ethics and Rules of the Council on Ethical and Judicial Affairs.* Chicago: American Medical Association.

Baker, Robert; Porter, Dorothy; and Porter, Roy, eds. 1993. *The Codification of Medical Morality: Historical and Philosophical Studies of the Formalization of Western Medical Morality in the Eighteenth and Nineteenth Centuries.* Vol. 1, *Medical Ethics and Etiquette in the Eighteenth Century.* Dordrecht: Kluwer.

Barber, Bernard. 1963. Some Problems in the Sociology of the Professions. *Daedalus* 92:669–88.

Brock, Lord. 1970. Euthanasia. *Proceedings of the Royal Society of Medicine* (July):661–63.

Brody, Howard. 1994. The Physician's Role in Determining Futility. *Journal of the American Geriatrics Society* 42(8):875–78, esp. 877.

Commission for Visiting the Universities and College in Scotland. 1837. *Evidence, Oral and Documentary, Taken and Received by the Commissioners Appointed by His Majesty George IV, July 23d, 1826; and Re-appointed by His Majesty, William IV, October 12th, 1830; for Visiting the Universities of Scotland.* Vol. 1, *University of Edinburgh.* London: His Majesty's Stationery Office.

Council on Ethical and Judicial Affairs (AMA). 1994. *Code of Medical Ethics: Current Opinions with Annotations.* Chicago: American Medical Association.

————. 1996. *Code of Medical Ethics: Current Opinions with Annotations, 1996–1997.*
    Chicago: American Medical Association.
Durkheim, Emile. 1958. *Professional Ethics and Civil Morals.* Glenview, Ill.: Free Press.
Farley, Margaret A. 1985. Feminist Theology and Bioethics. In *Theology and Bioethics:
    Exploring the Foundations and Frontiers,* ed. Earl E. Shelp. Boston: D. Reidel.
Gisborne, T. 1794. *An Enquiry into the Duties of Men in the Higher and Middle Classes
    of Society in Great Britain Resulting from Their Respective Stations, Professions, and
    Employment.* London: B. and J. White.
Gregory, John. 1765. *A Comparative View of the State and Faculties of Man with Those
    of the Animal World.* London: Printed for J. Dodsley in Pall-Mall.
————. 1770. *Observations on the Duties and Offices of a Physician; and on the Method
    of Prosecuting Enquiries in Philosophy.* London: W. Strahan and T. Cadell.
————. 1772. *Lectures on the Duties and Qualifications of a Physician.* London. W. Stra-
    han and T. Cadell.
————. [1774] 1821. A Father's Legacy to His Daughters. In *Letters on the Improve-
    ment of the Mind* by Mrs. Chapone [Hester Mulso]. *A Father's Legacy to His
    Daughters* by Dr. Gregory. *A Mother's Advice to Her Absent Daughters* by Lady
    Pennington, with Lives of the Author. Edinburgh: Printed for Fairbairn & An-
    derson; William Whyte & Co.; William Oliphant; James Robertson; and T. Tegg,
    London, pp. 145–94.
Holmes, Helen Bequaert, and Purdy, Laura M. eds. 1992. *Feminist Perspectives in Med-
    ical Ethics.* Bloomington: Indiana University Press.
Hooker, Worthington. 1849. *Physician and Patient: Or, a Practical View of the Mutual
    Duties, Relations, and Interests of the Medical Profession and the Community.* New
    York: Baker & Scribner.
Hughes, Everett C. 1963. Professions. *Daedalus* 92:655–68.
Jecker, Nancy S., and Schneiderman, Lawrence J. 1995. Judging Medical Futility: An
    Ethical Analysis of Medical Power and Responsibility. *Cambridge Quarterly of
    Healthcare Ethics* 4:23–35.
Little, Margaret Olivia, ed. 1996. *Feminist Perspectives on Bioethics,* special issue of
    Kennedy Institute of Ethics Journal 6:1–103.
MacIntyre, Alasdair. 1981. *After Virtue.* Notre Dame: University of Notre Dame
    Press, 180–81.
Pellegrino, Edmund D., and Thomasma, David C. 1988. *For the Patient's Good: The
    Restoration of Beneficence in Health Care.* New York: Oxford University Press.
Percival, Thomas. 1803. *Medical Ethics; Or, A Code of Institutes and Precepts, Adapted
    to the Professional Conduct of Physicians and Surgeons.* London: J. Johnson.
————. 1807. *The Works, Literary, Moral, and Philosophical, of Thomas Percival.* 2
    vols. Edited by Edward Percival, 1783?—1819. London: J. Johnson.
Roth, Russell B. 1971. Medicine's Ethical Responsibilities. *Journal of the American
    Medical Association* 215:1956–68.
Rush, Benjamin. 1981. *Lectures on the Mind.* Edited, annotated, and introduced by Eric
    T. Carlson, Jeffrey L. Wollock, and Patricia S. Noel. Philadelphia: American
    Philosophical Society.

Sherwin, Susan. 1992. *No Longer Patient: Feminist Ethics and Health Care.* Philadelphia: Temple University Press.

Todd, James S., Chairman. 1979. Report of the Ad Hoc Committee on the Principles of Medical Ethics [of the American Medical Association]. Unpublished report.

Veatch, Robert M. 1972. Medical Ethics: Professional or Universal. *Harvard Theological Review* 65:531–39.

———. 1995. Diverging Traditions: Professional and Religious Medical Ethics of the Nineteenth Century. In *The Codification of Medical Morality: Historical and Philosophical Studies of the Formalization of Medical Morality in the Eighteenth and Nineteenth Centuries.* Vol. 2, *Anglo-American Medical Ethics and Medical Jurisprudence in the Nineteenth Century,* ed. Robert Baker, 121–32. Dordrecht: Kluwer.

———. Forthcoming. The Isolation of Professional Medical Ethics: Why Physicians Quit Talking with Humanists at the End of the Eighteenth Century.

Wood, Paul B. 1993. *The Aberdeen Enlightenment: The Arts Curriculum in the Eighteenth Century.* Aberdeen University Press.

10

Medical Ethics as a Medical Matter

MARK SIEGLER, M.D.

In this chapter I address a difficult but circumscribed question: Who should control the scope and nature of medical ethics? The question requires us to focus on *medical* ethics rather than on the larger domain of *bioethics*. I will further narrow the issue to the ethics of medical *practice*, and will not discuss the ethics of medical *research*. But before deciding the "who" question, it is necessary to ask the "what" question: What is the appropriate scope and nature of medical ethics? What are its goals?

From the early days of the medical ethics enterprise, the specification of goals has not been easy. Daniel Callahan, cofounder and (until recently) president of the Hastings Center, recounted: "In the early 1970s, in one of my first articles on bioethics, I wrote that the principal aim of the field should be to help the medical practitioner deal with concrete cases" (Callahan 1996). In 1978 I wrote that "whatever else medical ethics is, it must have something to do with the practice of clinical medicine, or at least it should" (Siegler 1978).

Regarding this issue of clinical relevancy, we may ask what the track record of medical ethics has been in contributing to improving medicine or the quality of patient care; in building the compassion, empathy, and respect physicians have for patients; in strengthening the doctor-patient relationship, enhancing the content of doctor-patient communication, or improving the process of clinical decisions. Have ethics committees or consultants or required ethics courses improved patient care and outcomes? The short answer is "We don't know." There have been very few—almost no—studies examining the impact of medical ethics generally, or of specific medical ethics interventions, on the quality of medical care or on patient outcomes.

David Eddy (1996) enumerated a set of principles for deciding whether to invest scarce societal resources in a new treatment. The same principles could be applied to a new social or educational innovation like medical ethics. Eddy suggests that before a new approach is adopted

1. there must be convincing evidence that it works;
2. its benefits must be determined to outweigh its harms;
3. it must represent a good use of limited resources; and
4. the above determinations regarding efficiency and cost-effectiveness must reflect the preferences not only of the community encouraging the innovation but also of the individuals who are to be the nominal beneficiaries of the innovation.

Medical ethics has not met this four-part test.

In accordance with the dictates of his four standards, Eddy encouraged the development of evidence-based medical practice. In connection with that development, Eddy observed that the quality of medical evidence may be classified into three levels:

1. *the best* evidence comes from well-designed randomized controlled trials or cohort studies;
2. *fair* evidence is based on case control studies; and
3. *weak* evidence is based on expert opinion.

Until recently, traditional medical ethics has relied on the weak evidence of expert opinion.

A few years ago, in a similar vein, Leon Kass criticized the ethics movement for being too theoretical, philosophical, hyper-rational, and ideological, while at the same time failing to examine routine issues and to consider the habits and behavior of moral agents and moral communities. Kass considered the issue of outcomes and said, "Though originally intended to improve our deeds, the practice of ethics, if truth be told, has, at best, improved our speech" (Kass 1990).

Unfortunately, there is much evidence to suggest that Kass is correct and that the state of medicine and of ethical medical practices is not better in 1997 than it was at the birth of the medical ethics movement thirty years ago. During that time we have witnessed escalating healthcare costs, progressive deterioration in the doctor-patient relationship, and the steady decline in access to health care. Of course, it is not fair or appropriate to give medical ethics the entire blame for all of the changes in medicine that have occurred on its watch.

But what about the state of end-of-life care, a central preoccupation of medical ethics?

Despite hundreds of court decisions and many new laws about end-of-life care (and umpteen articles and seminars), the data from the SUPPORT Study are shocking in their demonstration of how badly we care for the dying—not only clinically, in failing to provide adequate pain medicine, but also ethically, in failing to respect the wishes of dying persons (SUPPORT 1995). I suspect the same findings would be uncovered if we did a SUPPORT-type study on informed consent in clinical practice or on other ethical aspects of medicine that we congratulate ourselves on having resolved in theory.

And so, in considering the idea that medical ethics should have something to say about medical practice, I return to Daniel Callahan's quotation from a recent essay entitled "Does Clinical Ethics Distort the Discipline?" Dan wrote: "In the early 1970s, in one of my first articles on bioethics, I wrote that the principal aim of the field should be to help the medical practitioner deal with concrete cases. While I would hardly want to overlook the needs of the practitioner, I now wonder if that is the right place to center our attention. . . . Does reality lie in the particularity of individual cases where most clinicians think it does—or in a more general, abstract and universal realm, no less real but just more hidden?" For an answer to his question, Callahan then turned to three respondents. All were ethicists, but there was nary a clinician, let alone a physician, among them (Callahan 1996).

What Is Clinical Ethics?

I think Callahan has it wrong, at least with respect to what clinical ethics is. Clinical ethics is more than individual cases, more than ethics consultation, more (and here I must offer apologies to my coauthor, Al Jonsen, and my old friend, Stephen Toulmin) than applied medical casuistry. To be sure, each of these—individual cases, consultations, and casuistic reasoning—are part of clinical ethics, but the field is larger than any one of these three and larger than all three together. In clinical ethics the case or its proper resolution is a mere example, a specification, of what the goal of clinical ethics is: to improve clinical care and medical outcomes generally.

Let me offer my view of what clinical ethics is, a view based on thirty years of practicing medicine and twenty-five years of reading and writing about clinical ethics. I will suggest four ways in which it differs fundamentally from traditional medical ethics or bioethics. In this short chapter, I can only sketch my argument.

Clinical Ethics Is a Subdiscipline of Medicine, Not of Legal, Theological, or Philosophical Ethics.

I begin with the assumption that good patient care requires that technical and scientific considerations be integrated with personal and ethical considerations. Ethical concerns have always been an essential part of medical practice—from Hippocrates to Gregory to Thomas Percival to Richard Cabot to Frances Peabody to the present. The past fifty years have witnessed extraordinary scientific achievements. These achievements are unparalleled in history. They include blood transfusions, antibiotics, new immunizations, open heart surgery, dialysis machines, transplantation, critical care units, protease inhibitors, and new reproductive technologies, to name just a few. And there are newer ones on the horizon. These achievements have increased the range, intensity, and frequency of ethical issues in medicine and have contributed to the emergence of clinical ethics as an important subdiscipline of *medicine*— not a subdiscipline of philosophical ethics or theological ethics or legal ethics.

The Teaching of Clinical Ethics

If clinical ethics is a subdiscipline of medicine, not of legal, philosophical, or theological ethics, then the teaching of clinical ethics, like any other subject in medical school, can only be justified by its contribution to the care of the sick. Therefore, the main goal of teaching clinical ethics, as with teaching anatomy, is not to produce junior ethicists or junior anatomists, but rather to improve the quality of patient care in terms of both the process and the outcome of that care (Pellegrino, Siegler, and Singer 1990).

These days, we teach clinical ethics because medical students and residents simply must know something about these subjects to practice competent, high-quality medicine. The modern standard of care requires a practical working knowledge about ethical subjects such as informed consent, truth-telling, confidentiality, end-of-life decisions (including DNR, advanced directives, and choices for palliative care), proxy or surrogate decision making for patients who are decisionally incapacitated, and physicians' ethical responsibilities within healthcare organizations, including managed care. All of these are ethics topics. Physicians cannot practice good medicine without some working knowledge of these issues. Patients and society expect physicians to have both technical proficiency and the practical ability to recognize and respond to ethical issues such as these.

The Philosophical Foundation of Clinical Ethics: The Doctor-Patient Relationship

In the vast majority of clinical encounters—in my clinical experience, certainly above 95 percent—the patient and physician are allies not adversaries. The reason for this remarkable level of agreement is not hard to discover: the goals of the patient, who seeks help, and of the physician, who offers help, coincide. The patient who is in pain with a fractured arm wants relief immediately. When the fractured arm mends, the patient wants an arm that functions as well as it did before the accident. The patient with two weeks of hacking cough and three days of blood-flecked sputum wants to know whether what he has is a bad viral bronchitis that will go away, or a pneumonia or tuberculosis that will benefit from treatment, or—and this may really be what patients want most to know—that he doesn't have cancer. The physician too wants to determine what is wrong with the patient in order to propose a reasonable approach that will help the patient. The physician-patient relationship—a generally cooperative and nonadversarial one—is at the heart of medicine and at the heart of clinical ethics.

Clinical ethics should not only focus on the quality of the decision for a particular patient. True, reaching a right and good decision has pretty much been the central concern of medical ethics for the past thirty years, and of the casuistical school of clinical ethics in particular. But clinical ethics is more than ethical casuistry. It must also focus on the ethos of the professional, and on the character and virtues of the physician, who is expected by the public to demonstrate integrity, loyalty, compassion, competency, thoroughness, and commitment. In teaching medical ethics, we must therefore not only teach our students cognitive information about ethics and develop their behavioral skills, but we must also remember to attend to their character development. Toward this end, the philosophical premises of clinical ethics must take account not only of Kant and Mill, but also of Aristotle's notions of practical knowledge and of the virtues (Siegler and Singer 1990).

In a still more fundamental way, the philosophical foundation of clinical ethics bears little resemblance to the philosophical and legal foundations of traditional medical ethics. The foundation of clinical ethics is the doctor-patient encounter, an encounter that meets universal and unchanging human needs and whose central goal has not changed very much from the time of Hippocrates. This goal is to meet the health needs of human beings who ask for help by using scientific and personal skills in an effective and efficient way.

What is needed in the future is a vigorous return to the traditions of medicine and a rebuilding of the vitality of the doctor-patient relationship. Clinical ethics aims to improve patient outcomes by supporting and defending a patient-centered focus in medical practice that encourages a process of nonadversarial, shared decision making between patients and physicians in the context of a patient-physician relationship and within the restrictions imposed by legitimate third-party interests. This voluntary, negotiated, nonadversarial process of shared decision making, which I have been proposing since 1975 (Siegler 1981), was strongly endorsed in 1983 by the President's Commission for the Study of Ethical Problems in Medicine (President's Commission 1983). In fact, one of the central goals of clinical ethics is to reestablish the alliance between patients and physicians that traditional medical ethics may have helped to weaken. Traditional medical ethics has artificially driven a wedge between patients and physicians by stressing the false dichotomy of autonomy and paternalism and by distorting the doctor-patient relationship by casting it as an adversarial one.

Research in Clinical Ethics

The research base of clinical ethics is very different from the legal-philosophical research of traditional medical ethics. Some of the research is descriptive: it shows us what current practices are and how the participants in such practices explain their intentions, motivations, and actions. This line of research helps clarify the ethos of professionals and the preferences and values of patients regarding a wide range of ethical issues in medicine. This is the line of research now being done by some of the brightest young ethicists, many trained in the discipline of clinical epidemiology. Excellent research in this area includes, to name just a few examples, Linda and Ezekiel Emanuel's work on end-of-life issues and advanced directives (Emanuel and Emanuel 1993); Joanne Lynn's work on good care for the dying (Scheel and Lynn 1988); Steve Miles's studies on justice and health care (Miles, Singer, and Siegler 1989); Bernard Lo's work on AIDS and end-of-life decisions (Lo 1995); Troy Brennan's studies on medical mistakes and malpractice (Brennan, Sox, and Burstin 1996); Susan Tolle's work on assisted suicide and end-of-life care (Buchan and Tolle 1995); Robert Pearlman's work on quality of life and patient decisions (Uhlmann and Pearlman 1991); John Lantos and Bill Meadow's studies on parental choice in neonatal intensive care units (Lantos, Mokalla, and Meadow 1997); Ellen Fox and James Tulsky's work on ethics consultations (Tulsky and Fox 1996); Chris Daugherty's work on patient attitudes and motivations to participate in cancer research (Daugherty et al. 1995); and Abigail Zuger's remarkable reports on caring for patients with AIDS (Zuger 1995). These are the promising next generation of clinical ethicists who are likely to establish the field as a vital medical discipline.

Another line of research is health services research, which increasingly focuses on ethical concerns. Some of the most important clinical ethics research of the past fifteen years has been performed by nonethicists who have explored aspects of the doctor-patient relationship, including communication, patient empowerment, and shared decision making. We have learned from health researchers such as Feinstein, Tarlov, Ware, Greenfield, and Kaplan (Kaplan, Greenfield, and Ware 1989) and Wennberg (1996) that patients who have good doctor-patient relationships and who interact actively with physicians to reach a shared healthcare decision have greater trust in their doctors and greater loyalty to the doctor-patient relationship. They cooperate more fully in implementing the shared decision. They tend to make financially conservative decisions, and they express greatest satisfaction with their health care. Most important, they enjoy better outcomes—at least for four chronic conditions: hypertension, diabetes, peptic ulcer disease, and rheumatoid arthritis.

My colleague Wendy Levinson (who recently joined us at Chicago as the Chief of General Medicine) and Deborah Roter from Johns Hopkins published empirical data showing that by practicing a few simple communication techniques in the doctor-patient relationship, one could improve patient satisfaction, improve patient involvement in care, decrease malpractice claims, and most important, improve patient outcomes (Levinson and Roter 1997). These communication techniques included such simple and ethically praiseworthy actions as alerting the patient about what to expect from the clinical encounter and checking with patients later to make sure they understood the doctor's instructions.

Recently, Dr. Jack Wennberg, in a statement that I think may indicate the future direction for research in the field of clinical ethics, said that "it is the job of the evaluative sciences to conduct technology assessment and outcomes research to estimate the probability for outcomes that matter to patients and to elucidate the importance of patient preferences in choosing treatment" (Wennberg 1996).

Conclusion

The future of medical ethics—that is, the ethics of medical practice—is up for grabs. During the past thirty years, we have seen little evidence that traditional medical ethics has improved the practice of medicine or the care of patients. There has been too much talking, philosophizing, legalizing, and reforming. The time is right for us to adopt a very different approach—the approach of clinical medical ethics—to see if this specialty, more closely aligned with medicine than ethics, can integrate some valuable insights of philosophical and legal ethics into clinical medicine.

First, it will be necessary to conduct the kind of empirical research that physicians require before they change their ethos—their habits, dispositions, and characters. That is the kind of research that ethicists should have been doing for the past thirty years and that a young generation of clinical ethicists is now beginning to do. Ironically, in pursuing these lines of investigation, contemporary clinical ethicists will increasingly draw upon the insights that traditional bioethics have contributed to the study of medicine over the last thirty years.

References

Brennan, T. A.; Sox, C. M.; and Burstin, H. R. 1996. Relation Between Negligent Adverse Events and the Outcomes of Medical-Malpractice Litigation. *New England Journal of Medicine* 335(26):1963–67.

Buchan, M. L., and Tolle, S. W. 1995. Pain Relief for Dying Persons: Dealing with Physicians' Fears and Concerns. *Journal of Clinical Ethics.* 6(1):53–61.

Callahan, D. 1996. Does Clinical Ethics Distort the Discipline? *Hastings Center Report* 26:28–29.

Daugherty, C.; Ratain, M. J.; Grochowski, E.; Stocking, C.; Kodish, E.; Mick, R.; and Siegler, M. 1995. Perceptions of Cancer Patients and Their Physicians Involved in Phase I Trials. *Journal of Clinical Oncology* 13(5):1062–72.

Eddy, D. M. 1996. *Clinical Decision Making.* Boston: Jones and Bartlett Publishers.

Emanuel, L. L., and Emanuel, E. J. 1993. Decisions at the End of Life: Guided by Communities of Patients. *Hastings Center Report* 23(5):6–14.

Kaplan, S. H.; Greenfield, S.; and Ware, J. 1989. Assessing the Effects of Physician-Patient Interactions on the Outcomes of Chronic Disease. *Medical Care* 27 (3 Suppl):S110–27.

Kass, L. R. 1990. Practicing Ethics: Where's the Action? *Hastings Center Report* 20(1):5–12.

Lantos, J.; Mokalla, M.; and Meadow, W. 1997. Resource Allocation in Neonatal and Medical ICUs: Epidemiology and Rationing at the Extremes of Life. *American Journal of Respiratory Critical Care Medicine.* 7:185–89.

Levinson, W., and Roter, D. 1997. Patient Communication: The Relationship with Malpractice Claims Among Primary Care Physicians and Surgeons. *Journal of the American Medical Association* 227(7):553–59.

Lo, B. 1995. Improving Care Near the End of Life: Why Is It So Hard? *Journal of the American Medical Association* 274:1634–46.

Miles, S. H.; Singer, P. A.; and Siegler, M. 1989. Conflicts Between Patients' Wishes to Forego Treatment and the Policies of Health Care Facilities. *New England Journal of Medicine* 321(1):48–50.

Pellegrino, E. D.; Siegler, M.; and Singer, P. A. 1990. Teaching Clinical Ethics. *Journal of Clinical Ethics* 1:195–98.

President's Commission for the Study of Ethical Problems in Medicine and Biomedical and Behavioral Research. 1983. Making Treatment Decisions. In *Deciding to Forego Life-Sustaining Treatment*, 13–118. Washington, D.C.: U.S. Government Printing Office.

Scheel, B. J., and Lynn, J. 1988. Care of Dying Patients. *Clinics in Geriatric Medicine.* 4(3):639–54.

Siegler, M. 1978. A Legacy of Osler: Teaching Clinical Ethics at the Bedside. *Journal of the American Medical Association* 239:951–56.

——. 1981. Searching for Moral Certainty in Medicine: A Proposal for a New Model of the Doctor-Patient Relationship. *Bulletin of the New York Academy of Medicine.* 57:56–69.

Siegler, M.; Pellegrino, E. D.; and Singer, P. A. 1990. Clinical Medical Ethics: The First Decade. *Journal of Clinical Ethics* 1:5–9.

Study to Understand Prognoses and Preferences for Outcomes and Risk Treatment (SUPPORT) Principle Investigators. 1995. A Controlled Trial to Improve Care for Seriously Ill Hospitalized Patients. *Journal of the American Medical Association* 274:1591–95.

Tulsky, J. A., and Fox, E. 1996. Evaluation Research and the Future of Ethics Consultation. *Journal of Clinical Ethics* 7:146–49.

Uhlmann, R. F., and Pearlman, R. A. 1991. Perceived Quality of Life and Preferences for Life-Sustaining Treatments in Older Adults. *Archives of Internal Medicine* 151(3):495–97.

Wennberg, J. 1996. Social and Economic Issues in Medicine. In *Cecil Textbook of Medicine*, 20th ed., ed. F. Plum and J. C. Bennet. Philadelphia: TOREW. B. Saunders Co.

Zuger, A. 1995. *Strong Shadows: Scenes from an Inner City AIDS Clinic.* New York: W. H. Freeman and Co.

11

Professionalism and Professional Ethics

ALEXANDER MORGAN CAPRON, J.D.

The question, "Should physicians determine the scope and nature of medical ethics?" provokes at the least two divergent responses. At one pole, Mark Siegler, who, as the director of the leading center for clinical medical ethics, has probably trained more physician-ethicists and spawned more doctor-run ethics centers than anyone else in the country, replies with a resounding yes. Not only is the physician's place at the center of medical ethics, he argues, but also ethics is the essential thread that holds the profession together, the obligatory commandments set by and for physicians that make medicine a profession. At the opposite pole one finds Bob Veatch, without doubt our most severe and persistent critic of medical paternalism. Since the early 1970s he has championed patients' rights to control their own care, while hacking away at the notion that physicians' technical expertise gives them any special claim to decide about matters bioethical. Rather than relying on their own particular religious, ideological, or economic views, physicians should look to the best philosophical thinking that has some claim of acceptance in general society.

The Law and Its Limits

Where does this chapter fit into this symmetrical picture? If Physician Siegler proposes leaving physicians in charge of medical ethics and Philosopher Veatch argues that philosophers understand ethics better than doctors, am I as a lawyer perhaps expected to claim, as one leading commentator has, that U.S. law, rather than medicine or philosophy, has been the dominant force in shaping the field (Annas 1993)? If so, I will disappoint, since I believe it is unrealistic and unwise to expect that the law should establish medicine's ethical code.

This is not to deny that the law has been a very important player in the process. Landmark court cases have had a major role in shaping the field's development in the past quarter century, and on a more routine level, the law's inductive methodology has provided a heavy counterweight to the "principlist" approach to medical ethics. Furthermore, the law's emphasis on correct procedures and its orientation toward rights have played a significant part in forming ethical discourse (Capron 1995). Of course, that influence may not always have been entirely helpful, as when the focus on procedures obscures the need to attend more carefully to substantive rules (is delegation of decision making to institutional ethics committees a good idea, unless we are confident of the standards they will employ?) or when, as feminist legal scholars have noted, the exaltation of rights downgrades the need to think in terms of relations (are rights defensible, and do they reflect our true feelings, if they are free of responsibilities to others?) (Glendon 1991). Thus, while the law certainly has a proper role in establishing normative behavior in medicine—because it draws lines whereby society establishes what is beyond bounds, aimed mostly at preventing conduct that is clearly harmful to others—I do not think that we can, or should, claim primacy for the law in answering the query, "Who should control the scope and nature of medical ethics?"

Why not? For both ontologic and instrumental reasons. I will turn to the latter in this chapter's concluding pages; however, to summarize, for the moment, I fear that assigning greater authority to the law will mean a diminution of physicians' professional commitment, a sense that the dictates of "medical ethics" are as foreign, and as resented, as those of medical law. Especially in the current era, when the present arrangement of health care leaves patients largely dependent on physicians for protection from economic forces aimed at reducing healthcare spending, things that undermine physicians' allegiance to the traditional professional obligations are likely to be harmful to patients. We should hardly want to give physicians the message that they can leave the exercise of ethical judgment to lawyers or others (Hyman 1990).

As to the former, constitutive limitations on law in this context, one can simply note that the law is a blunt instrument, not a surgeon's scalpel. Its dictates are of necessity broad and general, leaving many details to be filled in. (The same may be true to a lesser degree of much of "medical ethics," which at least is focused on the behavior of physicians and related matters.) Moreover, in liberal societies the law tends more to proscribe the forbidden than to command the good. Furthermore, when the law leaves citizens with a right to do something, that does not mean it is right to do that thing. This is where we must rely on other sources of rightness and other mechanisms, manifestations of what is sometimes referred to as the "private ordering" of life's affairs, which rest in turn on norms drawn from sources other than the law.

Private Ordering

There are many ways that rules are set, behavior is channeled, and societal sanctions are applied without direct legislation or governmental regulation. In traditional societies, norms were set and enforced by families, tribes, and communities outside any judicial context. Organized religion typically played a major role in those settings, as it does also in modern societies where institutions both commercial and nonprofit (such as schools and hospitals) also inculcate norms appropriate for the conduct within their own arenas, some based on general societal views and some on values and norms specific to the setting.

Another major form of private ordering is through the process by which contracts are set and private parties agree upon the rules that will govern their dealings. In the process, they in effect establish what is right and wrong in their relationships, even to the point that society will enforce those rules, with consequences not only for the immediate parties but for others as well. Some of the rules and expectations developed in this fashion may incorporate the general conventions within the field (so-called trade practices). But such rules may be far from general and can indeed be crafted individually or by agreements reached by a relatively small subgroup.

Is this enough for medicine? No, the rules that guide behavior in this field cannot be drawn solely from private ordering, enforced in turn by the law. And society has recognized as much: medical norms cannot be hammered out in the marketplace, in arms-length transactions among physicians, or between physicians and patients.

Expectations of Fiduciaries

The law, instead, regards the relationship of physicians to their patients as being comparable to that of other fiduciaries to the wards or beneficiaries for whom they are responsible. Fiduciaries must refrain from endangering the well-being of beneficiaries, and they may not engage in self-dealing vis-à-vis beneficiaries. When potential conflicts arise, fiduciaries are required to make full disclosure of the conflict.

But does that exhaust society's interest in the matter? Is the rest simply a matter of private ordering? And if so, is that ordering entirely individual case by case? Or does society expect at the very least a set of collectively formulated norms enforced by the group? Yes, more than private ordering is plainly needed, and certainly more than individually, contractually arranged rules.

Licensure and Professional Standards

Another possible source of medical ethics in the law might be thought to reside in the system of professional licensure. In licensing physicians (among many other professionals), the state is responding to the reality that physicians can wield great powers that could be especially dangerous in unskilled hands. Licensure also manifests the societal view that medicine fulfills the traditional norm of a profession—that is to say, it possesses the capability of establishing collective standards of skill and good behavior, of training and inculcating its members in those standards, and of implementing those standards within the professional group. Society recognizes this authority within the professions and also sometimes legally enforces the standards, such as by suspension or revocation of a professional license for a violation of the standards.

But that does not make the formulation of medical ethics a legal function, for legal institutions play a relatively minor role in setting the standards themselves. What then is the source of the standards? This volume celebrates the 150th anniversary of what most American physicians would probably regard as a sufficient answer to that question—that is, a physician-crafted code of medical ethics. Still, that code today cannot be understood as simply the basic seven principles of the AMA's Code of Ethics. Nor is it a brief description of the expectations of virtuous gentlemen, grounded on the underlying self-denying ordinance never to do anything with the purpose of benefiting oneself rather than one's patient.

Rather, it now extends through the opinions of the Council on Ethical and Judicial Affairs into the myriad of issues facing modern health care. The very existence of these issues, with their far-reaching reverberations, is one force that thirty years ago began the process of dethroning physicians as the sole sovereign in medical ethics. Or, if one prefers to say that they continue to control "medical ethics," then one would have to say that the ethics of the 1847 Code, or even its 1980 successor, became marginalized as the sole determinant of the full range of questions facing the field, which became instead the province of what is now referred to as bioethics.

Medical Ethics in Modern Dress

If medical ethics was the guidance relied upon by the conscientious physician in relationship to his or her patients, it was simply too narrow a basis for deciding about issues like the allocation of scarce dialysis machines or of organs for transplantation, the definition of death, the rules for research with human subjects, or the uses of new genetic and reproductive technologies. Moreover, the patients' rights movement beginning in the 1970s—part of the rights upsurge than started in the 1950s with the modern Civil Rights movement and extended to women's rights, gay rights, consumer rights, and so forth—added a political, power-focused challenge to the normative questions philosophers, lawyers, and social scientists had been raising about physicians' traditional dominance of the process of setting medical ethics standards.

The Self-Interest Inherent in the Traditional Disinterest

The central goal of those traditional standards was to ensure each professional's fidelity to the interests and welfare of his or her patients or clients. This injunction can be seen simply as an instance of self-denial, of adoption of a stance of disinterest in one's own welfare, or it can be seen to have an interpretation that would justify it to physicians' individual and collective self-interest. The self-interested justification for the medical profession's collective demand that individual professionals practice such self-denial in order to be allowed into the profession is that without the assurance of self-denial, the public would not leave self-governance to the profession, nor would patients entrust to individual professionals the enormous power they allow physicians to wield over their lives.

Yet for medicine, the promise of disinterest was linked with an assumption of superior knowledge on the part of the professional to act—in the language of the Hippocratic Oath—"[i]n my patient's interest as I see it." Furthermore, by the final third of this century, this ancient view was abetted by the changes in the financing of health care that increasingly insulated patients from financial responsibility for the choices made by physicians and hence further removed them from controlling how those decisions were made.

When a profession presumes to know the interests and welfare of its clients better than do the clients themselves, the result is a paternalism that not only denies the individuality of the client (and his and her right to make decisions) but also risks confusing the professionals' interests with the clients' wishes.

Reaction against this phenomenon in American medicine in the 1960s and 1970s, combined with the onslaught of new biomedical technologies that raised problems going beyond the individual physician-patient relationship, helped to create the bioethics movement. The ascendancy of the patient replaced the hegemony of the physician.

Can Ethics Be Left to Physicians?

The emergence of bioethics was, in my view, a good thing. It was right to insist that the difficult issues raised by health care and research are not solely matters for the consideration of the individual "ethical physician" but of necessity involve others, particularly the patients and subjects who are directly affected, but also society at large. Ironically, the idea that ethical issues cannot be left solely to physicians has become so firmly established over the last twenty-five years that the leading all-physician body that deals with medical ethics, namely, the AMA's Council on Ethical and Judicial Affairs (CEJA), has taken a back seat in establishing ethical norms on many important issues of medical practice.

Having said that, I should emphasize that it was critically important in the dissemination and acceptance of the new consensus on many important issues in medical ethics (such as on the withdrawal of life-sustaining treatment from patients near death) that CEJA addressed the issues and endorsed the consensus viewpoint. But in virtually every instance, the profession's official voice on medical ethics followed, rather than lead, the process of changing the norms of appropriate medical response to these difficult topics. More dramatically, when CEJA has attempted to depart from the bioethics consensus, it has had to retreat—as it did in 1994 on the issue of establishing a special "definition" of anencephalic infants as dead for the purpose of organ donation (Capron 1994). Therefore, paralleling Clemenceau's sage observation about war and generals, my conclusion is that medical ethics is too important to be left to physicians.

Ethics, Patients, and Ethicists

Yet medical ethics is also too important to be left to patients. Just as a profession without a "clients first" code becomes merely a business, a profession that is totally at the service of its clients and that is without a clear internal set of norms (and hence, of accepted and expected actions under certain circumstances) becomes merely a trade. The rights of patients must be framed by the ethical norms of the medical profession, or physicians become mere technicians without a claim to any ethical grounding.

Where, then, should one look for this guidance? Should the profession turn matters over to the Hastings Center or the Kennedy Institute of Ethics? No, because medical ethics is also too important to be left to ethicists. The grounding that the medical profession needs must arise internally. It may emerge from outside analysis and be checked at its outer limits by society, but it cannot be crafted solely by those—namely, the bioethicists (from the law and social science as well as from philosophy)—who can provide the useful commentary and analysis on ethics that can provoke further thought and revision of the underlying standards.

An Interdisciplinary (and Postmodern) Medical Ethics

What we need today is a socially situated, interdisciplinary medical ethics that seeks to protect professional judgment, not as an end in itself, but as a means to the end of furthering the interest of the patient. Such an ethics would have several characteristics. First, it would be dialectic not dogmatic. Just as uncertainty is the central unifying reality of all efforts to apply the storehouse of science to the needs of individual patients, so too, the application of ethical principles will always yield gray areas where thoughtful people will have to engage respectfully with one another across disciplines and, in our increasingly multiethnic society, across cultures, to address the complexity in each case.

Second, in this process physicians' superior technical expertise does not logically justify lodging control over ethical issues in physicians alone. Let's take a current example: although it would take a physician to clone a human being, it is not for physicians alone to say whether anyone should undertake such cloning. The harms that could arise in human cloning are limited neither to ones about which physicians can claim special expertise (though some of the harms may fall in this category) nor to ones that would befall the physicians or patients directly involved (especially if a physician regarded "the patients" to be the persons requesting cloning, rather than also being the product of any successful cloning procedure).

This is not to say, of course, that it would be inappropriate for physicians, at least in the present state of knowledge, to refuse even to allow their skills and expertise to be used in attempting to clone a human being. It is reasonable to expect that biomedical scientists in embryology, endocrinology, obstetrics, and related fields (the ones who would be capable of undertaking the experiments that would lead to human cloning) would apply, as a value drawn from the general culture but then instantiated in medicine itself, such a respect for human life that they would be committed not to act when doing so endangers the well-being of the subjects of their research. Therefore, they would not, at this time, be willing to attempt to create a human baby through somatic cell nuclear transfer (the method used by Scottish researchers to create the world-famous Dolly, the first, and thus far only, clone of an adult mammal). That is because such an attempt is in the present state of knowledge simply too risky: Dolly was produced only after 277 attempts, and even when other embryos were successfully produced, in the few that resulted in pregnancies that went to term, the lambs had problems that caused them to be stillborn or to die shortly after birth. Applying the standards used in all branches of medical research, investigators simply do not move from a single experiment in an animal directly to the clinic, but instead perform extensive experiments in the laboratory, typically over many years both with several types of animals and with human cells.

Society has adopted this risk-reduction norm and enforces it through regulations on federally funded research with human subjects. Most research centers also apply it to research that is not federally regulated, but it is a norm that medicine expects of its practitioners as well, independent of governmental stricture. The point is that the reasons why human cloning may be an unacceptable use of biomedical knowledge include reasons that would lead physicians to refuse to participate in the attempt, but are not limited to such reasons. For society may prove to have objections that go beyond concerns about safety, as the National Bioethics Advisory Commission (1997, iii) suggested in recommending to the president that a moratorium be placed on any attempt to create a human being through somatic cell nuclear transfer.

Third, and probably most important, the core value in the traditional medical ethics—namely, that the interests of the patient are paramount—must still shape the content and the reality of the new ethics. Physicians are understandably concerned over the erosion of their professional authority. There is an opportunity here to use the new interdisciplinary form of ethics that I recommend, because patients would gladly see a collaborative effort, given mounting dissatisfaction today with the direction of health care—particularly with the exigencies of managed care.

A Central Dilemma

That to me is the good news for physicians. The bad news is that there are at least two problems with their exploiting that dissatisfaction. The first is that some of the dissatisfaction is simply not justified. Of course, patients—at least insured ones—have come to expect full access to any services they deem them-selves to want. But that has nothing to do with good medicine or good med-ical ethics. That is a medicine of Nordstrom's, not of Johns Hopkins. It is fine for the marketplace, where "the customer is always right," but not for the med-ical setting—especially not for a profession whose activities are not governed by the normal checks of the market. Ultimately, even the public recognizes that too many resources have been consumed in medicine to produce results that too often are of marginal value, and that some reallocation of resources to lo-cations where they will produce the greatest benefits is needed. But the pub-lic knows, correctly, that it must have a say about what those uses are, both societally and more individually through their health plans. Rationing is jus-tifiable only if it is rational and participatory, only if it reflects the values and views of those who are directly affected.

Furthermore, reallocation of resources is justified only if it is guided by a greatly increased knowledge of the science of medicine, by a knowledge of what works clinically and when it works. The public is justified in being skeptical at the moment, not only because so much of medicine has proceeded without be-ing firmly grounded in demonstrated effectiveness, but also because of the ways in which profits have been made in health care, in which the incentives have inclined heavily toward over-utilization, particularly of ancillary facili-ties in which some professionals have had (disclosed or undisclosed) interests.

Some of the present public dissatisfaction with the new, resource-limiting structures is something that physicians ought to be able to exploit, but even then a second problem arises in trying to use it. One can, of course, point to the proportion of health insurance premiums that is spent on health care in some for-profit plans, which is as low as in the 70th percentile, the rest going for overhead and profit. But the dilemma is that in the view of many patients, physicians are to blame for this. That is to say, it is the physician with whom the patient interacts. Thus, if managed care is the devil, then some people think physicians have made a deal with that devil in order to hold onto their own share of the "insured lives" that make up the new way of describing one's pa-tients today.

The Hard Road Ahead: Reclaiming
Ethical Credibility

Furthermore, why is managed care even accepted? Why is it seen by many peo-ple, particularly those who pay the bills, as being necessary—albeit distaste-ful or disturbing? Many people believe managed care is necessary, or has been brought on, because of the excessive and uncontrolled growth in healthcare spending over several decades, growth that made the healthcare industry very profitable for all concerned without providing a comparable level of demonstrated benefit at the margin. This conclusion is linked with the suspicion that a good deal of this excessive spending has been driven by medical hubris and greed.

Of course, analysts can point out that physicians' income constitutes only a small part of our total spending on health care. But physicians control the overwhelming majority of the decisions that are made. Furthermore, the huge relative increase of physicians' incomes since 1965 (which curved ever upward, to be checked for the first time for many specialties in the mid-90s) suggests that the public's skepticism on this score has some justification. Thus, to regain authority, physicians must demonstrate that their authority will be exercised *on behalf of patients*, something that can no longer be taken for granted.

Some of this will involve addressing physicians' business activities much more candidly and forcefully. For example, the waffling that has occurred on the conflict of interest inherent in the ownership of healthcare facilities by referring physicians is not adequately resolved by CEJA opinion 8.032, as Arnold Relman (1992) has noted. It seems to me that physicians will need to forswear some profit if they want to reclaim the role of prophet or at least of advocate.

Physicians, individually and collectively, have received deserved credit and praise as advocates for patients regarding a number of important issues, like tobacco and violence. And they should also do the same about the greatest ethical issue facing our country: the lack of health coverage for one-fifth or so of our population. (It would certainly have been ironic if the Supreme Court had ruled that assisted suicide and euthanasia were constitutionally guaranteed rights: we would then have been the only country in the world to guarantee the right to die, but not the right to health care.)

Furthermore, the return to medicine's traditional fidelity to the patient must be informed by an understanding from the new, interdisciplinary-based ethics. This new ethics will draw from the insights of many fields to ensure that physicians are true to the patient as a person and not simply as an illness or as an opportunity for the application of technology. In this regard, I cannot help but note with some disappointment (not the least because I can see that it was very expensive to produce) that the cover photograph chosen by the AMA for its volume celebrating one hundred fifty years of medical ethics shows a young patient in the bed surrounded by physicians and nurses, yet at least three of these people in the room are not looking at the patient but at the machine to the right of the patient. This image is ironic for a book dedicated to medical ethics, because as important as technology may have been in contributing to medical results in recent years, it is looking away from the patient that has cost the medical profession some of the respect it has lost.

Plainly, society faces many value-laden questions beyond the allocation of healthcare resources, questions about acceptable uses of genetic and reproductive technologies, about how to obtain and distribute organs for transplantation, about the involvement of normal volunteers and of patients in research protocols, to name but a few. All of them will require a multidisciplinary reexamination of the goals of medicine. These are the questions that physicians involved in these respective activities face, so even if they are denominated questions of "bioethics," they are among the most important aspects of "medical ethics" for these physicians.

Beyond these particular challenges, the most obvious threat to medicine today is the risk that a profession guided by ethics will be replaced by a business guided by competition, with all of the implications of "devil take the hindmost" that go with that. The acquiescence of physicians to the demands both of payers and of patients animates such a movement. But the real threat is that medicine will either attempt to return to a physician-generated form of medical ethics or give up the fight and cede ethics to ethicists, when what is needed is the harder task of recognizing the indeterminacy of the whole field and joining with all who have a stake in the outcome—other professionals in health care, patients and their advocates, and representatives of society—to fashion a fluid and evolving ethics that is self-analytic but not self-contained.

This new medical ethics cannot be fashioned by physicians drawing on the most recondite philosophy, or by philosophers carefully scrutinizing medicine. Nor can it be carved into stone by legislators or regulators acting in the name of society. It must grow, instead, from a process in which no one party asserts control but also in which the medical profession plays an essential role. Only if the profession is willing and able to deal directly with the issues at the heart of modern health care—issues of access to care for all and of the goals that should define how resources are to be used to achieve legitimate ends— will the profession and its organs dedicated to "medical ethics" be able to participate in the creation of the new medical ethics. Certainly, this is a more noble—and for the survival of the profession, a more essential—role than simply refining its code by making filigrees around the border of the field.

References

Annas, George. 1993. *Standard of Care: The Law of American Bioethics*. New York: Oxford University Press.

Capron, Alexander Morgan. 1994. Ethics: Public and Private. *Hastings Center Report* 24(6):26–27.

———. 1995. Law and Bioethics. In *Encyclopedia of Bioethics*, 1329–35. New York: Simon & Schuster Macmillan.

Glendon, Mary Ann. 1991. *Rights Talk: The Impoverishment of Political Discourse.* New York: Free Press.

Hyman, D. A. 1990. How Law Killed Ethics. *Perspective in Biology and Medicine.* 34:134–51.

National Bioethics Advisory Commission. 1997. *Cloning Human Beings: Vol. 1, Report and Recommendations.* Rockville, Md.: National Bioethics Advisory Commission.

Relman, Arnold. 1992. Self-Referral: What's at Stake? *New England Journal of Medicine* 327(21):1522–24.

12

Who Needs Physicians'
Professional Ethics?

STEPHEN R. LATHAM, J.D., PH.D.
LINDA L. EMANUEL, M.D., PH.D.

Who needs physicians' professional ethics? Our response is that everyone does. Both question and answer require explication. We approach our claim in two steps. First, we offer an argument about what makes any ethic—including that articulated in the AMA's code—a distinctly *professional* ethic. We then set out a number of arguments by which we hope to show that professionals, patients, and society at large must all have recourse to specifically professional medical ethics as we have defined them.

What Makes Professional Medical Ethics "Professional?"

The assumption that there is any such thing as a distinctly "professional" medical ethic is not universal. In this very volume, for example, Robert Veatch argues that there is and should be no such thing as a professional medical ethic (chap. 9). Veatch rejects both what he terms the "ontological claim" that physicians are somehow licensed and able to invent the moral rules to which they are subject, and the "epistemological claim" that only physicians can understand enough about their work to discern the content of the moral rules that should govern it. These two claims, he believes, are the only plausible bases for a belief in a distinctly professional medical ethic. Finding them not very plausible, he rejects the claim that there can be a professional ethic; and this leads him to reject as misguided and dangerous all claims that physicians ought to control the scope and content of medical ethics.

We follow Veatch in denying both the ontological and the epistemological claims. With regard to the ontological claim, we agree that medical professionals may not and must not invent ethical values out of whole cloth. Medicine is and always has been a practice set within its social context, and the ethics of medicine have always been consistent, for the most part, with the ethics of society at large. Individual physicians live in society as the parents and children, the friends and siblings, the colleagues, servants, and employers of non-physicians; physicians as a group are recognized as one social body among others. The ethical standards of the medical profession are inevitably related to, and generally well integrated with, the common values of the people with whom physicians share their social world.

This is not to say that the ethics governing particular professions such as medicine will be the same as the ethics that govern persons in society generally. Professionals are engaged in particular occupations—occupations that place them in circumstances that others never face. This means that, at some level of particularity, they will be subject to moral rules that do not apply to others. Thus, to take a simple-minded case, a surgeon may open your chest and cut and sew vessels in your heart, but a school librarian may not—even in an emergency, even if you give him or her your permission. An attorney may conceal a confidence that a friend or even a stranger would be obliged to reveal. The fact that there are role-specific moral rules does not, however, imply that the persons playing the various roles are privileged to draft those rules—still less that they may draft them without consideration of broader social ethics (but cf. Arthur Applbaum's argument in chap. 8 of this volume). It means, rather, that people in different jobs have to do different things, and sometimes morally different things. This reality is generally accepted by society as a whole—though the acceptance is sometimes uneasy, and the extent of the divergence of occupational morality from common social morality is subject to constant renegotiation (Williams 1995).

As to our rejection of the epistemological claim: It is true that physicians' extensive training and clinical experience gives them a unique understanding of the technical content of their work. It is also true that physicians' repeated encounters with lived ethical dilemmas in clinical practice give them an invaluable and unique perspective upon, and appreciation for, the ethical dimensions of their work and may develop their powers of moral judgment. It does not follow from these truths, however, that only physicians can discern the formal content of the moral rules governing that work. (There are *some* things—not rules—that only physicians can discern, and that we shall mention briefly later.)

First, physicians' training and expertise cannot license them to determine, on their own, the moral rules that ought to govern in particular cases. As long as clinical encounters include patients, physicians' own experiences, as rich and extensive as they may be, cannot hope to supply the sole grounding for the ethical management of a particular clinical encounter. Patients, their relatives, and their friends in the community have essential and unique perspectives to bring to bear upon lived clinical ethics problems. Appreciation for this is reflected in the growing acceptance that ethics committees should include lay representatives and should provide processes pursuant to which patients' and others' views can be aired. Second, while the rich clinical and ethical experience of practicing physicians may shape their characters and hone their moral judgment, this alone does not make a physician able to articulate general ethical rules governing medical practice. Judgment, after all, involves determining the proper fit of general norms to particular circumstances, not the drafting of general norms. It is partly for this reason that the prescriptions and proscriptions of the AMA's Code of Ethics are written in a nontechnical language understandable by any literate layperson. Neither the special clinical expertise nor the ethical experience of the code's physician-authors needs to reveal itself explicitly in the code's pages. Nonphysicians understand the need for their physicians to be competent, honest, free from conflicting interest, capable of keeping a confidence, and so on; and at that level of generality, nonphysicians understand this need in the very same terms as physicians themselves understand it. At the level of articulation of the general rules governing medical practice, physicians' moral perceptions about medicine are not so different from nonphysicians' perceptions. Given that medicine is, as we have noted, a social practice, this should be no surprise.

In sum: Physicians are not empowered to invent, on their own, the moral law of their profession. Their specialized education and experience affords physicians a unique perspective upon, and appreciation for, the ethical elements of their practice, but it does not privilege them to compose, in a vacuum, the ethical rules that govern their own practices.

Having rejected both the claims that Veatch believes could ground a professional medical ethic, we nonetheless affirm the importance, even the necessity, of such an ethic. It is possible for us to affirm this because our conception of what makes an ethic *professional* does not turn, as Veatch's seems to, on professionals' alleged authorship of, or privileged access to, the ethical standards governing their occupation. On our view, an ethics is professional in virtue of the public commitment of professionals to the content of that ethic as the moral standard governing their occupation. The cleric is not a cleric in virtue of his having written "the Word," but in virtue of his vow to obey it life-long. Similarly, medical professionals are not professionals in virtue of any real or alleged power to author their own ethics, but in virtue of their pro-fession (their speaking-forth, their public avowal) of their willingness always to subject themselves to the authority of those ethics. The professional element of professional ethics is thus a matter of obedience rather than of moral authorship or authority.

This claim is consistent with the old sociological commonplace that professions can be distinguished from other occupations in part by the fact that they adopt their own codes of occupational ethics (Greenwood 1957; MacIver 1955). Many occupations recognized as professions, and many of those wishing to be so recognized, have written and published codes of ethics. Historians and sociologists alike have argued that part of the purpose in publishing such codes has been to establish the moral legitimacy of an occupational group in the eyes of the public and to distinguish the promulgators of the code from those who practice deceptively similar occupations. Codes of ethics, including the AMA's, have always been conceived of as public documents. They have been published in the full expectation that the public would immediately recognize and acknowledge them as articulating the proper standards of moral conduct for members of the profession in question (Freidson 1994, 174; and see Baker, this volume).

There could, of course, be no expectation of such immediate recognition— and ethical codes could lend occupational associations no public credibility— if the content of those codes were the idiosyncratic private constructs of professionals or if only trained professionals could understand them. The act of ethics codification and publication is thus the very opposite of an act of private moral invention in spirit and intent. There is no room for drafters of such public documents to make extravagant claims about their ability to invent moral standards independent of those of the broader community. Indeed, their act of codification constitutes a speaking-out to the broader community, not a gesture of moral independence from it.

If publication of a set of ethical standards is one mark of a profession, that is because it is one mode of pro-fession. A published code of ethics is a speaking-forth, a public promise by members of the occupation to the effect that they will live up to certain standards—standards that, significantly, society acknowledges as appropriate to the occupation.

Our account of professional ethics as public vows of obedience to socially acceptable standards also squares well with sociological accounts of the professions that stress professional autonomy. Professionals are often said to enjoy autonomy in determining the content of their work, an autonomy rooted in their privileged understanding of their highly specialized occupations. It may seem difficult, at first, to reconcile this fact with our claim that professionals have no privileged understanding of the moral rules that govern their work, but there is no real problem here. We need only distinguish between the ability to discern moral standards and the ability to assure compliance with them in particular cases. Physicians and other professionals are responsible for acting according to certain professional moral standards. As we have argued above, these standards are not of the professionals' invention; they are not, like a secret society's handshake, the private knowledge of the initiated.

Indeed, it is of the essence of these standards that they are generally accepted within the community as standards of practice for the profession in question. In the case of medicine, they include such general ideas as that physicians should be competent, that they should single-mindedly promote health, that they should act as fiduciaries to the sick, and so on.

The autonomy of the professions comes legitimately into play only when it is time to decide whether a given professional has complied with these profession-specific but also socially accepted moral standards. In many cases, only a professional can tell whether a fellow-professional has acted competently or has allowed conflicting interests to interfere with his single-minded pursuit of health or has failed in a fiduciary obligation. We thus affirm claims by sociologists that the professional has a privileged understanding of his or her specialized work, rooted in its complexity. This privileged understanding does not ground a right of professionals to invent the general moral standards to which they are subject, but it does place them in a privileged position with regard to judging themselves under those standards.

This said, it is not always true that "only a professional can judge a professional." Professionals, being human, are capable of committing numerous sins that are well within the powers of lay people to detect. The professional physician, for example, enjoys a privileged position with regard to judgment only in cases that involve the specialized content of the work: Was the procedure done competently? Was the explanation accurate? Was the more remunerative technique really the better one? Was the bad outcome the result of error or of bad luck? Nonphysicians cannot normally answer these questions for the simple reason that they do not have the specialized training to investigate them and for the more complicated reason that good medical outcomes do not dependably follow from good medical care, nor bad outcomes from bad care.

To summarize: we reject the claim that professionals have any unique ability to compose ethical standards for their work from whole cloth, and we accept the idea that professional ethics must be related to broader social ethics.

We reject the notion that professionals' training, experience, and expertise give them any special understanding of, or privileged access to, the moral rules that govern their work. We nonetheless assert that there is such a thing as a distinctly *professional* ethic. Such an ethic is professional in virtue, not of its having been composed by, or its being uniquely accessible to, professionals, but in virtue of its being professed by them. The act of pro-fession is a public commitment to obeying socially accepted moral standards governing one's work.

The publication of an occupational code of ethics can be an instance of such profession. The AMA's Code of Ethics is one example of physicians' professional ethics. But there are numerous others. These include, first of all, the professional codes of various specialty, state, and local societies. But they include also the host of journal articles that raise ethical questions explicitly and the angry letters to the editor that make implicit reference to a shared medical ethic; they include those inspirational speeches made at medical school graduations and clinic dedications, and the whispered assurances made to patients in wards or to friends in nursing homes; they include not only the hagiographic biographies of world-famous medical professors but also the everyday eulogies and obituaries that remark upon the decency and dedication of departed clinicians. Each of these is an act of profession—a public (re)affirmation of medical values (see Pellegrino and Thomasma 1981, 209–10, and Kass 1985, 211–23 for further accounts of such "acts of profession").

With this view of physicians' professional ethics in mind, we turn to our core question: Who needs this kind of public avowal from medical professionals, and why?

Who Needs Physicians' Professional Ethics?

Public avowals of fidelity are everywhere in our society, and indeed in most societies. People make public vows of fidelity to spouses in marriage ceremonies, to their constitutions and laws upon taking political office, to the aims of their professions upon being admitted to their practice, to their creeds on various religious occasions.

It is a common trait of every such public avowal that, while some instances of failure to live up to the vow can be detected, compliance with the vow can never be dependably verified. The avowed fidelity is essentially internal; it deals with intentions that cannot be externally monitored. Particular instances of violations of vows may go undetected. More important, some kinds of violation are undetectable even in principle. A politician may care not a whit for the Constitution but behave herself in office out of a Machiavellian desire to retain political power. A spouse may be unfaithful in her heart and may simply be awaiting an opportunity to act in violation of her former vow. Those without any vestige of religious faith may yet make their public observances.

But the fact that compliance with vows of fidelity is unverifiable does not make those vows useless. Indeed, it explains people's need for them. If a vow cannot be enforced, it can at least be acknowledged, repeated, and shared in hopes that the recitation of the outer word will inspire and support and nourish the inner fidelity. Public vows remind people of their shared past, allow them to celebrate their shared present, and constitute a promise of a shared future. If we conceive of physicians' professional ethics as consisting in a series of such public vows, it becomes clearer who needs them and for what reasons.

First, professionals themselves need their repeated acts of pro-fession. We do not now refer primarily to the need of professions to convince society of their pure motivation and high standards, though (as we noted above) that need has often been one motivation for one kind of professional act, the publication of an ethical code. We speak, instead, of professionals' internal need for acts of profession. It is widely accepted that repetition of our values and beliefs can help solidify them and bring our actions into conformity with them. It is for this reason that most faiths insist that worshippers engage in periodic repetition of prayers and creeds. To move from the sublime to the ridiculous, one may also think of the posters about commitment and values with which some business executives decorate their offices. Physicians need acts of profession because they serve to remind them of their core values; and this reminder may strengthen their resolve in times of moral trial.

Shared public recitation of moral sentiment also serves medical professionals by building their moral community. Such community building is not only socially pleasant for physicians but is also a condition of the possibility of any effective professional self-policing. A common complaint against professional associations (and against medical professional associations in particular) is that they are too "clubby" and that they do not adequately discipline their wayward members. We cannot dismiss this criticism. Nonetheless, we point out that the social solidarity constructed in part by acts of profession is a necessary vehicle for the regulation of medical practice quality. The very social solidarity that makes it difficult for professional groups to weed out those who go astray may prevent many others from straying. The kind of self-regulation that operates through identification with, and loyalty to, a community prevents breaches rather than punishing them, and is therefore unfortunately invisible. But its importance should not be underestimated. It would be best if physicians conformed their conduct to ethical precepts simply because such action was right in itself. But it is at least a valuable second-best if physicians conform their actions to ethical precepts out of concern for their reputation among their peers. Acts of profession may thus have direct and indirect efficacy: direct where they remind physicians of, and awaken or reawaken them to, their own ethical standards; and indirect where they serve to establish a community in which a reputation for conformity to shared ethical standards is valued.

This mention of effect upon physicians' conduct leads us directly to the category of persons whose need for professional ethics is normally most pronounced: patients. As was noted above, nonphysicians who do not share physicians' complex and lengthy training are not equipped to judge whether they are receiving quality care. They cannot reliably infer quality of care from satisfactory or unsatisfactory outcomes; moreover, they do not have the vocabulary or background with which to initiate an investigation into quality divorced from consideration of outcome. This means that patients cannot depend on markets or government regulators to weed out poor medical practices or practitioners. They must depend on physicians themselves to do that. They are, in other words, highly vulnerable as consumers of medical services.

And that is not all. There is a vulnerability deeper than the consumer's vulnerability in the context of market failure, a threat deeper than the threat of being sold poor services unawares. The complex knowledge of medical professionals is a double-edged sword: professional knowledge can be "guilty knowledge" (Hughes 1971). "Whoever is clever at guarding against disease is also cleverest at getting away with producing it," said Plato (1961, 333e); and this offhand pronouncement should remind us of the grave risk undertaken by anyone who gives his body to be acted upon by another. Professionals' use of their knowledge is not simply difficult to evaluate at the margin; it is deeply threatening at its core.

Physicians' professional ethics cannot make the market for health services work perfectly or remove the powerful air of vulnerability from every clinical encounter. Nonetheless, if we are correct about the personal and community-based forms of efficacy for acts of profession of medical ethics, then they can greatly reduce the problems. Physicians' acts of profession hold out the hope of (directly or indirectly) preventing most physicians, most of the time, from intentionally taking advantage of patients' vulnerability. Given that conflicts of interest can affect judgment and action at a level below the intentional, that hope is not everything. But it is a lot.

We have some evidence for the belief that physicians' repeated avowals of competence and of strict devotion to patients' interests have had some effect in reducing patients' sense of market and clinical vulnerability. In her contribution to this volume (chap. 5), Susan Lederer points out the ways in which the Hippocratic Oath (the recitation of which is another, and undoubtedly the best-known, act of medical pro-fession) has captured the popular imagination. The number of times we have seen angry patients invoke the Hippocratic Oath (without necessarily having an accurate notion of its contents) is itself a demonstration of the fact that patients take physicians' pro-fession seriously. It may even be fair to say that it is only physicians' history of professing ethics—their repeated collective vows to act competently, to avail themselves only of well-grounded medical practices, to avoid conflicts of interest, to police their fellows—that make bearable the uncertainties of the market for medical services, and the deeper and more fundamental uncertainties of the clinical encounter.

We have thus far attempted to show, first, that physicians need professional ethics in order to center themselves on the values of medicine and to create communities of persons devoted to those values; and second, that patients need physicians' professional ethics to the extent that acts of profession are efficacious in securing physicians' conformity with their ethics. But there is a third group that needs physicians' professional ethics, and that is the community at large.

We began by admitting, with Veatch, that medical ethics are necessarily a part of broader social ethics. This fact leads us to recognize the first of two ways in which the community needs professional ethics: acts of profession serve to keep the ethics of a tight-knit group of professionals from drifting too far from those of the society as a whole. In the case of medicine, physicians' repeated public profession of their values helps prevent confusion as to what those values are, and it also invites response from the public. Over time, the content of physicians' professions has often altered to fit more comfortably with prevailing community views on ethics. In recent decades in the United States, we have seen physicians' ethics move closer to those of the community at large, for example, with regard to the need for informed consent and the propriety of withholding and withdrawing of life-support in certain cases. This give and take is a natural part of the development of the ethic of any social subgroup. It is particularly visible in the development of medical ethics in this century, with its profound and rapid change in medical technical capacity and its great advances in public education and understanding of bioethical issues.

This is not to say, however, that the content of professional ethics will always tailor itself wholly to the prevailing social ethic. Medicine is, after all, the practice of preserving and restoring health. Its practice requires the acquisition of certain kinds of knowledge; it requires a willingness to approach the sick; it requires enough of an ethic of confidentiality and fiduciary responsibility to permit the truthful communication of private facts from patient to physician. The profession of medical ethics serves to remind the community of these core features of medical practice. It serves also to preserve them, to hold their place in the ethical consciousness of the friends and neighbors and lovers and employees of physicians, and of society as a whole.

The need for such preservation of medical values should not be underestimated. We should pause to consider that the public repetition of core medical values is even now serving to keep a place for those values in a community that sometimes seems willing to sacrifice them for the sake of consumerism and efficiency. Physicians all across the United States are objecting to management practices that interfere with their ability to tend to their patients' needs. Their most vehement objections are reserved for those practices that seek to control the cost of medical services by pitting physicians' financial self-interests against the health interests of their patients. The cynic may accuse them of being more concerned with the former arm of the conflict than with the latter. But the cynic should consider that physicians' professional ethics not only counsel physicians to avoid conflicts of interest when possible (Council 1996, Opinions 8.03, 8.031, 8.035, 8.061, 8.07) but also tell physicians how to resolve such conflicts when they arise: "If a conflict develops between the physician's financial interest and the physician's responsibilities to the patient, the conflict must be resolved to the patient's benefit" (Council 1996, Opinion 8.03).

In time of plague or natural disaster, no one objects when shopkeepers and gardeners and clerks flee and leave the sick and wounded behind. If the voice of medical professionalism were silenced, it might be that the new nonprofessional purveyors of health-related services would flee along with them. It is just possible that a physician who has vowed in public to place the interests of his patients above his own would find it harder to flee.

Bentham or Coleridge?

By now we will have raised the ire of critics who rightly point out that physicians often act in self-interested fashion. The noble sentiments expressed in physicians' professional ethics are not always matched by equally noble actions on the part of practicing doctors. What are we to do with this fact? What attitude should we take toward the claims of the 150-year-old institution of professional ethics, given the long history of apparently hypocritical disregard for it by individual practitioners? Two paths are available to us—paths that we might, following John Stuart Mill, denominate the Benthamite and the Coleridgean (Mill 1973).

According to Mill, Jeremy Bentham sought to "strip away" all claims that social institutions and customs were founded on moral principle in order to reveal what he regarded as their true foundation in human psychological motivation. We might join the chorus of contemporary critics of professional ethics who would like to follow Bentham by revealing the moral commitments of medical professionals as thinly disguised commitments to utility seeking. As Mill put it:

> Man is never recognized by [Benthamites] as a being capable of pursuing spiritual perfection as an end; of desiring for its own sake, the conformity of his own character to his standard of excellence, without hope of good or fear of evil from other source than his own inward consciousness. . . . If we find the words 'Conscience,' 'Principle,' 'Moral Rectitude,' 'Moral Duty,' in [their] Table of the Springs of Action, it is among the synonymes of the 'love of reputation.' (Mill 1973, 97–98)

We decline to join in this Benthamite unmasking, though we admit that there is much to be gained from exposing and reprimanding hypocrites. We find a grave danger in the Benthamite decision to treat as selfishly motivated—and therefore to condemn as useless—any professed ethical principle for which a selfish motivation can be imagined. For selfish motivation can be imagined always and everywhere. A physician may do her job well solely for the sake of economic gain; she may do good deeds solely in order to obtain reputation. A Benthamite destruction of the notion of professional ethics cannot be followed by a Benthamite reconstruction. There is no end to Benthamite unmasking, and Benthamites are left with nothing with which to replace selfish motivation as the "real" underpinning of professional ethics.

We believe that there is more in words like "principle" and "conscience" and "moral duty" than Bentham or his modern heirs can see. For this reason, we prefer to follow a strategy that holds out the promise of reinvigorating those words, rather than one that dismisses them as empty or deceptive. This strategy is the one associated by Mill with Coleridge.

"[T]o Bentham," Mill wrote, "it was given to discern more particularly those truths with which existing doctrines and institutions were at variance; to Coleridge the neglected truths which lay in them" (Mill 1973, 78). Where the Benthamite critic asks whether a given moral claim is true, the Coleridgean asks what the claim really means. Where the Benthamite points to hypocrisy and demands "the extinction of the institutions and creeds which had hitherto existed" (Mill 1973, 151), the Coleridgean points to hypocrisy and demands that those institutions and creeds be made a reality once again.

We urge that professionals take their professed ethics on their own terms and that they hold them up to one another as a critical standard. With Coleridge, we desire that medical professionals should "conceive the absent as if it were present, the imaginary as if it were real, and to clothe it in the feelings which, if it were indeed real, it would bring along with it" (Mill 1973, 94). It is precisely by thus setting in a clear light what a professional ethic *ought* to be, and what a commitment to it *ought* to feel like, that physicians will be able to offer the sharpest criticisms of what, in some sad cases, it has become.

That criticism too—provided it is undertaken in the spirit of Mill's Coleridge—will be an act of pro-fession: a public reaffirmation of professional ethics, and one that all of us—professionals, patients, and the community at large—need.

References

Council on Ethical and Judicial Affairs (AMA). 1996. *Code of Medical Ethics: Current Opinions with Annotations, 1996–1997*. Chicago: American Medical Association.

Freidson, Eliot. 1994. *Professionalism Reborn: Theory, Prophecy and Policy*. Chicago: University of Chicago Press.

Greenwood, Ernest. 1957. Attributes of a Profession. *Social Work* 2(3):44–55.

Hughes, E. C. 1971. *The Sociological Eye: Selected Papers*. Chicago: Aldine.

Kass, Leon. 1985. Professing Medically. In *Toward a More Natural Science*. New York: Free Press.

MacIver, Robert. 1955. The Social Significance of Professional Ethics. *Annals of the American Academy of Political and Social Science*, 297:118–24.

Mill, John Stuart. 1973. Bentham. Coleridge. In *Essays on Politics and Culture*, ed. G. Himmelfarb. Gloucester, Mass.: Peter Smith.

Pellegrino, Edmund, and Thomasma, David. 1981. A Philosophical Reconstruction of Medical Morality. In *A Philosophical Basis of Medical Practice*. Oxford: Oxford University Press.

Plato. The Republic. In *The Collected Dialogues of Plato*, ed. E. Hamilton and H. Cairns. Princeton: Princeton University Press.

Williams, Bernard A. O. 1995. Professional Morality and Its Dispositions. In *Making Sense of Humanity and Other Philosophical Papers*. Cambridge, UK: Cambridge University Press.

III

Current Challenges
to Medical Ethics

13

Codes Visible and Invisible

The Twentieth-Century Fate
of a Nineteenth-Century Code

CHARLES E. ROSENBERG, PH.D.

It is only fair to begin this chapter with a confession of my visceral sense that medicine is in some important dimension sacred, that although it functions in the market, medicine cannot be reduced to a series of market transactions. It still makes me uncomfortable to hear health care referred to as a product— and to see it advertised. I am not even comfortable with professional sports teams being referred to as products—let alone the work of men and women who diagnose and treat our ills, hear our most personal fears and anxieties, touch and observe our bodies. I am dismayed by the ubiquitous use of the term "healthcare system" when the presumably inclusive meaning of the word *system* is limited to bureaucratic and economic relationships. I feel, moreover, that my comments are neither idiosyncratic nor inappropriately nostalgic, but are an expression of a widespread, if not always well-articulated, social consensus. Whether our code of medical ethics is formal and written, inscribed at one moment in time or constructed step by step as we recognize new problems, it always reflects values that constitute de facto constraints shaping the actions of individuals, the profession, and the state. Our convictions about the nature and goals of medicine are one such constraint.

I first read the original AMA Code of Ethics many years ago when I sought to reconstruct a cross section of medical practice in mid-nineteenth-century New York City (Rosenberg 1967). I was struck at the time by the way in which the 1847 Code revealed so much about the world of medicine it sought to order. It was a world—at least in theory—of undifferentiated solo practitioners, a world in which the great majority of patients were treated in their homes and not in institutional settings. But it was also a world of sometimes brutal rivalry for the patronage of a less than adequate supply of fee-paying patients. Because every practitioner was a potential competitor, the code was structured around a need to control such competition. The code's emphasis on the etiquette of consultation and the responsibility of patient to physician—as well as physician to patient and among physicians—followed logically from this structure of practice. Fee-paying patients did not need to be "empowered"—to use late-twentieth-century jargon; they were empowered by their family's social position, by their often sophisticated knowledge of medical thought and practice, by their ability to judge a physician's character and competence, and—perhaps most important—by their ability to pay the fees that constituted the physician's sole source of income (Jewson 1974; 1976; Rosenberg 1977). It was a world in which face-to-face relationships both constituted and legitimated medical practice, a world—at least in theory—of relationships, not episodes, in which mutuality of obligation grew naturally out of long-term personal interactions.

Continuity of care was not simply a rhetorical embellishment but a commonplace reality—and one enshrined in a system of medical thought that construed disease and health as aggregate outcomes of lives lived over time. Lifestyle and social circumstance interacted with individual constitution to produce chronic disease and to predispose to acute disease. A particular physician was thus the appropriate monitor of each individual's health status, and his monitoring responsibility justified the code's emphasis on the continuity of relationship between a family and the physician who knew its idiosyncratic biological and emotional character. The 1847 Code (chap. I, art. II, sec. 3) urged, for example, that patients choose one particular physician, for a medical man acquainted with the "peculiarities of constitution, habits, and predispositions of those he attends, is more likely to be successful in his treatment than one who does not possess that knowledge" (Appendix C, 326). Similarly, the code emphasizes a patient's obligation to provide an explanation if he or she were to dismiss the attending physician.

The physician was a man—needless to say and thus my use of the masculine pronoun—of honor and humanity, and that notion of honor included a responsibility to respect and acquire the scientific knowledge that informed medical practice. The delivery of care in a hospital or dispensary was by definition an act of charity, as was the physician's contribution to the public health. But these institutional roles were in fact marginal to the lives of the great majority of medical men and their patients. (The impersonal and episodic world of hospital and dispensary medicine was almost exclusively urban in a still predominately rural society, and within America's cities it was limited to the "working and dependent classes.") The 1847 Code's focus on the doctor-family fee-for-service relationship was in good measure descriptive as well as prescriptive.

Much of the code's content can be, and has been, dismissed as mere ideology: invocations of honor, humanitarianism, and therapeutic necessity in the service of controlling and stabilizing the medical marketplace (see, e.g., Freidson 1970; Larson 1977; Rothstein 1972; Berlant 1975). From this perspective, the AMA's original Code of Ethics was no more than a body of guild etiquette. Profit maintenance, not moral commitment, explained its form and essence. And from a certain perspective, this way of thinking about the code and its social purpose makes descriptive and historical sense. The blackballing[1] of "deadbeats," for example, by local medical societies, or their forbidding of consultation with sectarian practitioners, were tough-minded practices designed to improve the physician's economic status; the relationship of such practices to traditional ethical norms and to the patient's interest was and is problematic.

But as a social institution, medicine had to be viable economically. And that viability depended to an extent on public and, I would contend, medical acceptance of a very specific moral and cultural history. Bakers and carpenters, silversmiths—even lawyers—could not call upon the same body of gentlemanly, humanistic, and moral reference in defining their social identities. Responsibility for life and death, for the touching of bodies and emotions, demanded such transcendent styles of self-presentation. The code would not, that is, have served as a public affirmation of a morally elevated professional role without invoking an historical tradition of selflessness and sacredness, of a gentlemanly commitment to learning and benevolence, as integral to the physician's identity. The status of knowledge and innovation alone, for example, constituted a significant, and seemingly selfless, element in the profession's collective social posture. Intellect and morality were necessarily linked.

In retrospect, such values were to prove a key change agent in the profession. Like many of the other selfless and gentlemanly values associated with medicine, this attitude toward knowledge would play an ultimately hegemonic role within the profession, at once rationalizing and constituting the status of social and institutional elites. And in the twentieth century, such elites have merged inexorably with elites defined by intellectual accomplishment.

As we are well aware, the medical profession and the practice of medicine have changed dramatically in the past century—as has the relationship between the historical code and the profession. The relationship had, in fact, already begun to change at the end of the last century as specialism, the shaping of an academic elite, and the growing role of clinic and hospital had already become apparent. None of these developments was entirely novel; even in 1847 there was a thriving consulting and academic elite, largely urban, that monopolized teaching and hospital positions. Such practitioners had also played a disproportionately prominent role in the profession's intellectual life, both as teachers and as writers. And specialism too had roots deep in the nineteenth century (Rosen 1944; Stevens 1971). The American medical profession had never been entirely undifferentiated.

The 1847 Code—with its several Progressive era revisions—was to become decreasingly relevant, however, in the twentieth century's ever more fragmented medical world. At the beginning of this century, the code could still play a role, serving as a justification, for example, in dealing with the perceived evil of fee-splitting (the practice of physicians receiving a portion of the fee collected by specialists—most frequently surgeons—to whom they referred a patient). The early twentieth-century campaign against such kickbacks was, in fact, a recognition of the reality of specialization and the linked insight that conventionally agreed-upon ethical standards could serve as a mediating and organizing mechanism in an increasingly differentiated profession (see chap. 4, this volume.)

In the years between the 1920s and 1965, however, the code of ethics played a less than central role. It was deployed most conspicuously, in fact, as a rhetorical weapon in organized medicine's consistent opposition to experiments in third-party payment and the organization of health care (Burrow 1963; 1977; Fishbein 1947). Such innovations could be and were assailed as undermining the centrality of the individual doctor-patient relationship and the fee for specific clinical service that structured this fundamental interaction. As medicine became inexorably more specialized, institutionally based, and highly capitalized, however, invocation of the sacredness of the individual doctor-patient relationship began to seem to many observers—including many academic physicians—increasingly narrow, self-serving, and politically short-sighted. It was certainly no accurate reflection of a pervasive social reality as it had been in the mid-nineteenth century. In fact, this widening gap between the code and a changed practice environment undermined its social relevance—just as the reality of an increasingly complex and differentiated profession was to undermine the AMA's ability to represent American physicians.

Problems such as those raised by the conflict over the integration of specialism into the profession (with its necessary recognition of differentiation among practitioners) were increasingly solved by bureaucratic means. In the case of specialism, these involved a by-now-familiar complex of linked mechanisms: specialty boards and board certification, reimbursement requirements, and hospital and residency certification. This was a strategy not necessarily inconsistent with an ethical rationale as well as an organizational imperative, for it could certainly be construed as protecting the patient's interest. But a web of credentialing practices is not easily related to an underlying moral justification—certainly not to an often-skeptical public.

Meanwhile, as we have suggested, the notion of a unified profession that informed the original code has become no more than a wistful self-indulgence. An ethical code based on the assumption of an undifferentiated—if competitive   profession and a practice norm based on long-term personal relationships has come to seem increasingly irrelevant to late-twentieth-century realities. Almost from the beginning of the century, for example, an academic elite in medicine grew increasingly distant from the concerns of everyday practice and increasingly absorbed by its own disciplinary goals. This was not unrelated, of course, to the extraordinary growth of specialism I have already mentioned and to the siting of so much medical care in hospitals and clinics. It was related as well to an increasingly basic-science-oriented style of academic research—with its subsequent reflection in clinical practice. Different social locations make for differing perceptions and interests; it is not always clear who speaks for medicine in late-twentieth-century America.

None of this is meant to suggest that contemporary medicine has not been shaped by ethical and value commitments. But those commitments reflect a tacit consensus around principles that have never been explicitly codified— and that are being continually renegotiated. Moreover, many of those negotiators are comparatively new players in the medical arena: local and central governments, civil courts, bioethicists, patient advocacy groups. And though they invoke a variety of points of moral reference, there is no consistent feeling that the historical code as such should be central to their ever-shifting debates.

I have just referred to "tacit values or points of moral reference." But what precisely do such words mean? Let me try to be more specific. Some aspects of a changing twentieth-century moral consensus have been general and not limited to medicine. I refer to the rights revolution, for example, and a developing notion of the state's responsibility for the preservation of individual rights. Access to health care is one such presumed right (and one, I should add, with strong historical roots. Americans have always assumed that even the poor should have access to care—though not, of course, equal care). The role of government in medicine has become increasingly important, if never explicitly—and consensually—conceptualized. Almost all of us have come to assume that government bears some responsibility for health care, in terms of both access and assurance of quality. Allied to this conviction is the working assumption that medicine is multidimensional—which implies the necessity of public support for research and clinical training, and, more ambiguously, for making technologically sophisticated care available to those in need.

Equally significant was the growing centrality of a new and more specifically medical absolute: the legitimating efficacy of an increasingly powerful body of scientific knowledge—even if that knowledge was not simply or easily translated into everyday clinical practice. Knowledge was an absolute good; it empowered all physicians, even if not in a consistent and symmetrical way. It made the physician something other than a mere profit maximizer on the one hand, or a sensitive caregiver on the other.

Such cultural—and inevitably political—assumptions have in the past half-century justified a cumulatively revolutionary change in American health care. I refer, of course, to a growing federal involvement in health, from the support of research through the National Institutes of Health, the support of hospitals through the Hill-Burton Act, the subvention of residency and fellowship programs, and administrative and fiscal responsibility for Medicare and Medicaid.

Technology, as exemplified in the capacity to intervene in disease, has become the key unspoken imperative in these developments. And, I would argue, our cultural faith in medicine's technical efficacy poses an ethical as well as an institutional and economic problem. We have come to accept a technologically mediated entitlement to care; that is, every American should have access by right to life-saving or life-enhancing technologies once such procedures become plausible clinical options. The history of dialysis illustrates this very well. Once the technology became available, it was difficult for American legislators to deny a "life-saving procedure" to individuals at risk. And thus began our quarter-century of experience with a novel clinical entity called "end-stage renal disease," the hybrid product of a union between bureaucracy and technical change (Peitzman 1992).

We have come to glory in, and suffer from, a peculiar kind of technological imperative: if a procedure can be done, the moral gradient demands, it should be done (paraphrased from Rosenberg 1987, 350). We have come, that is, to define entitlement to care in technological terms. Seemingly value-free and universal, technological entitlement has had a powerful effect in shaping the parameters of health care, definitions of quality, and the ethical assumptions legitimating the provision of care.

We have already seen aspects of this set of assumptions in public opposition to curtailments of service, which can be construed as rationing, and—most dramatically in the recent past—in morally framed and legitimated opposition to the de facto rationing of managed care. It has been illustrated as well in countless rhetorical endorsements of the quality of American medicine as compared to other societies. And "quality" is unquestioningly seen in technical terms, as the ability to intervene effectively in acute and life-threatening clinical situations. On the other hand, it has been difficult to see less technologically defined modes of care as equally worthy of support—especially if they are associated with the less-worthy poor and the far from value-neutral welfare system as opposed to the presumably value-free procedures of "scientific medicine." Similarly, chronic and preventive care have been comparatively neglected because they cannot be consistently defined and legitimated in terms of prestige-bearing technical procedures.

But if the tendency to understand and value medicine in reductionist terms has been dominant both within the profession and in the culture generally, the twentieth century has witnessed a continuing debate at the margins of this diffuse yet powerful consensus. Critics inside and outside the medical profession have articulated a variety of arguments assailing the narrowly technical and—often relatedly—commercial aspects of twentieth-century medicine. Perhaps most persistent has been a characteristic jeremiad bemoaning the depersonalizing consequences of reductionist medicine. In such critiques the solipsism of the laboratory and operating room parallels the moral solipsism of the market. From the very beginning of the century some physicians, many nurses, and a variety of social scientists and social commentators have expressed what might be called a patient-oriented holism, deploring the trend toward fragmentation and specialization within the profession, the tendency to treat organs and diseases, not men and women.

This familiar argument has been paralleled and in some ways duplicated by a sociological and social-medical critique warning of a narrow focus on acute care and technical procedures and of a self-aggrandizing quest for control of the medical market. Sociologists and planners—even historians—have invoked such arguments since the 1930s. They have ranged from advocacy for accessible health care and national health insurance in the 1930s, to sociological critiques of the late 1960s and 70s that tended in their most extreme form to reduce medicine's claims to social authority to a scheme for market domination. All these oppositional positions share a central rhetorical strategy: the underlining of a morally charged contrast between an "is" of impersonality and profit maximization (whether defined in terms of dollars or of status) and an "ought" of medicine as holistic, selfless, and community-oriented. Within this value-structured, bipolar narrative, organized medicine's demands for autonomy and control could easily be stripped of their selfless quality and construed in more sordid terms. From this critical perspective, the creation of bioethics and chronologically parallel demands for the securing of patient rights can be seen as but another attempt to create a framework for morally coherent social action in a fragmented and inward-looking medical world.

But none of these critical strategies has exerted a dominating influence; all have remained oppositional—drawing their energy and visibility from the continued centrality of the reductionist, impersonal, and acute-care-oriented medicine they deplored. The social science critique, as well as those drawn from medical humanism and left politics, has always remained marginal to mainstream trends in medicine.

Bioethics too has seemed incapable of articulating a contextual way of thinking about such widely felt dilemmas. Bioethics has in some ways remained a self-absorbed disciplinary technology itself, ironically mirroring in its defining concerns that self-absorbed and all-consuming technology it has sought to order and understand. Its authority and subject matter have been, that is, defined by the "bio" in its disciplinary title. The comparatively recent neologism, *bioethics*, implies, that is, an implicit focus on the isolated individual body and our increasing ability to manipulate it in one way or another. One might semifacetiously argue that bioethicists have focused narrowly on whether to pull the plug and paid comparatively little attention to the social and intellectual worlds that have produced and deployed the plug (Rothman 1991).

Contemporary practitioners of medicine feel beset by what they experience as the unfeeling pseudo-rationalities of bureaucracy and the callous pressures of the marketplace. Perhaps it is time to make explicit the tacit body of ethical commitment that has helped inform contemporary medical policy. It is not only the costs of medical care and the relentless pressures of demographic reality in an aging society that make us uncomfortable with contemporary health policies. It is more than petulance that makes physicians as well as patients uncomfortable with the contemporary realities of an ever more bureaucratized and increasingly market-oriented medicine. The crisis we are experiencing is one of authority and control, but also, inextricably, of values and orientations. In practical terms, it might be thought of as a crisis in maintaining the profession's appropriate and defining balance among a variety of not always consistent identities: medicine as humane caring, as applied science, as marketplace actor, and, more recently, as an aspect of public policy. How we configure these not easily compatible elements is in one of its dimensions necessarily a question of values as well as of institutional and political management.

Perhaps it is time for the fragmented profession to think about what binds its varied practitioners together, to examine and collectively affirm its often tacit and not always unanimous body of ethical commitments, and to recall that the wider culture has internalized, and acts upon, its own particular code of medical ethics. Such reasoning together might result in a new ethical code—or it might not. But I would like to emphasize, in conclusion, that no matter what the immediate future of medicine's consideration of itself in relation to society, the often rhetorically abused doctor-patient relationship must remain central to that consideration. The particular doctor-patient interaction is necessarily unique and circumstantial, yet in another dimension it is timeless and unchanging. Most important, an analytic focus on the doctor-patient relationship is the only way to precisely contextualize the goals of medicine and to understand how medicine functions as, and within, a social system. It is the nexus in which laboratory science, clinical application, market practice and motives, and government policy all interact to create the complex social reality that is medicine. Even if that focus can breed a delusive assumption of exclusive medical authority, it also preserves an overriding place in that relationship for the legitimating ideal of the physician as guardian of the patient's interests—as a kind of ombudsperson mediating between the patient and society.

We need to maintain our focus on the way in which medical care affects ordinary men and women, but we must be aware that to accomplish that end we cannot limit ourselves to the examination of ethical dilemmas at the bedside. The last century has made it abundantly clear that a variety of extraclinical factors have shaped the choices and understandings of individual actors in the healthcare system. If we limit our analysis to the bedside—that is, to the choices of individuals as moral agents in particular exemplary cases—we cannot understand what happens at the bedside. We must strive to see that unique social interaction within the broadest social context, yet not lose the clarifying focus on particular human outcomes. To achieve ethical ends, in other words, we must move from the individual to society and back again, to focus on the tensions between the general and particular, the structural and the individual—relationships that in the aggregate constitute the reality we call medicine.

Part of medicine's dilemma is the tendency to see itself—and for society to see it—as self-absorbed; it would be unfortunate if a renewed emphasis on the doctor-patient relationship should serve to justify that self-absorption. Our necessary ethical focus on the eternal dyad of doctor and patient must, that is, be social as well as individual if it is to be effectively moral. In this sense, moral issues become empirical as well as foundational questions: what people feel to be right and wrong helps define their public and private choices. This is perhaps a counsel of complexity, but it is the only one appropriate for the world in which we live.

Note

1. Blackballing was a practice often criticized by contemporaries. Some medical societies kept a list of patients who had failed to settle their accounts; society members were then obligated not to treat such patients.

References

Berlant, Jeffrey L. 1975. *Profession and Monopoly: A Study of Medicine in the United States and Great Britain.* Berkeley: University of California Press.

Burrow, James G. 1963. *AMA: Voice of American Medicine.* Baltimore: Johns Hopkins University Press.

———. 1977. *Organized Medicine in the Progressive Era: The Move Toward Monopoly.* Baltimore: Johns Hopkins University Press.

Fishbein, Morris. 1947. *A History of the American Medical Association, 1847 to 1947.* Philadelphia: W. B. Saunders.

Freidson, Eliot. 1970. *Professional Dominance: The Social Structure of Medical Care.* New York: Atherton Press.

Jewson, N. D. 1974. Medical Knowledge and the Patronage System in Eighteenth-Century England. *Sociology* 8:369–85.

———. 1976. The Disappearance of the Sick Man from Medical Cosmology, 1770–1870. *Sociology* 10:225–44.

Larson, Magali Sarfatti. 1977. *The Role of Professionalism: A Sociological Analysis.* Berkeley: University of California Press.

Peitzman, Steven J. 1992. From Bright's Disease to End-Stage Renal Disease. In *Framing Disease: Studies in Cultural History,* ed. C. E. Rosenberg and J. Golden, 4–19. New Brunswick: Rutgers University Press.

Rosen, George. 1944. *The Specialization of Medicine.* New York: Froben Press.

Rosenberg, Charles E. 1967. The Practice of Medicine in New York a Century Ago. *Bulletin of the History of Medicine* 41:223–53.

———. 1977. The Therapeutic Revolution: Medicine, Meaning, and Social Change in Nineteenth-Century America. *Perspectives in Biology and Medicine* 20:485–506.

———. 1987. *The Care of Strangers: The Rise of America's Hospital System.* New York: Basic Books.

Rothman, David J. 1991. *Strangers at the Bedside: A History of How Law and Bioethics Transformed Medical Decision Making.* New York: Basic Books.

Rothstein, William G. 1972. *American Physicians in the Nineteenth Century: From Sects to Science.* Baltimore: Johns Hopkins University Press.

Stevens, Rosemary. 1971. *American Medicine and the Public Interest.* New Haven: Yale University Press.

———. 1989. *In Sickness and in Wealth: American Hospitals in the Twentieth Century.* New York: Basic Books.

14

Alternative Medicine and the AMA

PAUL ROOT WOLPE, PH.D.

The 150th anniversary of the founding of the American Medical Association (AMA) and the writing of its code of ethics seems a propitious time to explore the history of organized medicine's relationship to competing medical practitioners. In the past, discussions of the code and its relation to competing practitioners of the nineteenth century have often been polarized. Some regard the code primarily as a self-serving attempt by physicians to monopolize medicine and to exclude competitors, while others suggest that the code represented all that is most noble in the medical profession and that it was unfortunate but necessary to exclude some possibly valuable therapies in its attempt to battle charlatans, undereducated physicians, and misguided therapeutics (see Young 1967; Kett 1968; Berlant 1975; Starr 1982; Baker, Porter, and Porter 1993; Baker 1995). The most extreme versions of both of these positions are, I believe, caricatures to some degree. Human motivations and human affairs are complex, and if the code had lofty goals, it also embodied the social relationships of its time.

Whatever one's perspective, it is clear that the 1847 Code of Ethics embodied and perpetuated a posture of orthodox medicine toward its nontraditional competitors and colleagues, both within, and external to, the medical profession, that it has (more or less) carried through until the late twentieth century. However we cast the tale, the history of American medicine, at least until recently, has clearly been characterized by the emergence of a powerful orthodoxy and a progressive attempt to marginalize competitors. While some may overstate the degree to which this process was for purely self-serving ends, it is clear that political and ideological battles between practitioner groups characterized the competitive atmosphere of the nineteenth and early twentieth centuries.

Many historians have written of these struggles. However, there is a tendency to see the ideological struggles of the nineteenth century as a unique product of their time and place and to assume that the strategies and postures of the time faded with the twentieth-century triumph of orthodox biomedicine over its competitors. As a sociologist, however, I am struck less by the differences between the attitudes of the founders of the AMA and their descendants 150 years later than I am by the similarities.

A powerful, institutionalized orthodoxy like biomedicine can use a variety of means to control internal and external competitors (Wolpe 1985; 1990; 1994). When an orthodoxy, or a group with aspirations toward one, confronts internal or external challengers, it will usually try to suppress, subjugate, or relegate those groups or practices to institutional or cultural spheres outside the orthodoxy. Professional prerogatives like self-licensure, control of the educational process, and exclusive access to the loci of professional activity (e.g., hospitals) serve, in part, to develop and maintain monopoly and thereby exclude potential competition. However, it is not enough to exclude competitors from institutional access or regulatory legitimacy; the orthodoxy must also deny challengers cultural legitimacy. By gaining control over the relevant discourse—by winning and retaining the right to define terms and to have the conversation cast in the language of the orthodoxy—the orthodoxy can more effectively paint themselves as the legitimate defenders of a discipline, and the challengers as misguided or charlatans. American medicine has done that quite successfully.

Modern American biomedicine has been singularly successful in excluding competitors from challenging its legitimacy. Its forebears, the "regulars" of the nineteenth century, established their strategy to deal with homeopaths, eclectics, and other competitors, and codified it into the AMA Code of Ethics of 1847. Those dynamics, with occasional modification, carried medicine through to its triumph in the early twentieth century and are still operative 150 years later. We can understand the dynamics of that strategy by describing it in terms of five major propositions. Each describes both the relationship of the "regulars" to their competitors in the mid-nineteenth century and the relationship of late-twentieth-century biomedicine to "alternative" or "complementary" practitioners equally well.

Proposition 1: *Science has been traditionally used by the American medical profession as a wedge (and sometimes a club) to denigrate, exclude, or deny the efficacy of alternative models of healing.*

It makes little sense to talk about "alternative medicine" in the early nineteenth century. Terms like "alternative medicine" and "complementary medicine" are terms of opposition. Medical forms are only "alternative" and "complementary" to an orthodoxy against which they are defined. That which makes a particular medical form alternative or complementary is the argument of people with the power to define disease for a society that such a form should be marginalized, opposed, subjugated, or relegated to institutional or cultural spheres outside that of the mainstream medical practice.

For example, Wallis and Morley (1976) have written that we can only talk of orthodox medicine, and hence alternative medicine, when (1) there exists an occupational group whose job it is to apply therapeutic procedures to the sick; (2) this group displays a high level of consensus about the causes and treatments of most ailments; and (3) its members are attributed a high degree of legitimacy by the client group, which regards them as peculiarly competent to treat the sick. In the nineteenth century there were many groups that claimed legitimacy as institutionalized healers, there was little consensus even among regulars about what caused disease and often how to treat it, and the "client group" used a variety of practitioners. In fact, some of the most prominent physicians, lawyers, businessmen, and politicians of the nineteenth century were ardent believers in spiritualism, phrenology, homeopathy, and the rest (Wrobel 1987). Homeopathy was the treatment of choice for the elite class. This makes sense given that the regulars' "heroic"[1] medicine consisted of bleeding and purging, which were as likely to harm the patient as help, while the homeopaths were administering highly diluted water solutions, which at least did no harm. The names of those who supported homeopathy or another of the "irregular" systems reads like a Who's Who of the nineteenth century: P. T. Barnum, Brigham Young, Andrew Carnegie, Thomas Edison, Henry Ward Beecher, Horace Greeley, William Cohen Bryant, James Fenimore Cooper, Charles Dickens, Margaret Fuller, Daniel Webster, Henry Clay, Harriet Beecher Stowe, Henry Wadsworth Longfellow, Louisa May Alcott, John D. Rockefeller, and Washington Irving. Writers such as Walt Whitman, Edgar Allen Poe, Herman Melville, Mark Twain, George Elliot, Nathaniel Hawthorne, and Charlotte Bronte all suffused their writings with spiritualist or phrenological concepts (Wrobel 1987).

There was thus simply no true orthodoxy to be an alternative to in the early to mid-nineteenth century. The reason we think of homeopathy, eclecticism, Thomsonianism, and the rest as alternatives is because the regulars won the battle for professional dominance; and it is the winners who write the history of the losers. Instead of orthodox and alternative medicine, the early nineteenth century is characterized by a stratified and diverse healthcare market in which different healthcare philosophies were competing. Within that field each group considered itself the legitimate representative of the future of medicine and others as pretenders.

Thomsonianism, for example, was started by Samuel Thomson in the early nineteenth century. It was a botanical movement that tried to promote natural cures that didn't carry with them the side effects of heroic medicine. It was the first movement to be considered a "sect" by the nineteenth-century regulars, who, as we will see, talked a lot about "sectarianism." Before Thomson, American medicine was primarily home-based care, with a hodgepodge of diffuse Euro-American, Native-American, and indigenous healing philosophies. Thomsonianism was the first to capitalize on the fear of the treatments of the irregulars, and in some ways, Thomson was the first to understand the medical spirit of his age.

Instead of offering therapy, Thomson began selling family rights to his system of natural cures, mostly derived from common roots and herbs. He claimed that by 1839 he had sold 100,000 family rights to his system at $20 apiece—$2 million worth of sales by 1839, an enormous amount of money at the time. He was a relentless critic of the regulars, and many of his criticisms would be shared today.[2] He abhorred the immediate tendency of the regulars to bleed patients and give them emetics, and part of his success was in convincing people (especially the poor) that there was another less harsh and equally "scientific" course.

Thomsonianism eventually was, in a complex manner, subsumed under eclecticism, a general medical movement focused on practical cures rather than on a particular philosophy of disease. The best among the eclectics practiced an empirical medicine that demanded validation of a therapy's efficacy, no matter its philosophical justification, and thus can be seen as encompassing the best science of the day. Certainly, quacks and undertrained practitioners hung on to the eclectics' coattails; yet at its philosophical core, eclecticism was a scientific movement.

Many other movements also based their philosophies on the science of the day, including phrenology, Mesmerism, and even American spiritualism, which tried to make a scientific argument as to the existence of spiritual forces and energies that could cure bodily and spiritual ills. These philosophies tried to understand the linkages between the mind and body, spirit and matter, a pursuit that was well in keeping with the intellectual currents of the nineteenth century (Wrobel 1987). (It is ironic that now, 150 years later, there is again an intellectual pressure to understand the connection between the mind and the body in human health.) There is no discernible sense in which the basic philosophies of these movements were antiscientific.

Despite these claims to scientific legitimacy, the regulars insisted that only their healing method was based on science. Yet the therapies that the regulars used were no more scientifically valid, even by the standards of their own day, than the ones used by their competitors. In fact, as Warner (forthcoming) demonstrates so well, it was the regulars themselves who vigorously cultivated an ideology bifurcated into "orthodoxy" and "otherness" in order to press their claims for exclusive legitimacy.

It was in no sense obvious or inevitable in the nineteenth century that those who practiced heroic medicine were going to win their claim to orthodoxy in the marketplace of ideas and that their competitors were going to become "alternative" medicines. Oliver Wendell Holmes (a vocal opponent of homeopathy, by the way) himself freely admitted that the regular medical therapeutics of the time were worthless. He said, "If the whole materia medica, as now used, could be sunk to the sea, it would be all the better for mankind, and all the worse for the fishes." Homeopaths were in no sense less scientific than regulars by the standards of the nineteenth century, and neither were the leaders among the eclectics. Homeopaths had their own scientific methodology, a system they called "proving," whereby they took scrupulous notes of all the symptoms and the remedies, and the way in which the remedies either did or did not cure particular patients, and they were used as empirical justifications of homeopathic validity. As Wrobel (1987, 3) has written, "in many ways homeopathy and hydropathy [a very popular water cure of the time] seemed to have greater claims to empiricism than did orthodox medicine, which was comprised of a motley, odd mixture of folk wisdom and intuitive approaches to healing." Homeopaths saw themselves supplanting allopaths and their dogmas, using terms like "Orthodox Theological Schools" to describe regular medical education (Warner forthcoming).

Homeopathy was not a pseudoscience of the nineteenth century; it was a science of the nineteenth century. The homeopaths, for example, were far ahead of the regulars in recognizing the need for an experimentally derived pharmacopoeia and creating systematic experiments to create one (Stoehr 1987). The fact that the AMA code of 1847 nonetheless excludes homeopaths and eclectics on the basis of not being "scientific" indicates ulterior motives at work, even though there were undoubtedly also noble ones. The inclusion in the code of the need to base all medical therapeutics on "science" was the very phrase used to exclude "irregulars" from participating in the AMA, as we will see in Proposition 2.

Let us try a thought experiment: Homeopathy, which was the main competitor of the upper end of wealthy, established medicine at the time, founded its American Institute of Homeopathy (AIH) in 1844, three years before the AMA was founded.[3] One year later, in 1845, the AIH restricted its membership to physicians who had received a regular medical education. The AIH was a professional organization; it was an exclusionary organization; it had all the trappings of what we think of as an elite, professional attempt to become the established medicine in the United States. Many homeopathic schools already had state charters, others were being developed, and many homeopaths held M.D.s from regular medical schools. They had begun their careers as regulars and had been "converted," to use the terminology of the time, to homeopathy. Homeopaths considered themselves members of a learned profession and had established their own professional journals, societies, and degree-granting schools. Some had ranked among the elite physicians in the United States before being converted to homeopathy, though most were then rejected by their former colleagues. Homeopathy was the medicine of much of the wealthy class—a largely urban, Northeastern, elite medicine—versus (for example) Thomsonianism, which tended to be a more rural, poor, Midwestern phenomenon.

Let us imagine, for a moment, that it was the homeopaths who had established themselves, that homeopathy became the dominant system in the United States, and that the AIH became the professional organization that dominated American medicine. It is unlikely that could have happened, for their numbers were much smaller, and, despite their elite status, they did not have control over the hospitals and other bases of institutional power. But let us imagine that the volume you are now reading was put together for the sesquicentennial of the AIH, that it was the regulars who faded away by the early twentieth century, and that today we are all homeopaths looking back at the regulars with the same critical eye that we in actuality apply only to the homeopaths. The authors of the volume would undoubtedly have essays expressing bafflement over why anyone would have gone to practitioners who bled them practically to death and who used blistering, puking, purging, cupping, bleeding, and mega-doses of mercury and arsenic. "How dangerous, and foolish!" we might exclaim. "How could they use methods so unscientific!" We might even fault the AIH for not excluding these "irregulars" from membership in their organization. After all, were they not "sectarians," holding fast to therapies that were often damaging to patients and ignoring empirical evidence of their inefficacy and side effects?

Yet throughout the nineteenth century and, except for a brief period at the turn of century, most of the twentieth century, it was their competitors' lack of scientific validity and lack of fealty to science that was used, again and again, as the excuse to exclude them from membership in the AMA and from the institutions that the orthodoxy controlled.

Of course, all this is behind us by the late twentieth century, as science has been consolidated into a coherent methodology. It therefore becomes much easier to determine scientific validity and exclude alternatives as unscientific —or does it?

American medical science in the twentieth century has accomplished what the regulars in the nineteenth could only dream of doing—it has created a monopoly over definitions of what is scientific and therefore can dismiss any system that either appears unscientific on its surface or subscribes to a scientific philosophy or methodology at odds with accepted American definitions. As the taken-for-granted definer of what is scientific in medicine, biomedicine can dismiss other systems as ipso facto unscientific, without even empirically examining their claims or efficacy.

In the 1970s and 1980s, when alternative medicine first began to gain adherents in sufficient numbers to concern orthodox practitioners, physicians often dismissed even the worth of doing validation experiments on alternative medicine. Many physicians in the late 1970s and early 1980s simply argued that the newly coined "holistic health" was quackery and thus unworthy of serious attention other than warning patients about it (Brown 1975; Brody 1980; Lange 1980; Kabler 1981; Fitzgerald 1983; Glymour and Stalker 1983). Nor has this attitude ceased. Those who practice or use alternative medicine are often accused of being "irrational" (Hufford 1995). Attempts to introduce modalities seen as foreign or alternative in mainstream journals often bring a host of letters, not urging serious scientific evaluation, but upbraiding the journal for considering publication at all (see, e.g., *JAMA* 1991). The National Institutes of Health Office of Alternative Medicine is still under attack as not being worth the resources donated to it (*JAMA* 1993a; 1993b; Kolata 1996).

As long as orthodox medicine has been able to dismiss alternatives as unscientific by their very nature, they could be relegated to marginal cultural realms. It is only now, when consumer demand has overwhelmed official jargon, that alternative medicine is getting any scientific scrutiny.

Proposition 2: *In pursuit of squashing their competition, orthodox medicine painted all alternatives as equally unscientific.*

In attempting to exclude competition, both in 1847 and in the twentieth century, orthodox medicine tended to paint anything that was not part of it with a broad brush of quackery. There was, indeed, an enormous amount of quackery in the nineteenth century, with nostrum salesmen, patent medicine salesmen, and practitioners pushing every therapy their imaginations could devise. In fact, concocting a potion was well recognized as a get-rich-quick scheme, if you could market it sufficiently well (Young 1967). Yet to suggest, as the AMA did, that the nostrum salesmen, many of whom were out-and-out frauds, and the homeopaths, who had regular medical education and scientific evidence for their therapies, were one and the same, was to simply ignore reality for political gain.

Baker (1995) has pointed out that one thing that drove the regulars at the founding of the AMA was a belief that medicine would only succeed if it became truly scientific. It is undoubtedly true that they valued science and believed that the future of medicine was a scientific one. In fact, the founders of the AMA were so committed to this ideal that they challenged not only the irregulars but also the entire system of medical education, including the most prestigious medical schools in the nation, to adopt a more scientifically rigorous training. Baker uses this point to explain the regulars' rejection of sectarians. He agrees with Kett (1968) that "it was [the AMA's] commitment to scientific medicine, to a scientific medical and pre-medical education, that forced them in to a reformist and exclusionary stance" (Baker 1995, 13). Baker quotes John Bell's introduction to the 1847 Code of Ethics (physicians are called upon to be "trustees of science and almoners of benevolence") as evidence of this perspective. More telling, however, is his attempt to further support his point through the comments of Nathaniel Chapman, first president of the AMA, as he welcomed the delegates to the first meeting of the AMA: "[Is not] the profession . . . environed by difficulties and dangers, arising mainly from the too ready admixture into it of individuals unworthy of the association, either by intellectual culture, or moral discipline, by whom it is abased?" The moral and intellectual elitism of this comment may portend another, less lofty motivation for excluding the irregulars from the AMA. To the regulars, science meant conforming, not to empirical validation of therapies, but to an existing system of therapeutics. Not methodological rigor, but ideological conformity was how they defined adherence to "science."

The inclusion in the code of the need to base all medical therapeutics on science was the excuse used to exclude irregulars. The lack of scientific justification for orthodox therapies themselves suggests that science was used at least as much as a club to beat over the head of rivals as an assessment tool in adjudicating therapeutic disputes. This was reflected in the fact that the AMA code was ambiguous about who was a physician but not ambiguous about who was not: homeopaths and eclectics, their main rivals for patients. "Scientific medicine" became synonymous with bleeding, cupping, and purging.

The resolution from the Philadelphia Convention of 1846 is explicit on this point: "That the certificate of no preceptor shall be received who is avowedly and notoriously an irregular practitioner, whether he shall possess the degree of MD or not." No mention is made of how scientific that "irregular" might be or how much empirical justification he might have for his practice style; the irregular practitioner was defined as unscientific.

Isaac Hays tries, at least, to point to a reason for rejecting irregulars in the Philadelphia Convention of 1846. His famous phrase, in which he denies irregulars the right to call themselves regulars or engage in consultation with regulars, states that "no one can be considered as a regular practitioner, or fit associate in consultation, whose practice is based on an exclusive dogma." Yet, what is an exclusive dogma? The regulars themselves ended up strongly defending the absolute truth of their heroic depletive therapeutics, as Warner (1987) so well describes: "Between the 1820s and 1850s [heroic depletive therapies'] standing as symbols of orthodox medicine became stronger and more rigid. Regular physicians praised their worth with unprecedented vigour, and avowed belief in their value became the central touchstone of orthodoxy" (246). "Sectarianism set up fidelity to the symbols of regular tradition as the cardinal test of orthodoxy" (252).

In other words, while the regulars tried to hold themselves above sectarianism, by almost any definition the regulars in the nineteenth century were as sectarian as those they opposed. Their practice also became based on an "exclusive dogma"—that only the standards of heroic treatment are valid and that questioning or rejecting them was grounds for being considered unfit for consultation. In fact, as time went on and the problems of heroic medicine became more obvious, and even as many regulars were abandoning the system at the bedside, its importance as an ideological dogma, as the symbol of that which separated the regulars from their rivals, only increased (Warner forthcoming).

The nascent AMA thus had a serious procedural dilemma. Who should be allowed to join? How was the convention of 1846 supposed to define a physician, when some people with M.D.s had passed eleven-week courses and were woefully ignorant and incompetent, while some elite, well-educated, and prominent physicians were practitioners of homeopathy or other therapeutics that the AMA officially rejected? The AMA did the only thing it could do under the circumstances: it defined a physician's eligibility to join primarily by the content of his beliefs (King 1982). One had to pledge allegiance to the heroic dogma in order to join the professional society opposed to exclusive dogmas. Protests by the elite that the exclusivity of the regulars and the AMA was entirely due to the desire to uphold science thus are simply not supported.

There were certainly many dangerous and useless therapies that populated the nineteenth-century landscape. The unregulated nature of medicine in the nineteenth century led to an explosion of homemade patent medicines and cures, most of which were little better than alcohol and water or some kind of combination of herbs or store-bought substances that were said to have some kind of curative power. Medicines with names like "Cure For Headache Brainfood" and "Raydol" (which billed itself as a "radium-impregnated" medicine on the heels of the Curies' discovery of radium) lulled the susceptible consumer into buying medicines with little or no efficacy (Young 1967). The same is true of a whole series of biomedical instrumentations, some of which used electrical charges or mysterious energies to heal ailments from lower back pain to hemorrhoids. The AMA was a very prominent advocate for regulation and often fought the good fight against these get-rich-quick schemes.[4] However, the AMA's suspicions of these charlatans was generalized into a general resistance to any medicine, any procedure, or any system of healing that was not born under the rubric of AMA-sanctioned methods, an attitude that still persists. The wholesale resistance to innovation or importation of ideas that came from outside insulated Western medicine from advances it might have made sooner, medicines it might have discovered sooner, and indigenous and foreign healing systems that had things to offer the general welfare of patients.

Ultimately, the attempt to paint all other practitioners as quacks weakened the AMA's fight against true quackery. It cast doubt on the orthodoxy's objectivity and its ability to distinguish between quacks and competing practitioners. Equally as important, it instilled in orthodox medicine itself a hubris that allowed it to dismiss for well over a century the insights and medical therapeutics of any system outside its sanctioned "science."

The absolutism of the AMA's rejection of alternative practitioners was to get the AMA in trouble again and again. The consultation clause, which threatened to expel any physician who consulted with irregulars, has a sordid history. For example, it played a major role in bringing down the president of the AMA, Morris Fishbein, who from 1920 to 1949 virtually personified the

AMA. In 1942 the California Medical Association (CMA) formed a committee to discuss the merger of medicine and osteopathy. Wielding the consultation clause like a club, Fishbein rode into town to stop the potential merger, claiming that osteopaths were "inferior" and that he would not let the AMA have anything to do with them. He so alienated the CMA that they generated an AMA resolution demanding Fishbein's removal, a resolution that failed, but that started a movement that ultimately succeeded (Campion 1984).

The tone set by the 1847 conference was to persist for almost 150 years. Modern medicine has until recently dismissed virtually all alternative systems wholesale, regarding all as equally unscientific and denying the need to empirically test them. Like their predecessors, they have appealed to science to justify an ideological agenda. Hufford (1995) has described how modern critics of alternative medicine use the term "quackery" to refer indiscriminately to all alternative treatments, describe users of alternative therapies as fools or naïfs being duped by greedy charlatans, cast orthodox medicine as "rational" and unorthodox as "irrational," use a neat circularity to dismiss scientific claims by alternatives as unscientific because "a rational person would know they couldn't work," and so on.

Proposition 3: *At the same time that a dominant medical system dismisses and condemns alternatives, it draws from them, is profoundly influenced by them, and changes its therapeutics because of models tried out by alternatives.*

Although it may seem that it would be to an orthodoxy's benefit to eliminate competitors, challengers serve an important social role for orthodoxies. Marginalized groups can be the testing grounds for new ideas that can then be co-opted by the orthodoxy once they show their efficacy or popularity. For example, the Catholic Church not only accepted subgroups (e.g., Jesuits) that disagreed with the mother church, but also carved out space within the church for them. By doing so, it defused their challenge to the church itself, created a space within the church for individuals who might otherwise leave or disdain the church, and strengthened itself by drawing on the innovations that groups such as the Jesuits developed and by claiming them as the church's own. Alternately, one might think of the 1970s in the United States, when new religious forms (Hare Krishna, the Unification Church) began challenging the mainline churches. In response, the churches co-opted the new spiritualism that made the challengers so attractive to a new generation. The meditation programs, spiritual and ecstatic movements, and revitalized liturgies of many churches were a direct response to the consumer demand identified and exploited so well by the new religious forms of the 1970s.

All of the competing practitioners of the nineteenth century routinely borrowed from each other. Though the ideologues who founded the AMA insisted on ideological purity, it is a mistake to think that the majority of regular physicians subscribed fully to the program. Most, being concerned healers, were more interested in effective therapies for their patients than they were in ideological fealty. In that sense, most nineteenth-century practitioners were eclectics. The medical competition provided a forum for testing therapeutic ideas and techniques, and many physicians drew from them. (If they had not, there would not have been such a strong need for a consultation clause). While this process did mean that many physicians tried out questionable techniques and nostrums, it also meant the regulars were constantly challenged by a wide variety of new ideas and therapeutic approaches.

The result was that even while the regulars were deriding homeopaths, eclectics, and hydropaths and writing consultation clauses, they were slowly moving away from heroic medicine toward the kinder, gentler therapies that those rejected alternatives practiced. For example, the regulars often claimed that homeopathic medicine was no more effective than sugar water, yet they still noted the homeopaths' successes and the fact that many patients got better despite not being given the noxious medicines that the regulars often administered. As one physician (no fan of homeopathy) wrote in 1857: "There is good in everything, and if Homeopathy with all of its fallacies has opened the eyes of all or at least of many to the evils of drugging patients, it has been of service." (quoted in Warner forthcoming).

The same process has been operative in the late twentieth century. Modern alternative medicine has profoundly influenced primary care in the United States. Over the last thirty years, as alternative medicine has increased its profile, many of the very therapies that were being continuously ridiculed by orthodox opponents have been finding their way into the orthodox regimen. The importance of nutrition, low-fat diets, and vitamin supplements; the concept of stress as a pathogen; techniques like meditation, yoga, massage, and biofeedback; the use of magnets to cure pain, acupuncture, and a host of pharmaceuticals drawn from traditional medicines—all were once marginalized ideas that were considered by many as quackery.

Another role alternatives can serve for the orthodoxy is to reintroduce or reinforce traditional orthodox values that have been neglected or trivialized (Wolpe 1990). Modern alternative medicine, for example, dramatically reemphasized such things as the need to establish a trusting, personal doctor-patient relationship, to tend to a patient's spiritual needs, and to listen to a patient's narrative, not only for clues to pathology but also as a subjective experience of disease that needs validation. In fact, a number of orthodox critics of alternative medicine reduced the entire phenomenon to a reminder to physicians to care more about their patients (Burstein 1979; Todd 1979; Candela 1982; Geyman 1984).

In the nineteenth century as in the twentieth, orthodox medicine looked to competitors for ideas and to discern consumer trends in medicine. Once the efficacy or popularity of an approach or technique was demonstrated, it was co-opted or incorporated into orthodox medicine. The best strategy for an orthodoxy, therefore, is to keep alternatives alive, but weakened, to serve as a gatekeeper for new therapeutic ideas.

Proposition 4: *In both eras, the alternative practitioners focused on the harm conventional therapeutics do, their rigid ideology, and their attempts to block competitors from practicing.*

The battle over medicine in the nineteenth century was not one-sided. Irregulars were vocal critics of the regulars, and their attacks were harsh and sustained. (They also spent quite a bit of energy attacking each other.) The remarkable thing about their complaints, however, is how much they resemble the critiques of conventional medicine by alternative medicine in the 1970s and 1980s. Nineteenth-century practitioners attacked primarily by focusing on three issues: the harm conventional therapeutics do, the rigidity of orthodox ideology, and the affront to liberty and individual choice that comes from the state's endorsing a single class of practitioners. Consider the following poem from 1836, written by Samuel Thomson, the founder of Thomsonianism (reprinted in Berman 1951, 411). Here is Samuel Thomson mocking the regulars' treatment of mental illness:

Recipe to Cure a Crazy Man

Soon as the man is growing mad
send for a doctor and have him bled:
Take from his arm two quarts, at least,
Nearly as much as kills a beast.

But if bad symptoms yet remain,
He must tap another vein;
Soon as the doctor has him bled
Then draw a blister on his head.

Next he comes, as it is said,
The blistered skin takes from his head;
The laud'num gives to ease his pain,
Till he can visit him again.

And lest the fever should take hold,
The nitre gives to keep him cold;
And if distraction should remain,
He surely must be bled again.

The bowels now have silent grown,
The Choledocus lost its tone;
He then, bad humours to expel,
The jalap gives with calomel.

The physic works, you well must know,
Till he can neither stand nor go;
If any heat should still remain,
The lancet must be used again.

The man begins to pant for breath,
The doctor says he's stuck with death;
All healing medicine is denied,
I fear the man is mortified.

What sickness, sorrow, pain, and woe,
The human race do undergo,
By learned quacks who sickness make,
I fear, for filthy lucre's sake.

Here the therapies of the regulars are mocked to great effect, creating a stark contrast with Thomson's comparatively benign botanical cures. Hahnemann and the homeopaths who followed him also regularly inveighed against what they perceived as the orthodox follies of their time: polypharmacy, heroic therapy with powerful drugs causing iatrogenic illness, and insufficient attention to the individual patient as a human being. The homeopaths and Thomsonians accused the regulars of the same transgressions that the regulars used to reject them: being tied to a particular healing philosophy and ignoring conflicting empirical evidence. Regulars are closed-minded, said the irregulars, in large part due to the desire to separate themselves from the irregulars. After all, if they admitted that homeopathy or botanical cures worked at all, they would lose their claim to dominance and their push for exclusive licensure. They therefore slavishly adhere to dangerous and ineffective therapies, which cause great harm to patients.

While attacking the regulars' therapeutics, irregulars also fought back politically. Worried that the state would solidify the regulars' power through licensing, the irregulars repeatedly stressed the rights of individuals to make their own healthcare decisions. The Thomsonians used antimonopoly rhetoric to great effect. In 1839 an anonymous editorial in a Thomsonian journal commented, "Every act which gives support to any particular class of practitioner is a violation of the sacred compact, and at war with the rights and liberties of the people" (quoted in Berman 1951, 412). The Thomsonians eventually persuaded virtually every state legislature to repeal its regulations of medical practice.

There is a remarkable congruence between those arguments and the complaints of alternative practitioners 150 years later. No longer true competitors, but now marginalized groups fighting a powerful, entrenched orthodoxy, alternative practitioners of the late twentieth century use arguments and approaches that closely echo those of their predecessors. Consider these quotes from physicians who considered themselves "holistic," recorded in the early 1980s (Wolpe 1987; 1990). First, the claim that medicine is ritualistic, ideologically adhering to conventions of treatment (echoing nineteenth-century claims of sectarianism):

> What conventional medicine does, to me appears often as convention more than scientifically-based. I know there are tomes of information, but a lot of times, the end result will be a choice for a medication, giving it and at the same time ignoring the likelihood of some of the harm it can do. You're making that choice. I know there's science in there, but in my perception, anyway, it's there with convention, and current custom as to what's done.

Next, echoing Thomson, biomedicine is claimed to cause iatrogenic harms:

> In orthodox medicine, so many things they use are harmful, and have bad side effects, and have questionable good results. A lot of the drugs are used temporarily and then taken off the market. There are many potent drugs that do horrible things to people. How can we justify that?

This physician, sounding like a modern eclectic, faults the orthodoxy for its therapeutic rigidity:

So I've become very open-minded. The philosophy of the holistic physician I think has come down to that we are willing to use any diagnostic and therapeutic modality, with reservation, if we see evidence that it can and may help our patient. However, safety to the patient is primary. And we are as interested in not destroying the patient as we are in helping the patient, with the drug or the modality. Therefore, if a modality is totally safe, we're very happy with it, if it is also effective. But if it's effective, but also kills the patient, what good have we done?

The conceit that keeps competitors and alternatives to the orthodoxy going is that the superiority of their system will inevitably win out in the marketplace of ideas. Certainly the followers of the major "irregular" systems of the nineteenth century, as well as the alternative practitioners of the twentieth, thought that was the case; and, as we saw from Proposition 4, they were not entirely wrong. While the orthodoxy won the political battle, it did so by ceding defeat to some degree, at least, to the claims of the alternatives, incorporating into their system many of the therapeutic and ideological correctives that the alternatives advocated.

Proposition 5: *In both eras, after a period of intense competition came a rapprochement.*

The goal of the AMA, both in its initial code and throughout the nineteenth century, was clearly to emerge as the exclusive and legitimated provider of medical care in the United States. The attacks on competitors were strong and prolonged. The writings in regular journals show the passion and approbation with which the regulars attacked the irregulars. After all the insistence on scientific legitimacy, the consultation clause, and the posturing and lobbying for exclusivity, the last thing the regulars seemed poised to do was to welcome the irregulars into their professional societies.

Yet by the end of the nineteenth century, the ideological purity of the medical orthodoxy was beginning to fray. Younger physicians were less tied to the fights for dominance of midcentury, and since the regulars had, to a large degree, won the struggle, they could afford to be more generous to their competitors. Advocating a true empiricism not blinded by ideological infighting, many physicians of the late nineteenth century refuted the idea that there were any important differences between ideological camps, arguing that empirical science was the only needed adjudicator. This resulted in an attack on the AMA code, particularly the consultation clause, which was seen as irrelevant and even insulting since science itself, not regulation, would be the arbiter of therapeutic legitimacy. A fight broke out between the older defenders of the orthodoxy and the defiant younger scientific libertarians. In his presidential address of 1882, P. O. Hooper, first vice president of the AMA (the president, J. J. Woodward, had taken ill overseas and could not give his address), defended the current order:

> I may be permitted to suggest that we should not retreat from our well-chosen lines of defense. One mistaken movement would involve us in a whirl of inconsistencies, tending to place us in a false attitude and bring dishonor upon the profession. The broad lines of demarcation between the irregular and true physician should never be obliterated. Our Association stands prominently forth in its high purposes, and its means of accomplishing these purposes are distinctly enunciated. In the discussion of all ethical questions, a spirit of liberalism has always mingled with a never-sleeping sense of imperative obligation to the established truths of science, of order, or law. I do not say that the time may never come—for there is no perfect work of mortal hands—when your organic laws will require modification and amendment; but until the time does arrive, when the impulse of the great heart of the profession shall be felt and radical changes demanded, in the light of a perfected knowledge, let us maintain without internal strife the unsullied standard of professional honor and morals, now "full high advanced" in our midst, and decline association with those who will not recognize that flag, or who, having once recognized it, have abandoned it. (Hooper 1882, 103)

Despite Hooper's impassioned plea, by the 1890s the opposition to incorporating eclectics and homeopaths into orthodox medicine had, for a variety of reasons, largely dissipated, and by 1903 the AMA code revisions say little about irregulars. Homeopaths and eclectics started being wooed by the very state medical societies that so strongly opposed them a few years before. As the sectarian rivalry diminished, physicians started writing tracts against partisan agitation and in-fighting. Homeopathy, no longer strengthened by its struggle for legitimacy, lost its distinctiveness, and it eventually disappeared into orthodox medicine. The last homeopathic medical school in the United States closed in 1939, and the assimilation (and virtual eventual elimination) of homeopathy was complete.

So too in the twentieth century. After years of grouping most alternatives as quackery, at least fifty major medical schools now teach alternative medicine, and even academic medical centers are providing in-house alternative medical services to patients (Vincler and Nicol 1997; Wilson 1996). The National Institutes of Health is funding research through its new Office of Alternative Medicine. Community hospitals and academic medical centers are opening new services such as the Division of Complementary Medicine (University of Maryland), the Center for Integrative Medicine (Thomas Jefferson University Hospital) and the Center for Alternative Medicine and Longevity (Columbia's Miami Heart Institute). The AMA is suggesting that perhaps doctors should know something about alternative medicine, though it recently pulled back from a commitment to publish a volume on alternative medicine, fearing a conservative backlash (Health Line 1997). Many states are loosening their laws as well. Washington state, for example, passed a law in 1996 mandating insurance coverage of alternative care, and conventional doctors and naturopaths are now working side by side in clinics and collaborating on the care of patients. The consultation clause is finally dead.

There is still resistance, however. In 1994 forty-two physicians, pharmacologists, scientists and others asked the FDA to crack down on the "homeopathy scam" (*JAMA* 1994), and there has also been vocal opposition to NIH's Office of Alternative Medicine (Kolata 1996). Yet the erosion of control of physicians over the healthcare system has allowed the usefulness of alternative medicine as an economic tool of healthcare administrators to override the still substantial resistance of many doctors. There seems a greater willingness of medical students to accept and learn about alternative medicine (Vickers 1997), and that will likely only increase as these services are further integrated into the healthcare system. The integration, however, may well come at great cost to alternative medicine. The routinization and medicalization of these technologies is the inevitable result of mainstreaming them. Alternative medicine today may follow the fate of homeopaths, who fell prey to the promises of establishment medicine, only to disappear within its clutches.

Conclusion

Medicine is a powerful cultural institution. Choosing a system of healing is as much a cultural display of ideology as it is a sober scientific judgment of what works. It should not be surprising to us that medicine follows certain patterns that repeat cyclically. A hundred years from now, long after the current rapprochement has been integrated into medicine, new rifts will have appeared, new power struggles will have been waged, and a new understanding will be forged between the orthodoxy of the day and its competitors.

Medicine's institutional form is determined by its internal ideological power struggles and its resonance with the cultural milieu in which it is embedded. Nineteenth-century sectarianism was successful because it was more in tune (at least in some ways) and more progressive than the "regulars." The middle 1800s were the time of the great reform movements: Horace Mann and public education, the temperance movement, abolitionism. Sectarians capitalized on the spirit of the times by saying that people have the right to choose their own medical care and by posing a system of knowledge that was scientific, rational, and egalitarian. In fact, if we look with an unbiased eye, it was the sectarians who were the progressives of their day. It was the sectarians who thought women had every right to be practitioners, who were nonelitist and democratic, and who believed in the participation of patients in their own care. They were also much better to the poor.

Noting the strength of competing modalities in the nineteenth century, Wrobel (1987, 1–2) wrote:

> The remarkable number of premises, methodologies, and teleological assumptions that [homeopathy, hydropathy, phrenology, mesmerism and so on] shared placed them squarely in the midst of major currents of 19th century thought. Their doctrines complemented the national belief that America occupied a special place in mankind's history; denied the distinction between body and mind, the material and the spiritual; gave credence to the message delivered by reformers that health and happiness are accessible to men; and presented a unified view of knowledge and human nature that seemingly accounted for the structure of nature and man's place within it. Rationalistic, egalitarian, and utilitarian, they struck familiar and reassuring chords that were pleasing to the ears of Americans.

Modern alternative medicine is also in some ways more in sync with the great reform movements of the 1960s and 1970s: environmentalism, peace movements, feminism, the ethic of individual liberty and autonomy, and multiculturalism. It is from that cultural coherence that orthodox medicine is beginning to draw some insights. As in the early twentieth century, two visions of medicine are merging; and the product, we can only hope, may incorporate the best insights of both the orthodoxy and its alternatives.

Notes

1. *Heroic* is the term often used to describe the philosophy of bleeding, cupping, purging, and other techniques used by many nineteenth-century physicians.

2. See Proposition 4 for more on Thomson's opposition to regular medicine.

3. It would be fascinating to see whether, and the degree to which, the founding of the AIH influenced the founding of the AMA. No one, to my knowledge, has yet checked through the correspondence of the founders of the AMA looking specifically for references to the founding of the AIH.

4. Ironically, in the midst of its campaigns against nostrums concocted by other practitioners, the AMA's own journal was filled with questionable advertising of the nostrums of its own physicians. It was not until the turn of the century that the AMA purged its journals of such advertisements.

References

Baker, Robert. 1995. Introduction. In *The Codification of Medical Morality: Historical and Philosophical Studies of the Formalization of Medical Morality in the Eighteenth and Nineteenth Centuries.* Vol. 2, *Anglo-American Medical Ethics and Medical Jurisprudence in the Nineteenth Century,* ed. Robert Baker, 1–22. Dordrecht: Kluwer.

Baker, R.; Porter, D.; and Porter, R., eds. 1993. *The Codification of Medical Morality: Historical and Philosophical Studies of the Formalization of Western Medical Morality in the Eighteenth and Nineteenth Centuries.* Vol. 1, *Medical Ethics and Etiquette in the Eighteenth Century.* Dordrecht: Kluwer.

Berlant, Jeffrey L. 1975. *Profession and Monopoly.* Berkeley: University of California Press.

Berman, Alex. 1951. The Thomsonian Movement and Its Relation to American Pharmacy and Medicine. *Bulletin of the History of Medicine* 25(5):405–538.

Brody, G. S. 1980. Holistic Medicine and Unscientific Cults. *Western Journal of Medicine* 133(2):172–73.

Brown, Helen. 1975. Cancer Quackery: What Can You Do About It? *Nursing,* 75:24–26.

Burstein, A. G. 1979. What the (W)hole is Hellism? *Pharos* (Fall):31.

Campion, Frank D. 1984. *The AMA and U.S. Health Policy Since 1940.* Chicago: Chicago Review Press.

Candela, L. J. 1982. Is There a Need for the Holistic Physician? *New York State Journal of Medicine* 3:301–2.

Fitzgerald, F. T. 1983. Science and Scam: Alternative Thought Patterns in Alternative Health Care. *New England Journal of Medicine* 309(17):1066–67.

Geyman, J. P. 1984. Holistic Health Care: Neither New Nor Coherent. *Journal of Family Practice* 19(6):727–28.

Glymour C., and Stalker, D. 1983. Engineers, Cranks, Physicians, Magicians. *New England Journal of Medicine* 308:960–64.

Health Line. 1997. AMA Backs Away from Alternative Medicine Book. 26 September.

Hooper, P. O. 1882. Address of P. O. Hooper, M.D., First Vice-President of the Association. *The Transactions of the American Medical Association* 33:103.

Hufford, David. 1995. Cultural and Social Perspectives on Alternative Medicine. *Alternative Therapies* 1:53–61.

Journal of the American Medical Association (JAMA). 1991. Maharishi Ayur-Veda (letters). *JAMA* 266(13):1769–74.

———1993a. Alternative Medicine Office Urged to Act Rapidly. *JAMA* 270(12):1400.

———. 1993b. Science Reporters Hear a Wide Range of Recent Data at 12th Annual Conference. *JAMA* 270(20):2413.

———. 1994. FDA Petitioned to "Stop Homeopathy Scam." *JAMA* 272(15):1154–55.

Kabler, J. D. 1981. Holistic Medicine. *Wisconsin Medical Journal* 80:13.

Kett, J. 1968. *The Formation of the American Medical Profession: The Role of Institutions, 1760–1860.* New Haven: Yale University Press.

King, Lester S. 1982. The "Old Code" of Medical Ethics and Some Problems It Had to Face. *JAMA* 248(18):2329–33.

Kolata, Gina. 1996. In Quests Outside Mainstream, Medical Projects Rewrite Rules. *New York Times,* 18 June, A1, B7.

Lange, R. H. 1980. Holistic Health: Is All Medicine Whole? *New York State Journal of Medicine* 1:996–99.

Starr, Paul. 1982. *The Social Transformation of American Medicine.* New York: Basic Books.

Stoehr, Taylor. 1987. Robert H. Collyer's Technology of the Soul. In *Pseudo-Science and Society in Nineteenth-Century America,* ed. Arthur Wrobel, 21–45. Lexington: University Press of Kentucky.

Todd, M. 1979. Interface: Holistic Health and Traditional Medicine. *Western Journal of Medicine* 131:464–65.

Vickers, A. 1997. A Proposal for Teaching Critical Thinking to Students and Practitioners of Complementary Medicine. *Alternative Therapies in Health and Medicine* 3:57–62.

Vincler, Lisa A., and Nicol, Mary F. 1997. When Ignorance Isn't Bliss: What Healthcare Practitioners and Facilities Should Know about Complementary and Alternative Medicine. *Journal of Health and Hospital Law* 30(3):160.

Wallis, Roy, and Morley, P. 1976. *Marginal Medicine.* London: Peter Owen, Ltd..

Warner, John Harley. (1987). Medical Sectarianism, Therapeutic Conflict, and the Shaping of Orthodox Professional Identity in Antebellum American Medicine. In *Medical Fringe & Medical Orthodoxy 1750–1850.* Ed. W. F. Bynum and Roy Porter, London: Croom Helm.

———. Forthcoming. Orthodoxy and Otherness: Homeopathy and Regular Medicine in Nineteenth-Century America. In *Culture, Knowledge, and Healing: Historical Perspectives of Homeopathic Medicine in Europe and North America,* ed. Robert Juette, Guenter B. Risse, and John Woodward. Sheffield: European Association for the History of Health and Medicine.

Wilson, R. 1996. Unconventional Cures. *Chronicle of Higher Education,* 12 January, A15–16

Wolpe, Paul R. 1985. The Maintenance of Professional Authority: Acupuncture and the American Physician. *Social Problems* 32:409–24.

————. 1987. Shamans of the Metropolis: Holistic Physicians and Cultural Movements in Modern Medicine. Ph.D. diss., Yale University.

————. 1990. The Holistic Heresy: Strategies of Ideological Control in the Medical Profession. *Social Science and Medicine* 31:913–23.

————. 1994. The Dynamics of Heresy in a Profession. *Social Science and Medicine* 39:1133–48.

Wrobel, Arthur. 1987. Introduction. In *Pseudo-Science and Society in Nineteenth-Century America*, ed. Arthur Wrobel, 1–20. Lexington: University Press of Kentucky.

Young, James Harvey. 1967. *The Medical Messiahs.* Princeton: Princeton University Press.

15

The Challenge of Serving
Both Patient and Populace

CHRISTINE K. CASSEL, M.D.

During this time of turbulent change in health care, we are surrounded by much discussion focusing on population health. Some of this discussion stems from an increasing awareness of the importance of using a population framework to evaluate preventive needs, to initiate preventive interventions, and to assess outcomes of preventive measures. Some is a consequence of the managed-care framework that allows health plans, at least theoretically, to take responsibility for the health of populations, thus focusing analysis on health issues within specific population groups. Much of this talk is rhetorical, used for marketing purposes or as superficial, poorly understood descriptions of what some hope may be advances in the cost effectiveness of health care; yet the concept of population health offers real promises and poses real challenges and risks to the medical profession.

Leaders of healthcare organizations, including many physicians, are excited that we are now thinking about populations and about promoting healthiness. Yet we must view the new managed-care opportunities with a completely open mind and seriously ask ourselves whether this development is good or bad. On the one hand, we might think that surely no one could be opposed to a population approach to health care. It seems to be an unquestioned, affirmative duty; and it offers new potential for measurement and thus new, higher, and better standards of accountability. On the other hand, a population approach may appear to pose problems, in part because it requires drastic changes in the fundamental tenets on which the traditional medical-ethics model is based (Pellegrino 1996). Some may view a population approach as a challenge to the fiduciary relationship between physician and patient because a focus on population health inherently suggests choices made on behalf of the group rather than on behalf of the individual, especially in cases of limited resources. However, this fiduciary trust is not necessarily threatened by population health, since all individual patient care is an outgrowth of the scientific study of populations. In addition, the goals of these two models—to improve health and the quality of care—are congruent.

Another, more serious division between the two models emanates from the broad perspective of a population context in which resources that might have been available for one patient may, instead, be more effective if reallocated to benefit many more people. Such reallocations may be, by a utilitarian ethic, seeking the greatest good for the greatest number. The traditional ethics of clinical medicine, however, have grown, not from a utilitarian base, but from one that emphasizes rules and duties to individuals. Public health, in contrast, has always explicitly incorporated a utilitarian framework. This conflict is fundamental and needs to be explicated more thoroughly and understood more profoundly before we can decide whether a transition to a population-based medicine with its utilitarian ethic is good or bad.

Most physicians do not understand population medicine. They do not even know how to measure, evaluate, or conceptualize population health. One reason for this is a longstanding split between the disciplines of public health and medicine. This absence of expertise and lack of availability of relevant information are also barriers to a serious approach to population health by practicing physicians. In European countries the situation is quite different. Physicians and public health professionals interact much more closely. They train in the same schools and take the same courses. In practice, these physicians work closely with public health departments not only in reporting infectious and communicable diseases but also in arranging healthcare delivery for a particularly needy population during times of epidemics or simply when it is more efficient to work through public-sector organizations. In the United States public health and medicine diverged at the end of the nineteenth century at approximately the same time that the American Medical Association (AMA) was approaching a crisis over its nature and definition (see chap. 3, this volume). At that time, practicing physicians began to view themselves as more of a private-sector "guild" than as public servants engaged in political activity. Interestingly, in Europe during approximately that same time period, the legendary Rudolf Virchow prophesied that "politics is but medicine writ large," understanding the extent to which socioeconomic factors, affected by political decisions, have a dramatic impact on the health of individuals in populations (Rosen 1958, 254–58).

In the early twentieth century in the wake of the Flexner Report (Ludmerer

1985), when medical education was dramatically restricted and improved, medical schools began to develop separately from schools of public health. Since then medicine has been primarily, often exclusively, focused on the individual doctor-patient relationship (Barondess 1991). Any social or common role—if present at all—has been merely an afterthought. The 1847 AMA Code of Ethics had a section on the physician's responsibility to the community, but this was abandoned in the "reforms" of 1903 and was reasserted only in the late 1950s. Even now it is a vague exhortation rather than a scientifically based description of responsibilities to population health (AMA 1997). Medical students have limited exposure to the science of epidemiology, and most remember it as a course they either skipped, or to which they paid little attention, because it did not weigh heavily toward their grade and was not considered a "core" topic by their professors.

Yet now, as a consequence of the managed-care revolution, we find ourselves using the language of population health. Although this language is not new, it does have new force and relevance. If we were able to give physicians the tools to truly understand population health, would it then be easily incorporated into the practice of medicine in managed-care organizations? Would it be practically possible to integrate population medicine into managed care? The answer is not an easy one. The concept of population health requires a stable population for which one is held accountable or in whom one is interested. In every other Western country, universal healthcare insurance allows information to be collected about entire populations and then analyzed geographically. In the United States, however, even managed-care plans that have an adequate information base do not reflect any coherent population. Furthermore, in the churning of the marketplace, people frequently change health plans; thus, the effect of preventive measures over time, for example, is difficult to evaluate. The overlap of public health departments, their data bases, and their at-risk populations is not identical to that of any particular managed-care plan; therefore, promoting a closer collaboration with a public health authority is complex and does not immediately solve the problem at hand.

Population health care requires a conception of a "population." Who are we referring to in our discussion of population health? Is a population limited only to a managed-care physician's own patients? Are these only his or her patients at that particular time but not those last year or next year? Are these only patients enrolled in a given managed-care plan? Can we overcome the privacy and confidentiality issues inherent in having a single kind of identifier for all citizens regardless of their managed-care plan? While population health is, in theory, a good idea, one must certainly define the population at risk before it makes any sense. Until this occurs, physicians who are committed to science and rationality will be unable to engage in any meaningful way with the concept of population health. They will not be able to effectuate goals of population health without understanding for which population they are responsible.

Population Health Measures

If population health is our goal, what are the appropriate measures of success or failure? The traditional information that a physician obtains about his panel of patients usually does not include an epidemiologic database. Most physicians are not trained in public health or epidemiology and are much better at "numerator medicine"—the treatment of individual patients—but lack an understanding of the "denominator"—the workings of disease within the population as a whole. At its simplest, physicians should understand the existing prevalence of a given disorder within their population.

A misunderstanding of population health care is also reflected in the public controversy over screening-test recommendations. For example, in 1997 the nation witnessed a solid mathematically based recommendation that women over fifty should be screened by mammography for breast cancer at least every two years. The recommendation was exceedingly important because many women, particularly those in older age groups, are not adequately screened. Yet many members of the public, and Congress as well, failing to understand the difference between "screening" and "case finding," viewed this recommendation as somehow neglecting women under fifty. Subsequently, when public pressure led Congress to overturn the recommendations of the NIH, and the NIH—in an extraordinarily unscientific piece of public policy—caved in to that pressure, we witnessed one of the most painful political diversions of health policy. Totally disdainful of science, Congress and many physicians supported NIH's retraction of its recommendation.

To offer a classic "utilitarian" argument: It makes better sense to focus a recommendation for universal testing on a population where the risk is greater, namely those over fifty, than those at least risk, namely those under fifty; but this does not mean that a younger woman with a family history of breast cancer or any other reason for concern should not be tested by her physician. Urging unnecessary testing in younger women will just make it more difficult to pay for testing in older women—who are, moreover, already underserved and for whom cancer risk is much greater. Yet physicians did not speak out meaningfully in this debate.

The United States will be unable to work within a framework of population health in any rigorous or meaningful manner until physicians themselves are educated well enough to assume a leadership role and educate the public to accept these sound policies—policies that will have a greater impact on public health than those based simply on public opinion and interest-group politics.

Population Health and Medical Ethics

The problems discussed thus far are conceptual and logistical, but are they ethical? The moral issue is partially one of honesty and integrity, derived, in part, from our inability to really mean what we say when we state that we are concerned about "population health." Are we being hypocritical when we talk about population health and yet do nothing to create a health system that makes it possible to even begin to achieve population health measures?

The most important moral problems that ensue from a population-health framework for health care come from the nature of the fiduciary relationship. Although it is possible to focus on population-health outcomes in a context of unlimited resources, this is not the reality that we face. Throughout this century population health, as a focus of public health policy, has been used to make difficult decisions about the most cost-effective use of limited, usually public resources in the pursuit of health. An example is the decision to invest in increased access to prenatal care in an attempt to reduce the cost of expensive premature and complicated deliveries.

The ideals of population health take on new significance in the context of so-called managed care. Managed care is taking hold in the United States in part because it promises to reduce healthcare costs. While many believe that managed care provides better care, especially the capitation models, the primary interest of employers who purchase managed care for their employees is in cost, not quality. Savings go to profits for shareholders rather than to expanding access (Cassel 1996). Managed care may improve access to preventive measures for those individuals enrolled in that health plan at a particular moment in time, but that is an exceedingly constrained view of the concept of population health. The diverse types of managed care that are available do not expand access and thus do not substantially improve the health of the uninsured population.

The context of resource constraints exists within any of these models, and thus tests or therapies that are only marginally effective are often unavailable or less available than they might be in an unfettered fee-for-service system. This type of decision making is not inherently unethical. Indeed, it may be viewed as even more ethical, because unnecessary tests and procedures do not necessarily contribute to an individual's health. Every medical intervention, moreover, has some associated risks, and overtreatment can be just as risky as undertreatment. This was part of the argument to constrain unnecessary mammography.

Nonetheless, insofar as managed care is "population health care," it necessarily affects the physician-patient relationship. The patient becomes a member of a broader community or "population" for whom the physician is responsible. In the 1970s, when medical-ethics literature began to confront the problem of resource constraints, almost every ethicist counseled the same dogma—that the physician should do everything possible for the individual patient and that society should somehow determine how to handle the problem of resource constraints (Hiatt 1975). Today, however, the same advisors require physicians to challenge a "faceless government" or the "corporate bureaucrats" making healthcare decisions—even though, ironically, the ethicists of the 1970s recommended that physicians stay away from rationing decisions. Thus most physicians today want a greater role in resource allocation.

We will have to take seriously the dramatic paradigm shift that these conflicts bring into the patient-physician relationship. The physician still must have a professional fiduciary relationship with each patient and do whatever is best for that patient, within reasonable limits, however those are set. Should the patient be informed about those reasonable limits before entering the healthcare plan? A recent study by the Commonwealth Fund suggests that more than 50 percent of people receiving health care through their employers are offered only one health plan, and the vast majority who do have a choice are offered only two (Davis, Schoen, and Sandman 1996). What kind of "choice" exists for patients in this type of setting? Can the caveat emptor model work here? Even if it could (e.g., for federal employees and Congresspersons, who have a wider range of choices), this is still not a comfortable role for physicians. Are we to say to our patients, "If you choose this lower-cost model, you are accepting the limits that it implies"? In fact, we may even be implying something stronger: "If you accept this lower-cost model, you are asking me to exercise prudence in the use of healthcare resources." Few people view their doctors as directly responsible for what they pay for their health care, but perhaps a more explicit link would create a more honest and, in the long run, more beneficial relationship between doctors and patients in this new paradigm.

Under the premise of capitated managed care, physicians are responsible for managing the care and spending their patients' money (and, just as importantly, the employers' money) as prudently as possible. Inevitably, this means rationing decisions—preferably at the margin of extremely ineffective or experimental treatments. It is important to point out here that what is extremely ineffective in one population may be far more relevant in another. To take an extreme example, needle exchange as a way of preventing AIDS would not be as effective in a population whose AIDS risk is predominantly based on sexual exposure. The scientific and epidemiologic base of population health and the limits thereto are also directly relevant to the moral context we are discussing here.

Rationing: The Physician as Prudent Purchaser

The clarity afforded us before Medicare and Medicaid, when we implicitly used ability to pay as a rationing principle, is now gone. This is not to say that we do not ration by ability to pay. Indeed, we do. Extensive research indicates that the poor and the uninsured receive worse care and have less access to high-quality care than those with better forms of insurance (Blumberg and Liska 1996).

We ration by ability to pay rather than by what most likely will help the individual patient, and we often do this covertly. We depend on "the market," but we do not explicitly ask patients what they can afford. One of the most astounding findings of the SUPPORT Study was that many families lost all of their life savings during their dying family member's final episode of illness, yet the physicians involved in the patient's care had no idea of this cost to the families (Covinsky et al. 1996). As physicians, we should be ashamed of these findings and should be working hard to determine how to even the playing field. But we cannot do this until we first learn how to take the concepts of population health seriously and how to make difficult choices within a rigorous and substantial epidemiologic framework.

Perhaps, when enrolling in a managed-care plan, patients should sign an informed consent form stating that they understand they are placing their medical care into the hands of this specific physician and health system, who are responsible for prudently managing the healthcare dollars, which may, in turn, make certain treatments unavailable. What should a patient know before making such a decision? Is there an accountability for quality as well as for costs? And can we also claim an accountability for prudence? If we did this, we would need to seriously consider, among other things, alternatives to traditional liability law, such as enterprise liability or no-fault insurance.

The physician-patient relationship in our society has traditionally been based on an expectation that the patient was significantly vulnerable, both because of potentially being ill and therefore in need of care, and also because of the physician having a significantly disproportionate amount of information about the technical medical issues involved. Thus, the physician had a responsibility to act in the best interests of that patient and put that patient's interests above all others. This tradition was grounded in the ethical responsibilities of beneficence and was strongly rooted in the Hippocratic tradition. In the modern world we have many different factors influencing the doctor-patient relationship and potentially changing it in fundamental ways. These factors include the following:

- We understand that medical science operates within a good deal of uncertainty. We have many more diagnostic and therapeutic options for every patient that we see, and therefore the costs of medical care have grown enormously.
- Concerned about the rising costs of medical care, employers and public funders have put pressure on providers to find ways to reduce those costs. But it is not only the third-party payers who are concerned. Patients themselves, who have now come to be called consumers, are concerned about growing costs because their out-of-pocket expenses have grown enormously.
- Thus, these "consumers" share the concern of employers and public funders about rising costs and are increasingly choosing health plans (when they have a choice) where more services are covered at lower costs. These plans tend to be managed-care plans in which some degree of choice is restricted to keep costs down.
- Within provider groups striving to keep costs down, one important target is to reduce the use of services that are not documented as truly contributing to positive health outcomes. Much of what is done in medicine cannot be precisely justified, for example, by expensive and extensive randomized clinical trials that provide conclusive statistical information about efficacy. Much of medical diagnosis and treatment is based on smaller sample sizes, on personal experience, and on so-called clinical judgment. While it is important that we invest in more research to understand the scientific basis for outcomes, we must also understand that we will never have 100 percent statistical confidence about everything we do. Clinical judgment will remain important.
- But there are many medical interventions that have only marginal utility and where a legitimate and wise purchaser (the consumer), understand-

ing the nature of these marginal interventions, might select a health plan that does not offer those services of marginal utility or unproven utility, in exchange for expanded benefits known to be more efficacious.

- If the consumer were given this responsibility, the physician would then be charged with being a prudent purchaser on behalf of that patient. It would be necessary for that physician to be well-versed in epidemiologic science and the principles of population health, as well as in cost-effectiveness management.

- For this model to work, the physician's responsibility would have to be legally redefined so that a decision not to use an experimental and unproven treatment, for example, could be justified based on the greater benefit to the population served by that physician. Currently, physicians are still held responsible for decisions they make in the context only of the individual patient, not of the population. The individual patients involved would have to be willing to accept this kind of model.

The pitfall of such a physician-as-purchaser model is that it changes the traditional Hippocratic doctor-patient relationship. The strengths of the model are that it reflects in a scientific way what is happening in the marketplace and that it does not make the physician's decision strictly based on an economic self-interest model—a model that worries so many commentators who see physician rewards for undertreatment as a serious threat to the quality of medical care. It recognizes the commercialization of medical services and gives the patient certain responsibilities as a consumer. The corollary of these responsibilities would be a set of consumer rights that the President's Advisory Commission on Consumer Protection and Quality in the Health Care Industry is currently discussing.

This role of prudent purchaser poses great anxieties and indeed threats to physicians, but it is an increasingly important role for them to play. As scientific advances increasingly offer improved function and effective treatments for diseases related to aging—such as osteoarthritis, osteoporosis, Alzheimer disease, heart disease, and cancer—the success story of the aging of our population will come to sit firmly on the shoulders of whomever is doing the rationing. This could be physicians, bureaucrats, or a combination of the two, perhaps even including community members, similar to what occurred with the Oregon Plan. If the federal government decides to look to managed care as a means of handling the exploding costs of the Medicare program, this challenge will become increasingly acute (Morgan et al. 1997). To date, roughly 15 percent of Medicare patients are under some type of managed-care plan, and many experts doubt that under the current arrangement these plans will be popular among those at higher risk of illness (Davis, Schoen, and Sandman 1996).

Politicians can, however, change the incentives so that traditional Medicare becomes more costly out-of-pocket, or HMOs become more attractive, or both. If this occurs, we may be talking about rationing not only marginally effective treatments but also treatments known to have some effect. To do this on a firm moral base would require an interaction between the physician and the community for whom this financing is intended. Here again, we face the importance of a stably defined population who would themselves delineate a set of priorities for healthcare spending. This can only occur in a setting where health care is universal or at least where marketplace competition does not lead to rapid and frequent turnover.

But even in such an ideal, Oregon-like situation, with a true democratic or even communitarian approach to population health and health-spending priorities, we will be forced to rewrite the Hippocratic Oath and add some new chapters to the AMA Code of Ethics. Even the one component of the code that mentions the health of the community does so obliquely. All the other features of the code refer to the physician's responsibility to the profession, to colleagues, or to individual patients. The complexities of real responsibility for population health have not yet begun to be addressed by any of the traditional codes of ethics.

Furthermore, judging by recent legal settlements, the law still holds the individual physician responsible for doing whatever might benefit the patient, regardless of the patient-payment category or of how slim the chances of success. Attempts at enterprise liability or no-fault approaches to medical malpractice (American College of Physicians 1995) remain minimal, and organized medicine has yet to embrace anything other than the traditionally taught model, while at the same time trying to reduce risk by enforcing caps on awards. Medical liability may need a new conceptual framework as dramatically different as that of medical practice in an environment where the goal is population health. This is the brave new world in which we must be accountable not only for quality but also for cost.

Conclusion

When William Carlos Williams practiced medicine before World War II, ability to pay was a clear rationing principle. His stories reflect the difficult decisions he put before his patients, knowing that their ability to pay was a major factor in determining what would get done (Williams 1984). Williams practiced before Medicare, Medicaid, or any other health insurance was available to most people. He took for granted that poor people could not afford much that might be available to them, and the tragedy that implied accounts for much of the vitality of his stories. The limits of what he might do for them, however, did not intrude upon his sense of loyalty to his patients, and he frequently provided his own treatment without payment to those who could not otherwise afford to receive it.

Population health is a major shift from Hippocratic medicine. How can the traditional Hippocratic ethic of unwavering and selfless responsibility to one's patients be combined with a utilitarian judgment in which one decides to do the greatest good for the greatest number? Many political and bioethical analysts believed this conflict could be resolved by including "the community" within the broader allocation frameworks (Emanuel 1991) or even by specific rationing decisions such as the Oregon Health Plan, which was remarkably successful at constraining some Medicaid expenditures in order to expand coverage to the working uninsured. If we are to involve the community in these frameworks, we must define *community*. Does it include all Americans or only those with private insurance? Or is it only Americans with insurance this year? Until that is determined, it is extremely difficult to generalize about the role of the community and the allocation of resources.

With universal coverage, the concept of community underlying population health goals is much more meaningful. This would be an ideal moral framework in which to construct a benefit structure that would be flexible enough to change with scientific advances and that would reflect the values of both the enrollees and the healthcare providers. The argument is both moral and practical. First, morally, we have ample evidence that being uninsured leads to worse health outcomes; therefore, goals of population health must work from this fact. Second, only universal systems allow coherent health data and geographic descriptions of populations that make epidemiologic measurements accurate enough to assess which health issues should be given priority. The transition to a utilitarian ethic will be difficult enough for U.S. physicians to do, and to do well. Lack of a universal commitment to access and to a broad population base will make it much more difficult. Anything in between is simply population rhetoric, not population health.

References

American College of Physicians. 1995. Beyond MICRA: New Ideas for Liability Reform. *Annals of Internal Medicine* 122:466–73.

American Medical Association (AMA). 1997. *Code of Medical Ethics: Current Opinions with Annotations.* American Medical Association: Chicago.

Barondess, Jeremiah A. 1991. The Academic Health Center and the Public Agenda: Whose Three-legged Stool? *Annals of Internal Medicine* 115:962–67.

Blumberg, Linda J., and Liska, David W. 1996. *The Uninsured in the United States: A Status Report.* Washington, D.C.: Urban Institute.

Cassel, Christine K. 1996. The Patient-Physician Covenant: An Affirmation of Asklepios. *Annals of Internal Medicine* 124:604–6.

Covinsky, Kenneth E.; Landefeld, Seth; Teno, Joan; Connors, Alfred; Dawson, Neal; Youngner, Stuart; Desbiens, Norman; Lynne, Joanne; Fulkerson, William; Reding, Douglas; Oye, Robert; and Phillips, Russell S. 1996. Is Economic Hardship on the Families of the Seriously Ill Associated with Patient Surrogate Care Preferences? *Archives of Internal Medicine* 156:1737–41.

Davis, Karen; Schoen, Cathy; and Sandman, David R. 1996. The Culture of Managed Care: Implications for Patients. *Bulletin of the New York Academy of Medicine* 73:173–83.

Emanuel, Ezekiel J. 1991. *The Ends of Human Life: Medical Ethics in a Liberal Policy.* Cambridge: Harvard University Press.

Hiatt, Howard H. 1975. Protecting the Medical Commons: Who is Responsible? *The New England Journal of Medicine* 293:235–41.

Ludmerer, Kenneth. 1985. *Learning to Heal: The Development of American Medical Education.* New York: Basic Books.

Morgan, Robert O.; Virnig, Beth A.; DeVito, Carolee; and Persily, Nancy A. 1997. The Medicare-HMO Revolving Door—The Healthy Go In and the Sick Go Out. *The New England Journal of Medicine* 337:169–75.

Pellegrino, Edmund D. 1996. Ethics. *Journal of the American Medical Association* 275:1807–9.

Rosen, George. 1958. *A History of Public Health.* New York: MD Publications.

Williams, William Carlos. 1984. *The Doctor Stories.* Ed. Robert Coles. New York: New Directions.

16

The Challenge of Universal Access to Health Care with Limited Resources

ROBERT M. TENERY JR., M.D.

There are a multitude of problems facing our healthcare delivery system that must be addressed if it is to serve this country in the twenty-first century: the exploding costs of health care services that consume an ever-increasing portion of our national, state, and local expenditures; the decreasing amount of resources and increasing waits for services that are being endured by our growing indigent and underprivileged population; and the overwhelming number of regulations, coupled with decreasing reimbursement, faced by those who deliver health care services, to name just a few.

However, this country is where it is today, not because of how poorly, but because of how well the healthcare system has performed. Led by the physician community, hospitals, teaching and research institutions, and drug companies all joined together to develop the highest level of health care in the history of mankind. But all these accomplishments have come at a price. This country also has the world's most expensive healthcare delivery system.

Until recently, providers of healthcare services have been able to make up for much of the loss of reimbursement on patients who could not afford to pay by what is widely referred to as "cost shifting." However, due to the decreasing level of reimbursement for all covered services, this is no longer possible. Thus, many in our disadvantaged population are forced to seek care only through publicly funded programs. In increasing numbers, many get no care at all except for emergency conditions.

In other words, the advances in medical technology have outstripped this country's ability to pay for health care and to make it available to the majority of our population. Thus, one of the major challenges facing our elected leadership and the medical community is how to properly allocate and fund the limited resources that are available so that the citizens of this country receive the most benefit.

The answer to this most difficult problem may be found by asking the right question: Where can we, as a just society, best put this country's healthcare dollars and limited resources? Traditionally, much of that funding has been used in the last three months of life, instead of in the first three months of life. Much of it is used to treat patients who have no chance of meaningful survival, instead of on the 33 percent of the children in this country under the age of two who are not adequately immunized against infectious diseases. Unfortunately, an increasing amount goes to pay for the salaries of the growing number of regulators of healthcare services, instead of to the care of our disabled, disadvantaged, and uninsured.

These are allocation problems. These are access problems that strike at the very core of the American ethic. Who gets care and who does not? Only by bringing the various elements of our society together can there be any hope of solving these issues. Access to, and allocation of, the limited healthcare resources will be at the center of the ethical dilemmas that will challenge our generation and many generations to come.

Society is a product of a social contract among its citizens, who follow mutually agreed-upon rules in order to gain benefits. Certain obligations are thus assumed by society for those individuals included within its social contract. One of those obligations is access to a basic level of affordable healthcare services. According to policy established by the American Medical Association (AMA 1994), no patient should be deprived of necessary care because of inability to pay for that care (Policy 140.75). These obligations, however, create conflicts not only between groups of patients vying for limited healthcare dollars, but between individual patients as well.

Traditionally in this country, we have focused on taking care of one patient at a time. Virtually all available resources have been directed toward overcoming each patient's malady, regardless of the cost or the patient's ability to pay. However, with the rapidly increasing expenditures for healthcare services and the growing financial restraints being placed on funding, this era of unlimited access is coming to an end. No longer can patients assume that everything medicine has to offer will be made available to them in their time of need. Rationing, or allocation of resources, as some call it, is a reality.

The practice of rationing is not new. It is seen every day with the allotment process for organ donation and allocation of the limited number of intensive care beds to those individuals who are most likely to obtain benefit. What *is* new, however, is that this cost-benefit rationing approach is becoming the norm, even for some of the basic healthcare services. Thus, a balance is evolving in which we weigh the needs of individual patients against those of the rest of the patients within the particular healthcare delivery system. The number of services available to all patients within that system is being limited to fit within the funding allocation—for example, the pool of funds in a capitated system. This not only creates potential discrepancies between individual delivery systems, but it also creates potential conflicts among individuals competing for services within each system.

Although it is considered to be a more efficient means of dividing up the healthcare dollar, this approach subordinates the rights of the individual patient to the group. At peril of bankrupting the funding system in which they participate, physicians are forced into the role of "playing God"—mediating between the interests of the patients under their care. While this role is not new to physicians, in the past it rarely required compromising the care of one patient for the sake of others.

Secondarily, there are concerns about whether patients enter into these arrangements of their own free will and whether they are adequately informed about the consequences of their actions. In a larger sense, however, when dealing with healthcare systems with limited resources, one could question whether individuals have the right to make allocation decisions in the first place (Tenery 1996).

Two ethical principles confer an obligation to provide access to adequate health care (CEJA 1994). The first is the ethical principle of *collective protection*: society assumes a duty to protect its citizens from general threats such as crime, fire, foreign and local military aggression, and disease. In general, the obligation of collective protection derives from the social contract and applies in the public domain, not to particular individual patients. However, since the health of the community is no better than the health of its individual members, the principle implies that at least some of the healthcare needs of individuals must be met. Failure to adequately protect the health of the individual can potentially lead to serious public-health problems, such as epidemics created by exposure to individuals with highly contagious diseases. The obligation of collective protection thus also extends to providing a safe water supply, clean air, building codes to ensure sanitary conditions, and inspection of the food supply. Public funding is widely accepted as a means of support for the construction and maintenance of our medical teaching and research institutions. These symbolize the extension of society's obligation to provide charity care for the indigent and to extend advances in medical science and technology to everyone in society.

A second ethical principle, *fair opportunity*, upholds society's obligation to provide its citizens with access to an affordable level of basic healthcare services. The ethical principle of fair opportunity states that a just society helps its citizens to "counteract the lack of opportunity caused by unpredictable bad luck and misfortune, over which the person has no meaningful control. Insofar as injury or disease creates these profoundly significant disadvantages and disturbs our moral capacity to function properly, justice suggests that resources be used to counter the disadvantaging effects" (Beauchamp and Childress 1989, 277) Under this principle, each individual within society should be allowed to cultivate his or her talents, develop skills, and pursue goals without unjust interference from others. This is accomplished by providing each citizen with access to adequate amounts of the basic goods that will allow these individuals to survive and to flourish if they are so inclined. The basic goods are usually considered to be food, shelter, and clothing; but the concept is easily extended to include education and effective healthcare services. For without the latter, the individual's ability to succeed is greatly diminished.

The argument for providing access to a basic level of health care is justified because illnesses may diminish an individual's ability to pursue goals and take advantage of opportunities. Although access to adequate health care can never ensure freedom from illness, such access does, at the very least, contribute to the chances of maintaining good health. Thus, through the principle of fair opportunity, society's obligation to provide its citizens access to an affordable level of basic healthcare services is upheld.

A second obligation under the principle of fair opportunity is to insure that potential opportunities for individuals to succeed are not affected by traits and circumstances over which they have no control. Thus, discrimination on the basis of race, gender, and physical characteristics such as height and weight would clearly be unjust.

In general, the onset of illness can be considered to be an undeserved circumstance over which individuals have little or no control. Some may claim that many illnesses are a consequence of unhealthy behavior, such as smoking, alcohol and drug abuse, poor dietary habits, or inadequate exercise; however, this does not necessarily mean that individuals should always be held responsible, since such behavior is often a consequence of an addictive disease or of lower socioeconomic status, over which individuals have little control.

Although access to adequate healthcare services is no guarantee against ill health, society's fulfilling of its obligations under the principles of fair opportunity and collective protection would at least make it more likely that individuals would have an opportunity to enjoy life. Thus, these arguments seem to support the view that every citizen is entitled to a basic level of healthcare services. The benefits of this entitlement would also accrue to the larger segment of society with whom these individuals might come in contact. By addressing the medical problems of the individual citizen, the exorbitant social costs that result from delay of appropriate services for our disadvantaged and uninsured could conceivably be lessened.

Once the argument for the right to a basic level of health care has been made, the next question that must be resolved is whether that right is to be realized through universal coverage or through universal access. Such questions concerning funding mechanisms brought down the healthcare reform debate raised by the Clinton administration several years ago.

When discussing health-system reform, the terms *universal access* and *universal coverage* are frequently used interchangeably. This leads to confusion. *Universal access* is a method of making health care available and affordable to all our citizens. *Universal coverage* is a required funding mechanism for universal access. They are clearly not the same, and they have totally different financial consequences.

Universal access can be achieved either through federal takeover and control of the healthcare delivery system or through major changes in the health-insurance industry. After observing the effects of a government-controlled single-payer system in countries like Canada, most of our elected leadership seem to prefer the latter.

Universal access through health-insurance reform would involve requiring insurance companies to combine their resources, forming large funding pools to spread their risks. This would then allow them to offer an affordable package of medical benefits that would be community-rated and portable, and would have limited exemptions for preexisting conditions. The benefits package developed under universal access by itself would not be mandatory; thus, those who elected not to avail themselves of the coverage would have that right.

Universal coverage, on the other hand, would require all individuals to obtain healthcare coverage by one of several possible methods. With this concept, the availability of services is taken for granted. The problem then becomes how to accomplish the necessary funding.

There are three potential funding mechanisms for universal coverage: a single-payer system, an employer mandate, and individual mandates. In a Canadian-style *single-payer system*, there would be federal control, and funding would most likely be accomplished by levying a general revenue tax of some type. Besides being unpopular, this option raises the question of the government's ability to control costs without affecting the quality of health care. *Employer mandate* requires funding by employers, creating an unfair burden on this sector of society. Although many large corporations would benefit, many smaller companies would suffer an additional financial burden, even with assistance from the federal government. This option creates a potential loss of jobs or at least a hiring slowdown. A third option is the *individual mandate,* in which individuals would be responsible for obtaining and funding their own coverage. Penalties would be levied on those who chose not to participate. Coverage could be paid for with personal funds, medical savings accounts, or payroll deductions, with a federal subsidy for those who could not afford to purchase health insurance.

A healthcare system that offers universal access has difficulties beyond those of funding. First, many individuals, trying to save money, may not acquire the coverage until they need it. It is thus possible that there would be more uninsured citizens than there are currently. In addition, since illness is often unpredictable and can come on suddenly, a system of universal access will force these uncovered individuals to rely heavily on more costly emergency care. Finally, these uncovered individuals will probably not utilize to the same extent preventive care services shown to be effective in controlling health care expenditures over time that are available to covered individuals (Tenery 1994).

With the failure of the health-system-reform debate and increasing costs with the fee-for-service healthcare delivery, the employers in this country said, "We've had enough." Their status in the world market was threatened by the increasing burden of covering the costs of the healthcare services for their employees. They demanded a change, and the private sector responded.

At first, the private sector response was discount pricing, where individual physicians or groups of healthcare providers would agree to supply services, but at a lower rate of service. They were hoping to offset the losses on individual cases by increasing volume. Insurance companies and hospital corporations joined in realizing that they could become the middlemen between the employers and the providers—and that was the birth of *managed care.*

Realizing that even more decreases could be squeezed out of healthcare services, delivery models were established in which all services were covered for a fixed fee as long as the patient groups were large enough. Hence, the birth of *capitated healthcare systems,* which were very similar to Canada's single-payer system, except these were multiple single-payers.

Where does this leave the patients in the United States today? In many ways, not too much better off than before these radical changes started taking place just a few years ago. This country still has 43–45 million people who are uninsured each year. There are still 10 million children who have no healthcare coverage at any one time. One-third of the children under age two are not adequately immunized. And the United States still ranks twenty-fourth—in the bottom tier of industrialized countries—for infant mortality (Guyer, MacDorman, Martin et al., 1998).

If the United States is to meet its moral and ethical obligations and allow all its citizens access to an affordable level of healthcare services, it must deal with the massive problems created by the numerous and diverse entitlement programs. There is simply not enough money in our present system to cover the current obligations to the millions of citizens who are currently without adequate healthcare coverage. Hence the evolution of the concept of shifting the responsibility for healthcare costs back to the patients themselves, but only to the point that each patient can afford (Goodman and Musgrave 1992). This plan calls for shifting the incentives for not over-utilizing the system onto the patients by rewarding them—in other words, making them prudent purchasers of their own healthcare services.

The key word is *incentives*. Exactly how those incentives are structured will determine the long-term success or the downfall of any future healthcare delivery system. Only three groups control the size of healthcare expenditures —the payers, the providers of care, and the patients. In any delivery system, payers would always have the incentive to spend less. In the unconstrained fee-for-service system, providers were rewarded for doing more; while in managed care under capitation, the incentives encourage the providers to do less. Even this latter system has not effectively stemmed the growth of overall expenditures. The reason is that the incentives are still structured so that patients are encouraged to utilize the system more, not less. Thus, it seems that only a system that creates incentives for the patients, the users of the system, to do less will effectively control healthcare spending. It would be preferable if these incentives to limit utilization were remunerative and self-directed, rather than perverse and mandated.

Making patients fiscally responsible for at least a portion of their own care seems to be the preferable way to create incentives not to over-utilize healthcare services. This concept is not a delivery system in itself, but a funding mechanism for payment of health care that can be incorporated into most existing systems. It allows patients to make the judgment—frequently referred to as cost / benefit analysis—as to whether the medical services in question justify the costs. Who can better make that analysis than the patients themselves (Tenery 1997)?

To be successful, however, those who cannot pay for the necessary health-care services would still be funded through one of the established assistance programs. Those citizens who could afford to purchase services or coverage for those services would no longer be eligible for the assistance programs even if they were qualified by age, as is currently the policy under Medicare. Only in this way can funds be freed up to expand the current programs to cover those who are currently without coverage. In addition, supplemental funding would be brought into the healthcare system from the private sector to continue to grow and advance our current healthcare delivery system.

In looking for solutions to the problems of access and affordability of our present healthcare delivery system, one vital concept has been lost. We have become so embroiled in cost-containment accountability that we have forgotten to whom the system belongs—to the patients. It does not belong to the government, to insurance companies, or to employers. In our attempt to control the problems created by their country's advances and discoveries, we have literally taken the system away from its citizens.

Only if citizens are allowed to come back into the system and make some of the difficult decisions on allocation and access that pertain to their own care, can we hope to meet our moral and ethical responsibilities of providing adequate and affordable health care to all.

References

American Medical Association. 1994. Policy 140.75. In *Policy Compendium of the American Medical Association,* 125. Chicago: American Medical Association.

Beauchamp, T. L., and Childress, S. F. 1989. *Principles of Biomedical Ethics.* New York: Oxford University Press.

Council on Ethical and Judicial Affairs (CEJA). 1994. Ethical Issues in Health Care System Reform. *Journal of the American Medical Association* 272(13):1056–62.

Goodman, John C., and Musgrave, Gerald L. 1992. *Patient Power.* Washington, D.C.: Cato Institute.

Guyer, B.; MacDorman, M. F.; Martin, J. A. et al. 1998. Annual Summary of Vital Statistics, 1997. *Pediatrics* 102 (December):1333–49.

Tenery Jr., Robert M. 1996. Commentary—Our New Health Care Systems May Not Be Fair. *American Medical News* (4 November):21.

———. 1994. Commentary—Don't Confuse Universal Access with Universal Coverage. *American Medical News* (9 May):21.

———. 1997. Commentary—Sen. Gramm May Be Right About Medicare Incentives. *American Medical News* (7 April):21.

IV

**Future Challenges
to Biomedical Ethics**

17

Future Challenges to Medical Ethics and Professional Values

ALBERT R. JONSEN, PH.D.

The future has as yet no facts to discover and relate, as history does. The future has no pressing problems that call for analysis, as the present does. The future is by definition not yet in existence, and those who are invited to talk about it must thrust their imagination ahead, using the past and the present to invent the world and its problems that might be. This is, for me, an enjoyable task, for unlike historians or analysts of the present, it is difficult to prove the futurist wrong, at least at the moment of prophecy. Condemnation must always be retrospective, and by the time it comes, the prophet may be gone. Still, the futurist does have a moral obligation, if not to truth, at least to plausibility. A responsible prophet has the duty to prepare the minds and hearts of those who must live out the future as it comes. A prediction does not merely imagine the future; it prepares for it in the present.

With these responsibilities in mind, I will attempt to articulate the future challenges to medical ethics and professional responsibility. I must begin in the past because futures, however novel, are usually designed against a background of what has preceded. I will dwell briefly in the present because it is the launching ground for any recognizable future. Then I will travel into the genuine future. Any journey into the future is faced with a map of infinite routes because the future, being yet unformed, is infinite possibility. So I can choose, out of the infinity of guesses, only a few that seem to me particularly important. My treks into the future will follow the parabolas of genetics, cultural pluralism, and institutional structures as these will affect medicine and health care in the next century. Each of these routes is fraught with ethical questions.

As I start this trip into the future from the past, I have a personal image about ethics in America. All peoples profess moral beliefs and praise moral practices, but each people in each era does so in its own way, and all these ways show differences and similarities. Ethics done in the American way—that is, in the culture that began in the colonies and spread into the states populated by diverse ethnic and religious groups—has a peculiar pattern. My image of that pattern comes from a scene that tourists can see when they visit the extant churches of colonial America. They will often see, behind the altar or pulpit, a board blazoned with the Ten Commandments, those verses from the book of Exodus that proclaim the moral laws at the heart of Judaism and Christianity. Imagine parishioners staring at that sign Sunday after Sunday and generation after generation. My fantasy is that those ten rules, or at least the form of those rules, was imprinted on the conscience of the nation. As the nation became religiously plural, skeptical, and secular, Americans still believed that ethics means rules of right and wrong. Indeed, the rules might change greatly in content, but rules there must be. The second commandment, as delivered from Yahweh by Moses, ordered, "Thou shalt make no graven image or any likeness of any thing that is in heaven." Today it might be "Thou shalt make no clone." Ethics, as we think of it, is a list of rules.

Imagine again that the preacher in that colonial church lifts the Bible and reads a verse only a few lines away from the Commandments: "Behold, I will send my Angel before thee, to keep thee in the way and to bring thee into the place which I have prepared." The preacher, taking those words as his text, would inform his parishioners that God had given them a destiny: to make a new land, to create by covenant fresh societies, to subdue nature to human purposes, and to bring unimaginable riches out of the wilderness, all for the glorification of God. This sermon was heard again and again by early American settlers, and it convinced them that their exploration and exploitation of the land was a divine destiny. I believe that this message too marked American ethics: the ethical was an exploration into new ways of being human. Rules faded before bold and benign creativity.

Americans, in this fantasy, think of ethics in two fashions—as commandments and as exploration—which, while they may seem complementary, are often in conflict. The major American moral philosophers, from the puritan Jonathan Edwards, through William James and John Dewey, and even down to today's John Rawls, exhibit both themes, often weaving them together but also leaving them in opposition. Medical ethics, as it has developed in the United States, bears the marks of these two themes.

The AMA Code of Ethics of 1847 was composed very much in the commandment tradition. Even its title, Code of Ethics, announces this. It contains imperatives, exhortations, and admonitions. Indeed, as it went through emendations, it even took on the literal form of the Ten Commandments. Ethics, even medical ethics, consisted of rules. A Judicial Council was formed to adjudicate violations. The code, during most of its history, was commandment without destiny. The ethics of the code also reflected only a tiny slice of the moral world in which it was composed. 1847 was in the middle of the abolition debates, the contentious Mexican War, the expulsion of Native Americans from their lands, the persecution of the Mormons, and many another national turmoil. In that very year, 1847, the flood of impoverished, starving Irish into American cities peaked. Yet the code has hardly a hint of that moral turbulence. It speaks only to the sedate behavior of doctors among themselves and with their patients. Even the brief mention of the duty to care gratuitously for the poor, and the injunction not to flee epidemics, appear as sober moral advice rather than fervid exhortations to correct rankling social crises.

In the 1960s bioethics came into being. Medicine had moved with breathless speed after World War II. Its technologies, techniques, drugs, and delivery systems leapt ahead in efficacy and complexity and left in their wake unprecedented problems. Life support by ventilators and dialysis, for example, saved lives but sometimes sustained bodies drained of their human qualities. Physicians and scientists confessed concern about these problems. Philosophers and theologians saw in these medical problems material for their reflections. Meetings were organized, debates held, articles written, and slowly a new ethics of medicine emerged with many medical outsiders as participants. Those outsiders were, in large part, theologians and philosophers, with a scattering of lawyers and sociologists, some of whom were invited by the scientific and medical community to join their discussions, and others who looked in from without on the interesting spectacle. Some were appointed to government commissions and the committees of professional bodies. Many of these outsiders were hired into medical faculties to become the teachers of the new medical ethics. While the medical establishment showed some puzzlement, even disdain, for these newcomers, they were tolerated and, in time, judged to be helpful colleagues. The theological and philosophical ethicists brought no definitive ethical theory to medicine. Indeed, those years were particularly arid ones in moral philosophy. Most of the philosophers were students, not of ethics, but of more vital areas, such as philosophy of science. The theologians were recently liberated from doctrinal constraints and were seeking an ethic rather than preaching one. Thus, these medical outsiders came to medical ethics with an open mind about ethical theory.

They did not come, however, without ethical convictions. They had been the student protesters against the war in Southeast Asia, the student marchers for civil rights, the advocates of gender equality. They were the teachers of those concerned young people, pressed by them to bring their speculative knowledge of ethics down to the turmoil of ethical decisions. They saw morality and immorality in the world that was swarming around their universities. Most of the medical ethicists of my generation were activists in one cause or another. Thus, as they formed theoretical views about ethics, they reflected on rights, autonomy, skepticism about authority, risk, and responsibility. They were heirs of the ethics of discovery, destiny, and exploration rather than the ethics of rules and commandments. Yet, like most Americans, they could not completely abolish ethics as rules from their minds. The first titans of bioethics, the theologians Joseph Fletcher and Paul Ramsey, exemplified the duality: Fletcher was an ethicist of exploration; Ramsey was committed to commandments. Most of their serious readers were drawn to find a middle ground.

This double mind became evident during the first major public enterprise in medical ethics, the work of the National Commission for the Protection of Human Subjects of Biomedical and Behavioral Research, established by Congress to formulate the principles and policies that would protect the rights and welfare of human persons involved in research. During its four years, 1974–78, the commission invited many philosophers and theologians to bend their intelligence to issues that had never before entered their minds. Many original studies contributed to the commission's official reports. Among the reports one, called the Belmont Report, stated the ethical principles that should govern research. Three principles were noted: respect for persons' autonomy, beneficence/nonmaleficence, and justice.

Principles look a bit like rules, but they are not rules. They are guides into the future, anticipating problems that will have to be resolved in new circumstances. These three principles came to mind almost unbidden as the commissioners and their consultants thought about the ethics of research. *Autonomy:* research imposes risk on persons, not for their good, but for a future good for future persons; thus, research should never use subjects, but must invite consenting volunteers. *Beneficence/nonmaleficence:* research must minimize its risk of harm and must never confuse the good of individuals with the good of society and scientific progress. *Justice:* research must never exploit the vulnerable who had often been its subjects—the dying, retarded persons, the medically indigent, uneducated rural black sharecroppers. These principles, natural to research, also were reminiscent of the moral experience of the ethicists who conceived them. The principles were not intended to set definitive rights and wrongs but to give general direction to policies that could be applied to research of various sorts.

Those principles, created for research ethics, were easily translated to another major ethical problem of modern medicine: the technological imperative and the paternalism of those with technical expertise. Autonomy, beneficence, and justice could guide thinking through the dilemmas raised by these features of modern medicine. Before long, scholars deepened their meaning, reshaped their definitions and applications, and gave them the place of primacy in bioethics. Bioethics, then, was an American ethic of the second sort, of discovery, destiny, and exploration, recognizing the possibilities of a new medical science and practice and encouraging it to move ahead, like those led in a straight path by the angel of Exodus, under the guidance of principles.

It may be time to admit that the bioethics born in the 1960s is showing the signs of aging. Bioethics must be refreshed as the future opens. The principles that worked very well for research ethics, and rather well for paternalism and medical technologies, may have to be enlarged to meet the emerging medicine. The principles are not wrong; rather, they are defined and expressed in ways that render them clumsy instruments for the ethical analysis of the future as it arrives.

I said at the outset that I would travel into the future of medical ethics along three routes. The first of these is the scientific road toward molecular medicine. This is the medicine of the future. Molecular medicine, rooted in science of molecular biogenetics, will gradually introduce diagnostics and therapeutics that will revolutionize medicine as much and even more than did the germs of the last century and the antibiotics of our times. However, these will be diagnostics and therapeutics with a difference. The diagnostics will reveal diseases not only of the individuals but also of their kinship. Disease will be seen as rooted in the physical propensities of clans and will be predictable for generations. Therapies, when they come, will modify the genomes of beings yet unborn. These future features of medicine challenge the principle of *autonomy* as we now know it.

The bioethicists created the principle of respect for autonomy out of some venerable pieces of moral philosophy and theology, as well as out of their own moral convictions about personal freedom. In the venerable pieces, autonomy seldom held primacy of place. In earlier moral philosophy, it was a prop for arguments about moral accountability and responsibility: how could persons be held morally accountable unless they had free will? In moral theology, autonomy was a prelude to salvation: how could God's grace save from sin unless the sinner could accept it freely? Some philosophers, like Immanuel Kant, put autonomy in a central place, but only to prove that humans must be makers of a universal law that they impose upon themselves.

The bioethicists knew this, but they saw in autonomy a useful antidote to the exploitation in research and to demeaning paternalism. In their hands, it came to mean the moral right of individuals to choose for themselves, in accord with their own values. As we move into the genetic world, where humans are seen as linked in communities by their chromosomes, the principle of autonomy is still needed to assert that persons are more than their genetic destiny. At the same time it needs to be deepened; it must be taken back to its philosophical and theological genesis, as an argument against genetic determinism. It needs also to be broadened by situating the autonomous person in a community of similarly autonomous persons who share a common property. The venerable thinkers knew that autonomy was not a proclamation of isolated individualism. The theologian Martin Luther opened his ringing tract entitled *Christian Liberty* with the words "The Christian is a perfectly free person, yet the Christian is dutiful servant of all" (Luther 1915–32, 2:312) Almost three centuries later, the philosopher Immanuel Kant proclaimed, "A rational being belongs to the kingdom of ends as a member and as its head, for he makes the universal laws to which he is subject" (Kant 1964, 101). Both of these great thinkers realized the conceptual and political tensions that surround any claim to human autonomy. The bioethicists of the future, pushed by the progress of science and medicine, must restore the tension that has slackened in our one-dimensional principle of autonomy. A deepened and broadened principle of autonomy must shed light on the genetic science and molecular medicine that is coming into being.

The second route I shall take into the future is through cultural pluralism. Bioethics was born in the United States but rapidly had siblings in many nations. Those siblings were not clones; they resembled the cultures in which they were born. Bioethicists are beginning to talk with each other over national borders and to learn that, while we share many views, the American way of conceiving ethics differs remarkably from that of other cultures. As persons from those cultures come into our medical world more frequently, we are forced to think seriously about how to respect their values within our values. This challenges the principle of *beneficence* as we have known it.

Beneficence means, to us, effecting good rather than evil. So far, so good: this is a principle known to moralists since time immemorial. St. Thomas Aquinas begins his treatise on ethics with the words, "The first principle of ethics is to do good and avoid evil"(Aquinas 1964, 28:77). The ethics of commandment listed some quite definite goods—worship of God, honor to parents—and evils—killing, lying, theft, adultery; and the moralists embroidered around those goods and evils many others. The American ethos of exploration became more tentative about specific goods and evils. Be brave in forging ahead, it urged, and you will discover a better world. It is hard to say what it will look like, but you will know it. So the principle of beneficence became somewhat fickle. It became an appendage of the principle of autonomy. Doing good, it came to say, was doing to others what others choose for themselves. A few goods of the old sort remained—better to be healthy than sick, independent rather than dependent—but most of the particulars of the Decalogue melted away into the free choices of free persons.

Multicultural ethics summons us to another world. Many cultures retain strong concepts of obligation. Doing good means doing what is commanded as right. The good is an imperative challenging freedom, not an invitation to freedom or one option among many. When the American ethic encounters some of these obligations, it should, in accord with its own principle of respect for autonomy, simply respect them and let them be. Yet sometimes they appear irrational, abhorrent, hateful, silly: life saved by transplanting another's heart is unethical; a sick baby prayed over by a shaman is better treated than by antibiotics; useful information about illness is repudiated as a threat; one person's choice is subsumed in the choice of another, more authoritative person; bodily mutilations are sought as signs of pride and proper submission. Such things, by the American ethic, should be respected, not rejected. Yet we are extremely uncomfortable about such practices. How does our desiccated principle of beneficence deal with obligations that we do not appreciate? May we not need a stronger sense of obligation and commandment ourselves if we are to criticize the customs of others? We need a more defined meaning of good and evil. Multicultural ethics reminds us of that need.

My third road into the future is along the paths of structural and economic changes in the delivery of health services and in the work of physicians and other health professionals. Bioethics, from the beginning of its career, spoke about the principle of *justice*. Bioethicists participated in the discussions about the allocation of scarce medical resources, the barriers to access to care, and the exploitation of the charity patient for research. These issues were all framed within the definitions and arguments of the ethical theories of justice. The principle of justice that bioethics has espoused urges that every patient have the right to speak and demand. It also urges that the benefits of health care be distributed to all who need them, not to those who can pay for them or who have, by good fortune, the power to command the resources. As the medical world is evolving into a highly complex system of investment and production, this principle of justice will be challenged. The medical act is no longer produced only by a compassionate doctor serving a needing patient. The instruments of compassion are costly, and their delivery requires many coordinated steps. The needing patient is a covered life, a cost center, a financial risk. Surrounding the medical act, a cohort of those who produce it by their taxes, their investments, and their planning and managing also assert their rights and claims to justice. The work of assessing these claims is now imposed on the principle of justice.

My speculation about the future of medical ethics, then, suggests that the future's genetics, multiculturalism, and institutional forms will challenge the standard principles of autonomy, beneficence, and justice. I could, given time, find other challenges or elaborate on those I have mentioned. These three areas of change entail challenges to each of the three principles, and the three principles are challenged by many coming changes other than those three I have mentioned. The challenges I have described call for conceptual revision of principles. That is a challenge posed to the bioethicists but also, in reality, to all who work in medicine and health care. The bioethicists create bioethics in their heads and write it in their books. Physicians discover ethics in the circumstances of their work. They should read the books of bioethicists, and bioethicists should be intimately familiar with the work of doctors. The expansion of the standard principles must come from their collaboration. I assume that the AMA's Institute of Medical Ethics will promote such collaboration.

Beyond the bioethicists and the physicians stands the multitude of American people within whose morality the bioethicists and the physicians live. Ethics is not made from scratch. Whatever formulation ethicists give it, ethics needs as material the moral life of a people. Professional ethics, too, is enveloped in the general moral life of a culture, which is difficult to define. I have offered a simple image of commandment and exploration. Yet today it is more than difficult to discern the commandments that the people acknowledge and to describe the directions for the exploration. Will an ethics that bioethicists design and physicians desire fit the moral life of the people? Will a principle of autonomy that acknowledges community have any resonance in the minds and hearts of individuals? Will a demand for justice be heard in a competitive commercial world?

These are great challenges. The ethicists and physicians of the next generation, and the next generation itself, must take them on with intelligence and prudence. Yet the best advice I can give to the next generation of ethicists comes from the distant past. My favorite moralist, Michel de Montaigne, once wisely wrote, "Those who have attempted to correct the world's morals by new ideas, reform the superficial vices and leave untouched the serious ones" (Montaigne 1965, 3:615). The challenges I have mentioned go, not to any serious vices, but to the serious questions for medical ethics in the coming century.

References

Aquinas, Thomas. 1964. *Summa Theologiae. Latin Text and English Translation.* New York: McGraw-Hill.

Kant, Immanuel. 1964. *Groundwork of the Metaphysics of Morals,* ed. H. J. Paton. New York: Harper and Row.

Luther, Martin. 1915–32. *Treatise on Christian Liberty.* In *Works of Martin Luther,* ed. J. H. Eyster and A. Spaeth. Philadelphia: A. J. Holman.

Montaigne, Michel de. 1965. *Complete Essays,* ed. Donald M. Frame. Stanford: Stanford University Press, 1965.

18

Can Ethics Help Guide the Future of Biomedicine?

ARTHUR L. CAPLAN, PH.D.

One of the challenges facing any code of ethics meant to govern medical practice is whether or not it can keep pace with the rapid advance of biomedical progress. There seems to be no doubt on the part of scholars and students of the AMA Code of Ethics that it exerted a powerful influence over medical practice over the past hundred years (Baker 1995; chap. 2, this volume). But there is tremendous skepticism in the United States that the AMA Code, or any code—or, indeed, any set of moral values—could have any impact whatsoever in guiding the future direction of biomedical research and medical practice. This skepticism was very much in evidence in reactions to the announcement of the first somatic cell cloning of a mammal using DNA from an adult cell— Dolly, the sheep (Adler 1997; Powers 1998). But it is also present in the commonly voiced concern of politicians, policy makers, and scholars that ethics seems always to trail behind the latest scientific or medical breakthrough (Fox and Swazey 1992).

The phenomenon of the "ethics lag" is simply taken for granted. All one need do to see the depth of this belief is track any story about the ethics of any major new breakthrough in biology or medicine. It will not be many paragraphs before the writer notes either that ethics always seems to be lagging behind scientific advances or that biomedicine has outstripped the capacity of ethics and the law to keep pace. The "ethics lag" is a powerful presumption in American, European, and Japanese assessments of the future of biomedicine (Adler 1997; Weiss 1998).

Why Bother with Ethics: The Case of Cloning

The worry about the "ethics lag" was never more evident than in the announcement in March 1997 that an adult sheep, Dolly, had been cloned using the DNA of a cell obtained from the udder of an another adult sheep (a long-dead progenitor!). This announcement set off a frenzy of concern and worry that ethics could not possibly hope to keep up with the rapid pace of change soon to be flowing from cloning (Caplan 1998; Powers 1998; Stolberg 1998).

One way to respond to the worry that ethics was lagging was to create bans on human cloning. The president of the United States moved quickly to ban the use of federal moneys to support research into human cloning. This was followed by many calls for Congress to enact legislation banning human cloning. Germany, Britain, and France quickly banned human cloning, as did the European Parliament, the Council of Europe, and the World Health Organization. But there was and is a great degree of doubt that bans will have any impact (Kolata 1998).

Many people believe that it is a simple matter to evade a ban and conduct human cloning research secretly or in a Third World location. Some believe not only that it is simple but that it is inevitable. This is the only way to explain the elevation of Dr. Richard Seed, a retired Chicago physicist who announced at a conference in Chicago on December 5, 1997, that he intended to clone human beings, from obscurity to a figure capable of inspiring national anxiety. Seed was the most obvious manifestation of the belief in the ethics lag. But in the months after Dolly's birth became public knowledge, there were many other manifestations of doubt that ethics would make any difference whatsoever to the future of the genetic revolution.

Commentators and pundits went bonkers over the appearance of Dolly. Some fretted about the national security risk posed by clone armies in the hands of rogue regimes. Others wrung their hands over the use of cloning to create hordes of clones who might be mined to supply tissues and organs to those in need of transplants. A few commentators speculated on the societal implications of immortality achieved by means of cloning oneself sequentially. These sorts of speculations made little scientific sense, but they did reflect deep public doubt and mistrust of advances in the realm of genetics and genetic engineering (Caplan 1998).

One legislator who spoke out very vociferously about human cloning on the basis of the Dolly experiment was Senator Tom Harken of Iowa. In hearings on cloning, he expressed the view that once science had started down the path toward new knowledge there was nothing anyone could do to stop its progress.

He ventured the opinion that no law or moral rule or set of values had ever deterred biomedicine from doing anything, and that the best the world could hope for was that those working on cloning would choose to do so in an ethical fashion (Lane 1997; NBC News 1997).

The view that biomedicine cannot be stopped, shaped, or changed by ethics might well be called "Harkenism." The position holds that biomedical progress moves under its own momentum. It also maintains a fatalistic and skeptical view about ethics—once science has made a key breakthrough and gets rolling, there is nothing anyone can do to stop it.

There is something terrifying about Harkenism. If accepted, it means that there is really no point in debating or arguing about the ethics of the future of any biomedical advance. That future will be what it will be, and there is nothing anyone can do about it. Worse still, if the unscrupulous or the crazy get their hands on biomedical advances, there is nothing anyone can do to deter or stop them. The only problem with both the ethics-lag thesis and Harkenism is that they are wrong.

Has Ethics or Bioethics Ever Stopped Anything in Medicine?

Many years ago, in the late 1970s, when I was a graduate student just beginning a position at the Hastings Center, the nation's most influential private bioethics institute located just north of New York City, Daniel Callahan, then the director, and I had a standing bet. We would ask the various scholars, physicians, and researchers who came to the center to give talks or participate in seminars to name a single technology that had been stymied, blocked, or destroyed as a result of a bioethical objection or argument. Our bet was that no one would be able to do so. We agreed to provide a free lunch for all staff if someone ever came up with a single case of a technology that had been stopped because of ethical concerns or reservations. No one ever did.

Dan and I would use the inability to identify any scientific application or technology that had ever foundered on the rocks of ethics as a way to calm the worries of physicians and researchers that if they even talked about ethics they might somehow wind up being responsible for hindering inquiry. No act could have been seen as more treasonous, more incompatible with being a member of the biomedical community, than to permanently hinder scientific progress for ethical reasons. Reassured that they could not do permanent damage to their own research programs or those of colleagues, the visitors would then almost always dig in for a dialogue on bioethics, since they felt certain that talk of ethics would not really put the practice of science at any real risk.

I have come to think that Daniel Callahan and I were wrong about the power of ethics. The problem was that when we asked for case examples, we were looking for instances in the very recent past where someone's bright idea had gone down in smoke forever due to ethical worries. However, seeing the impact of ethics on science is more akin to detecting the processes of evolutionary change, being aware of barometric pressure, or being alert to the presence of gravity. Evolution is difficult to observe because it goes on very slowly all around us. It is hard for anyone to be aware of the weight of air or the pull of gravity because they are present in our lives at all times. These forces are a part of our environment. We adjust to them. It is only in their absence, when humans travel into space or deep into the sea, that we realize the powerful force they constantly exert on us.

Similarly, ethics is most noticeable with respect to the role it plays in shaping science when it is not present or when it is present in a very different form. The inhumane experiments conducted in the German and Japanese concentration camps by competent scientists and physicians and public health officials during the Second World War show how very different scientific behavior is in the absence of the normal ethical restraints that dominate the practice of science and medicine. Nineteenth-century research conducted in the United States and other nations on serfs and slaves, who were not seen as persons or even as human, or on animals in the eighteenth and early nineteenth centuries, give more tragic evidence of the role played by ethics in biomedical research today (Caplan 1998).

It is simply not true that ethics has not had or cannot have an impact on what biomedicine does or what biomedicine becomes. While the influence is not always obvious or even detectable, once one looks closely it can be found. For example, we presume that doctors will reveal to potential subjects the nature of experiments they might want them to serve in and that they will obtain their permission before studying them. The requirement of informed consent in recruiting subjects to biomedical research is, however, a relatively recent innovation. As recently as the 1930s and 40s, subjects were routinely lied to or deceived about the nature of human experimentation, and consent was often not sought.

Prohibitions on research on retarded children and on fetuses, except when it might be for their benefit, have been in effect for decades, as have prohibitions against embryo research and fetal tissue transplantation. These moral bans have had the effect of bringing these areas of inquiry to almost a complete halt. Research on the total artificial heart and the use of animals as sources of organs for transplant was halted for more than a decade as a result of moral objections. The inclusion of women in clinical trials is a direct response to moral criticism. The decision to halt research involving recombinant DNA work in the 1970s until sufficient oversight could be applied to experiments was fueled by moral doubts on the part of basic scientists (Singer 1977). It is hard to maintain a strong allegiance to either the ethics lag or Harkenism once one takes a close look at the history of biomedical research.

True, ethics cannot always restrain or curb biomedicine's drive to know. Nor can it always provide a reliable safeguard against the actions of a fiend or a nut. But the fact that ethics is not omnipotent should not blind us to the fact that it is not impotent either.

Oddly enough, one powerful piece of evidence in favor of the power of ethics is the AMA's own code. When efforts were made in the 1990s to modify the code to permit the use of anencephalic infants as sources of organs for transplant, the proposal drew such heated opposition that the effort of the AMA's Council on Ethical and Judicial Affairs had to be abandoned. The code still prohibits the use of these children, and whether the policy makes sense or not, no anencephalic infants have been used as organ donors in the United States since 1989 (AMA 1996).

Similarly the code is very explicit about conflicts of interest, noting that "under no circumstances may physicians place their own financial interests above the welfare of their patients" and noting that "avoidance of real or perceived conflicts of interest in clinical research is imperative if the medical community is to ensure objectivity and maintain individual and institutional integrity" (AMA 1996). Not only is the code of ethics frequently cited when companies or private entities propose relationships with researchers that would appear to create conflicts, but also it is often an effective basis for changing the nature of those conflicts. When in 1997 the AMA negotiated an arrangement to endorse certain products made by the Sunbeam Corporation in return for payments to the AMA's educational outreach programs, the organization itself was taken to moral task by many of its own members, and not a few outsiders as well, for violating its own moral code. The code was of sufficient power that the AMA had to change its arrangement at a cost that included the resignation of many top executives and many millions of dollars.

The power of ethics in steering and even prohibiting certain kinds of conduct is not always easy to see. Just as Jane Goodall spent fifteen years observing chimpanzees without seeing them engage in killing before an all-out war broke out in the groups she had known and written about as peaceable, ethics may not be much in evidence until a true conflict of interest or scandal sends everyone scrambling for their code of ethics.

What's in Store in Genetics?

If it is true that bioethics and ethical values can and do have influence over the actions of researchers and scientists, then what area of biomedicine is likely to prove most in need of moral attention in the years to come? Many might nominate human cloning or human genetic engineering as strong candidates. Yet the state of scientific understanding in these areas, and the technical skill required to apply them to human beings, is at such a rudimentary level that it is not likely they will prove ethically pressing in terms of human application before well into the next decade. Much more likely to pose a moral challenge are the advances in mapping and sequencing the human genome and the consequent possibility of applying this information to the testing and screening of human beings. The easiest way to see why bioethics and medical ethics need to attend closely to this area of biomedicine is to look at the issues raised by the testing of young children for genetic differences and diseases.

The Ethics of Genetic Testing of Children

In the early days of mining, canaries were used to determine whether a dangerous gas leak might be present. The tiny birds were more susceptible to the adverse effects of mine gas than were humans. When they had trouble breathing, or when they simply stopped breathing, they gave miners advance warning of a serious problem.

One way to understand the nature of the problems and challenges raised by genetic testing is to assess the impact of testing on an especially fragile and vulnerable population. An examination of the impact that genetic testing may have on young children, who are more susceptible to problems and risks due to their inability to protect their own interests, sheds important light on the ethical challenges that require a prophylactic ethical response.

Children and babies come up frequently in contemporary discussions of genetic testing. Nearly every week an advertisement appears in the *New York Times Magazine* from the Genetics and IVF Institute, a famous infertility clinic located in Northern Virginia. The basic thrust of the ad is to solicit new clients who seek treatment for their infertility through the use of in vitro fertilization. The ad suggests that the Genetics and IVF Institute is the optimal place for the manufacture of embryos because every embryo made at Genetics and IVF undergoes preimplantation genetic testing. This means that every embryo has a cell removed early on in its development. The DNA from this cell is extracted, copied (or cloned), and then analyzed to detect genetic problems such as markers for breast cancer. Only embryos known to be free of markers for genetic disease need be used by couples undergoing infertility treatment. Other clinics in the United States and England offer similar embryo biopsy / genetic testing options (Caplan 1997; 1998).

Infertility is a very competitive field. Clinics are always on the watch for a marketing advantage. In the case of embryo biopsy, some clinics have realized that the promise of a healthier child might provide an edge over the competition. But the questions of what constitutes a genetic disease, what risks are worth testing for, what sort of counseling patients ought to receive about the meaning of different genetic susceptibilities, and what expectations are created in parents and children when genetic testing is a part of the creation of a new life remain morally very murky.

What is a disease to some parents is merely a difference to others. What is an obsession for one couple may strike some physicians doing genetic testing as minor or irrelevant in thinking about the health of a potential child. And what might get a person to use one IVF clinic as opposed to another in terms of genetic testing possibilities for embryos might strike some persons with disabilities or unusual capacities as at best bigoted and at worst blatantly discriminatory.

Genetic tests for newborns have become an accepted part of the process of the birth of a child, despite the fact that these tests involve almost no informed consent on the part of parents and little assurance of confidentiality, and they are not done with prior education or counseling. How can this be? It is because for nearly every one of the currently used tests for conditions like PKU deficiency, there are therapeutic options that are available if something is detected. It is also the case that the sooner the existing therapies are started, the better for the health of the child. The moral rationale for current widespread forms of mandatory genetic testing of children is that the best interest of the child requires that routine screening be done. Other considerations take a back seat to the need to provide therapies quickly to prevent damage, disability, and death.

A new area where genetic testing is being done with young people is the detection of risk among young athletes. Not too long ago I got a call from a friend of mine about a young boy of eleven who wanted to play basketball at his school. He was very tall for his age and a good player. But his pediatrician was concerned because he thought the boy had the appearance of someone with Marfan syndrome.

Marfan syndrome is a condition that causes connective tissue in the body to behave abnormally. Ligaments and tendons stretch inappropriately, leading to joint and muscle pain. Connective tissue lines the insides of the major blood vessels like the aorta. If a major vessel like the aorta stretches under the demands of high blood pressure, a fatal aneurysm can result causing death. There have been a number of deaths due to aneurysms among basketball and volleyball players suspected of having Marfan syndrome.

The boy wanted to play basketball. His parents had seen in a national magazine that a test was available for Marfan syndrome, and they wanted the test done. The boy was not sure whether he wanted the test, since a positive test result might prevent him from playing basketball. But his parents were adamant, and ultimately the pediatrician decided to perform the test despite the boy's ambivalence. He proved positive for Marfan syndrome and so, despite his heated protests, his parents brought his burgeoning basketball career to a rapid end, though he stills plays in pick-up games at the playground whenever he can.

The case of the young man who for whom a genetic test meant the end of his basketball activity reveals a number of important facts about genetic testing. Some forms of genetic testing are done for children even without their assent or consent where the goal is prevention or treatment. A genetic test may reveal a risk associated with a lifestyle or behavior that might pose grave risk to the person with a particular genetic constitution. And genetic testing may be seen as disempowering by the person getting the test, even though the motives of those providing the test are to do good rather than to harm.

Still another case in which genetic testing is being done for children involves a new genetic test for albinism. A physician who had discovered the marker for a hereditary form of albinism suddenly found himself swamped with requests for information about how to detect its presence in the fetus. The requests were coming from Japan. Why Japan?

Japanese physicians wanted the test in order to help couples who wished to have more children prevent the tragedy of having a white child. Couples who have had a white child want the assurance that it won't happen again. In Japanese society being white carries stigma for both child and parents—a stigma that is severe enough that some couples will only try to have another child if they have some reassurance that their future children will not be albino.

The physician sought advice from an ethicist—me. The question was whether the test for albinism should be made available for clinical use to the

Japanese who were inquiring about it. It so happened that a man who was an albino worked in a lab near my office. He was then a postdoctoral fellow in biochemistry. I sought him out and asked him, "Are you sick?" He said, "Are you nuts?" After this bit of enlightening dialogue, I explained that I was trying to understand whether albinism was a disease and dysfunctional in light of the request of Japanese doctors to test fetuses for this condition. He told me that he did not feel sick or disabled in any way. At most, his vision gave him some problems, and he had to stay out of the sun, but that was about it.

I also found out from the postdoctoral fellow that at least two Nobel prize winners have been albino—both in chemistry, his chosen field of science. While some Japanese may consider a lack of skin pigment a disease, it has not been such a burden that many people who are albino cannot enjoy life. Those with albinism have made, and certainly will continue to make, important contributions in science and in many other fields that greatly benefit society. The issue of what counts as a disease is one that is seen very differently through the eyes of parents in a particular culture than it might be through the eyes of someone with the same condition in another society.

The last and perhaps most typical case in which genetic testing is already starting to appear is with respect to young children at risk of genetic diseases for which some sort of screening test has been created. There are many families in which a hereditary form of breast cancer is present. In some of these families, parents are very concerned about having their young daughters tested to see if they have inherited the genes that put them at high risk of this form of breast cancer (Lerman and Croyle 1994; Geller et al. 1997). While the only available therapy for this disease is the surgical removal of the breast, many parents still hope that by having their daughter tested they will know once and for all whether they face a high risk of acquiring breast cancer. In many instances where requests for tests are made, it is the parents, not the child, who are eager for the test to be done.

Why do genetic testing? One reason is that in Western societies, at least in the United States, information is thought to be good, and more information is thought to be better. "Know thyself" is an old moral maxim in both religious and secular traditions in the West. Part of the reason that genetic testing is seen as attractive is that, in a society committed to autonomy and self-determination as core values, information is valued for its own sake.

But not every society sees information as a good. Nor does every cultural and ethnic group within U.S. borders see information as a good. This particular normative stance—that information is in itself valuable—is generally accepted in America society, but not in all of our society's constituent subcultures.

Obviously there is also some value in genetic testing that allows for planning and preparation (Geller et al. 1997). Depending on what you find out about your genes, if you know that you are at risk of getting a genetic disease, or if you can establish through testing that you have a genetic disease, you can then begin to chart a course with it. You can buy life insurance, or you can get a funeral plot, or you can think about whether and whom you might marry, or decide many other things.

There is also the value of finding out that you are not at high risk. A negative test result can bring relief from worry and anxiety. Of course, no one should take too much relief from a negative genetic test result. There is a growing perception that if you pass your genetic test then you must be immortal. Unfortunately, even those who pass a particular genetic test will still die eventually. Part of the drive to do genetic testing is the fantasy that if we can dodge the different genetic bullets that a test can detect, then we will live forever.

Why not do genetic testing? Self-knowledge can be harmful—harmful to your self-image. You might feel yourself flawed. You might feel guilty that you have passed on a lethal disease to your own child. Or, if you are the child who does not test positive, you may feel that you do not deserve to have escaped the dread disease that has cut down other family members. Genetic testing can cause damage to relationships with others, with your own family. People may come to view a child differently who has been found to have a risk associated with a genetic disease.

More concretely, positive results on genetic tests or even taking a genetic test can be the basis of discrimination or underwriting exclusions from life, health, or disability insurance (Caplan 1997; Geller et al. 1997). It is not at all inconceivable that a nation that allows risk rating for all forms of insurance and that links health insurance to employment could find itself excluding entire categories of persons found to have certain genetic dispositions from employment or stigmatizing them as "costly" or "sick."

The ability to empower a child by genetic testing, I would submit, is not as great as it might be for an adult, since some of the goods realizable through testing—enhanced self-image, self-understanding, and so forth—are not the sort of goods that a newborn or a child can benefit from. The ability of a child to decide the value of self-knowledge for itself is poor; thus the very information that can be invaluable to an adult may be valueless to a child.

Prospects for rash behavior, however, may be greater for children. Children thus need to have decisions made for them by surrogates and other third parties. It may be that those people, because of the complicated emotions that they have when they deal with their children, or when picking the traits of their potential children in the case of embryos and fetuses, may act less rationally than they might otherwise act in pursuing their own self-interest.

The prospects for coercion where children are concerned are certainly greater. There is no more desperate creature in the universe than a parent who has been told that his or her child is at risk, or could be at risk, and that it was not detected because no genetic test was done. And the ability of parents to impose a choice about genetic testing on a child who may someday wish they had not done so is enormous.

Moral Principles and Values That Might Help

What sort of ethical principles might help guide decisions about when to test a child or fetus? One principle that seems important is *primum non nocere,* the principle of not causing unnecessary harm—in this case, not causing harm to the person being tested, not making the person worse off than he or she otherwise would have been. The "do no harm" principle that has long dominated professional codes of medicine would seem to be of special importance in trying to decide whether to use genetic testing on a child who cannot consent and for whom there is no prospect of therapeutic intervention if the test result is positive. If the child being tested is disempowered, disenfranchised, or otherwise damaged, testing should not be done (Caplan 1997; 1998). This principle may dictate saying no to a parent if a child might be harmed by knowing the results of a test and there is no remedy or prophylaxis to offer.

A second principle is that testing should only be done in children or fetuses or embryos if it will permit the creation of a person healthier than otherwise would have been created. Is the goal of medicine to indulge parental whim or to indulge parental choice, or is the goal of medicine to battle against disease and dysfunction? It may be that parents want genetic testing to avoid having an albino child or a female child or a short child. But unless the states for which testing is being sought are clearly dysfunctional or disabling, genetics testing should be avoided.

Third, there should not be testing without choice. Testing involves risks, so there ought not to be testing without the permission of the person being tested. If a person cannot consent due to age or incapacity, then someone must be appointed to do so for them. This person must try to act in the best interest of the person for whom they are choosing, not from their own interest or society's interest or medicine's interest in a particular disease or research question.

If these three simple principles are valid, they could have direct and significant implications for the practice of genetic testing in the future. Children would not be subjected to testing simply at the whim of their parents. Clinics would not advertise testing for any and every possible trait or characteristic in which parents might be interested; they would try to orient their testing of embryos, fetuses, and children to dysfunction and disability prevention. Finally, genetic testing would not proceed full tilt without some attempt to ensure that employment and insurance access are not contingent on the results of the tests.

Will these ethical principles form the template against which genetic testing evolves? It is impossible to say. But whether these principles are adopted and put into public policy is a matter of choice. The technology that is genetic testing is not going to go where it will, whatever we think or no matter what ethical values and rules we impose, in some Harkenesque manner. The only question is whether we have the political will to ensure that ethics and the law do not lag behind where we can see that genetic testing might be going.

References

Adler, Eric. 1997. What's Next? Technology Inspires Wonder and Worry. *Kansas City Star,* 2 March, A1, 5–6.

American Medical Association. 1996. *Code of Medical Ethics: Current Opinions and Annotations.* Chicago: American Medical Association.

Baker, Robert, ed. 1995. *The Codification of Medical Morality: Historical and Philosophical Studies of the Formalization of Medical Morality in the Eighteenth and Nineteenth Centuries.* Vol. 2, *Anglo-American Medical Ethics and Medical Jurisprudence in the Nineteenth Century.* Dordrecht, Kluwer.

Caplan, Arthur L. 1997. *Due Consideration.* New York: John Wiley.

———. 1998. *Am I My Brother's Keeper?* Bloomington: Indiana University Press.

Fox, Rene C., and Swazey, Judith P. 1992. *Spare Parts.* New York: Oxford University Press.

Geller, G.; Botkin, J. R.; Green, M. J.; et al. 1997. Genetic Testing for Susceptibility to Adult Onset Cancer. *Journal of the American Medical Association,* 277:1467–74.

Kolata, Gina. 1998. With an Eye on the Public, Scientists Choose Their Words. *New York Times,* 6 January, B12, F4.

Lane, Earl, Senator. 1997. Human Clones OK / But Scientists Tell Panel: For Animals Only. *Newsday,* 13 March, A08.

Lerman, C., and Croyle, R. 1994. Psychological Issues in Genetic Testing for Breast Cancer Susceptibility. *Archives of Internal Medicine* 154:609–16.

NBC News Transcripts. 1997. Senator Tom Harkin Discusses His Views on Human Cloning. *TODAY Show,* 13 March.

Powers, William. 1998. A Slant on Cloning. *National Journal* 30 (10 January):58.

Singer, Maxine. 1977. Historical Perspectives on Research with Recombinant DNA. In *Research with Recombinant DNA.* Washington, D.C.: National Academy of Sciences Press.

Stolberg, S. G. 1998. A Small Spark Ignites Debate on Laws on Cloning Humans. *New York Times,* 19 January, A1, A11.

Weiss, Rick. 1998. Fertility Innovation or Exploitation? Regulatory Void Allows for Trial—and Error—Without Patient Disclosure Rules. *Washington Post,* 9 February, A1, 16.

19

Bioethics in the Developing World

National Responsibilities and International Collaboration

FLORENCIA LUNA, PH.D.

Medical science and technology challenge medical ethics simply by their sheer inventiveness. Modern genetics challenges our conception of illness and our conception of the physician-patient relationship. It offers us the technology of cloning, and we puzzle over whether it should be permissible. Intensive care technologies challenge our very conception of life and of death, forcing ethicists to address issues of medical policy and law. The public and the press are intrigued by these issues because they demonstrate the human power to alter the future and transform the nature of birth and death through scientific and technological ingenuity.

These questions preoccupy bioethicists, but despite their intrinsic attractiveness, I do not address them in this chapter. My concern is with another challenge that bioethics must face, a challenge with respect to some of the most vulnerable people on the planet, the people in the developing countries, especially the less-privileged, less-educated, less-literate members of these countries. I discuss the question of how bioethics applies to these people and, more generally, the relationship between bioethics in developing countries and in the international community. For as the world becomes a "global village," we need to discuss the links that should be forged between international bioethics and the national bioethics, especially those in the developing world.

As an Argentine bioethicist, I naturally write from the perspective of my own and other South American countries, but I believe that what I say is relevant to many other countries in the developing world—especially those in which scientific medical practitioners must deal with a scientifically unsophisticated and often illiterate population. In the first part of this chapter I focus on the strong paternalistic physician-patient relationship and the correlatively weak theory of patients' rights in my own and other developing countries. I also consider a very common argument offered by physicians in such countries, "the argument from illiteracy," which states that because patients are illiterate, they lack the capacity to participate in decisions about their own health care.

In the second part of this chapter, I turn from the national to the international community, outlining the case that developed countries have certain responsibilities toward the developing countries. I use as an example medical journals' policies about publishing unethical research and argue that the international medical societies and the editors of medical journals have a responsibility to develop standards that protect the subjects of medical research who reside in the developing world.

National Problems and Responsibilities in the Developing World

In the most recent edition of *Principles of Biomedical Ethics* (1994), Tom Beauchamp and James Childress note that the *Oxford English Dictionary* "dates the term 'paternalism' from the 1880s, giving its root meaning as 'the principle and practice of paternal administration, as by a father; the claim or attempt to supply the needs or to regulate [a] life . . . in the same way a father does those of his children.'" They observe that "the analogy with the father presupposes two features of the parent's role: that the father acts beneficently (that is, in accordance with his conception of the interests of his children) and that he makes at least some of the decisions with respect to his children's welfare, rather than letting them make these decisions." They observe that to apply a paternalist model in health care is to envision the health professional as a "loving parent with dependent and fearful children" (Beauchamp and Childress 1994, 273–74).

In the developing world, healthcare professionals' predilections toward paternalism tend to be reinforced by what I call "the myth of illiteracy." I use the word *myth* because, in developing countries like Argentina, rates of illiteracy are not high. A comparison between Argentinean censuses in 1980 and 1991 reveals that elementary-school attendance increased from 90.55 percent to

95.69 percent, while secondary school attendance went from 41.85 percent to 59.24 percent. Illiteracy in the *literal* sense seems to be a marginal problem at best, if over 90 percent of the population is receiving a primary education and over half a secondary education. Yet as I have shown elsewhere (Luna 1995), Argentine healthcare professionals commonly claim that because they have to deal with illiterate patients, they are justified in assuming paternalism as their normal stance in their relationships with their patients.

This all-too-common justification for paternalism, however, rests on a fundamental confusion; for even with respect to the minority of patients who actually lack the ability to read, the presumed need for paternalism confuses illiteracy with incompetence or decisional incapacity—that is, it confuses the inability to understand written information with the inability or incapacity to understand information that has been properly communicated. Undoubtedly, in some circumstances there might be difficulties related to capacity or competency since an illiterate person may suffer from psychological problems, fear, addiction, and so forth; but the same could be said of educated and literate people. In such cases, when we notice problems of impairment in communication or in understanding, it is valid to raise the question of competence, whether the person is literate or not. But to assume, a priori, that illiterates are incompetent is to commit what philosophers call a category error—mistaking one kind of thing for something entirely different.

It is, of course, convenient for healthcare professionals operating in the developing world to presume that, unless they have evidence to the contrary, their patients are incapacitated by their illiteracy. Paternalism *appears* efficient. It is quicker and easier to issue doctors' orders than to take the time to explain carefully the nature of a problem and then to consider the preferences and beliefs of the patient. Generally speaking, of course, patients who are actually illiterate require more time for explanations, since one needs to adapt technical medical language into a simple and clear language. Actual illiterates, moreover, are unlikely to have the means to compensate physicians for this extra time and effort. So Argentine healthcare professionals find it natural and convenient to adopt a paternalistic stance toward the average patient and to justify it by the argument from illiteracy.

The position I have outlined is widely held by a majority of Argentine physicians, who use it to show why paternalism in our country is justified. The argument is usually directed against the principle of respect for persons, which is understood as "foreign" and irrelevant to Argentina because it originates in countries where health professionals can presume that there is no illiteracy.

Autonomy, it is said, may be appropriate for North Americans; but it is not considered useful in light of the social realities of Argentina and other Latin American countries.

One might expect that Argentine health professionals would reject the principle of autonomy and adopt a paternalistic stance only toward their illiterate patients, but in fact they extend paternalism and reject the principle of autonomy when dealing with the majority of their patients. Their rationale is that patients are like "infants" who could be scared by the information about their illnesses and about possible treatments. Hence, the argument for paternalism that was initially advanced because of the presumed pervasiveness of illiteracy is generally extended to apply to most patients, irrespective of whether they happen to be literate.

Informed Consent and Refusal of Treatment

Informed consent is just beginning to develop as a legal doctrine in Argentina. It is required for sophisticated surgery, plastic surgery, and new reproductive technologies. But quite often in these cases, surgeons secure consent to protect themselves or their institution from legal problems, not to inform the patient or to respect the patient's wishes. This is not a trivial or accidental phenomenon. It seems to cohere with the pattern of neglecting patients' rights and the principle of autonomy described in the preceding section.

Even to speak of "patients' rights" in the Argentine context is problematic. There is no official "Patients' Bill of Rights" in Argentina. There is no document hanging in the hospital corridors informing patients about the possibility of refusing treatment or of asking for information about alternative treatments. Moreover, there are no laws concerning refusal of treatment, withholding life support, or anything similar.

There is a general law governing the practice of medicine (law 17.132, article 19) that (with some exceptions for unconsciousness, incapacity, and so forth) establishes the need to respect the patient's will when he or she refuses treatment or intervention. This requirement is even stronger in the case of mutilating surgery. The problem is, the law is not clear; its terminology is ambiguous and obsolete. These normative failures favor indiscriminate intervention and the paternalistic tradition mentioned (Kraut 1997, 212). Nevertheless, in September 1995, there was a truly important advance in the consideration of patients' rights, or at least in recognizing the significance of a patient's values. For the first time ever, the Argentine judicial system ruled that a patient could refuse a treatment. A 63-year-old competent man with diabetes, who had had one of his legs amputated, refused a second amputation for his other leg. This was the first time that a refusal based on the autonomy and dignity of a person was accepted by an Argentine judge. There has since been an attempt to pass a law regarding end-of-life refusal of treatment, but it was not accepted and is not currently being debated in the Congress.

The wishes of members of religious minorities like Jehovah's Witnesses are not respected in Argentina. Paradoxically, in this supposedly religious country, the possibility of refusing treatments on religious grounds has generally not been accepted by the judiciary, except in a few recent cases. In 1995 a 30-year-old woman, a practicing Jehovah's Witness suffering from leukemia, petitioned a judge to recognize her right to refuse blood transfusion before her condition necessitated it. Her petition was accepted, but only if her husband would not oppose it. Despite this last constraint, the court's decision could be considered the first step toward recognizing the rights of religious minorities. Unfortunately, in January 1997 a court issued an order obliging a 48-year-old Jehovah's Witness woman to undergo a blood transfusion. This last decision ignored the previous one, threatening to restore the old paternalistic model.

In the area of respect for persons and patients' rights, there is much work to be done in Argentina. Bioethicists need to analyze the arguments currently accepted in Argentine culture and demonstrate the underlying fallacies, not only to their own satisfaction, but in a way that can be appreciated by health providers and patients. There is even harder work to be done in the legislative arena—not only in relation to the right to be informed about treatment, to consent to treatment, and to refuse treatment, but also with respect to end-of-life issues and questions about the beginning of life and reproductive freedoms.

I believe we have a basic national responsibility to address the kinds of problems that are deeply entrenched in our society. This does not mean that some international collaborative work could not be done, but there are certain changes that have to be promoted from within a particular society, and the main responsibility lies on the locals.

The Importance of the International Community: The Case of Unethical Experimentation

While there are some activities that are properly the prerogative and the responsibility of local bioethicists, there are others for which the international bioethics community should play a responsible role. The international bioethics community can assist by fostering educational programs and initiatives, as well as by providing advice about the importance of various ethical codes and legal regulations affecting patients' rights. International policies may also help to change national attitudes. These are sensitive issues that are very difficult to deal with abstractly, so I will shift the subject slightly and present a specific example that may allow us to think reflectively about an international approach to bioethics. The example I have in mind is the decision about whether or not to publish morally tainted experiments. What attitude should the international bioethical community adopt toward unethical research?

The dilemma that an editor faces when he or she has to decide whether to publish a manuscript that describes research that he or she believes to be unethical is whether to: (a) publish the research; (b) publish it with an editorial explaining why the research is morally suspect, or with an editorial explicitly condemning the methods used; or, (c) reject the article on moral grounds. Prudence suggests a combined policy. For cases in which the ethical problems are serious—where basic human rights have not been respected, where consent has been given without complete or proper information, where voluntary participation by subjects is dubious, or where deceit has been practiced—I would support the strong policy of rejecting the article on moral grounds. Maintaining a strong deterrence policy is important because no matter how important the knowledge revealed in an experiment may be, the way this knowledge is obtained is also important to medicine and to the future of medical research.

For dubious cases, where the risk assessment can be doubted or where there are suspicions of ethical problems, I argue for a policy under which the article is published along with a serious discussion of the ethical problems suspected, allowing a rebuttal by the authors. I recognize that sometimes it is not clear whether the research was unethical, but I suggest that in such cases a measure of deterrence is preserved if we publish the article with an editorial exploring the ethical issues.

The debate over publishing unethical research has been closely connected to the question of publishing the Nazi's altitude, burning, and freezing experiments. In my opinion, however, these examples are misleading because the Holocaust hypothermia experiments represent a unique situation, a historical aberration that we hope will never be repeated. These experiments are related to issues of anti-Semitism, war, and totalitarianism. Therefore, they do not provide examples that seem applicable to democratic societies in peacetime.

The problem that editors face today is not whether to publish an experiment in which a scientist has killed his research subjects in concentration camps, but rather whether to publish the results of experiments in which researchers appeared willing to deceive their subjects or promised impossible benefits or hid the actual risks to induce people to think they were receiving therapy when they were really being used as research subjects. As Marcia Angell, editor of the *New England Journal of Medicine,* points out, unethical experimentation today is more likely to reflect thoughtlessness than callousness (Angell 1990). Intentionally or not, researchers disrespect persons and act in ways that do not allow them to make an informed decision about whether or not to enter a research program.

More important still, at least to bioethicists and patients in developing countries, is the fact that researchers in developing countries, and researchers from developed countries who are working in developing countries, may often be tempted to engage in morally tainted experiments by the easier conditions that are common in the developing world. A long history of political authoritarianism and medical paternalism has made this population accustomed to obedience. Moreover, it is often difficult to implement proper safeguards in developing countries, in part because of a lack of adequate level of respect for persons, especially for the lower classes, for minority groups, and for women. Complicating matters further, most research is carried out in public hospitals whose main population is poor people—a population with little education and little awareness of their basic rights. They often do not know what research is and do not understand that they can refuse participation or can leave a research program whenever they wish.

To make matters even worse, scientists in developing countries are often not educated about the ethical aspects of the human subjects research. Education in biomedical ethics and research ethics is just beginning in the developing world; often there is very little teaching or research on these subjects at the national level. Local "IRB's" (institutional review boards) are confused with clinical ethics committees—which, in some countries, are just starting.

Even though there are differences between countries, this is an accurate picture of the situation of many countries in the developing world, particularly in Latin America. And this brings me back to the question of the responsibility of international bioethics toward bioethics in the developing countries. Consider, for example, some cases:

In "Editorial Responsibility: Protecting Human Rights by Restricting Publication of Unethical Research," Marcia Angell (1992) describes the study of virus X, which, while harmless in normal adults, can cause devastating, often fatal disease in premature newborns. The authors of this study were conducting a randomized clinical trial of a method to make seropositive blood —that is, infected blood—safe for premature newborns who require blood transfusions. The study was conducted in a developing country. All infants received blood from untested donors. In half of the cases the blood was treated. As expected, some of the patients in the control group received infected blood and became sick. Some even died. Angell points out that the *New England Journal of Medicine* refused to publish the study on the grounds that the researchers knowingly exposed some of their subjects to unacceptable risks. I would add that the experiment also demonstrates the lack of respect for the importance of human life, in this case infant life, by some researchers working in developing countries. One must also question whether these researchers really had any respect for the persons upon whom they were conducting experiments. One wonders what sorts of "informed consent" forms were signed by these parents? How was the research explained to them? Were they informed that there was a safer and not very complicated alternative (transfusing tested blood)? Could this research have been conducted in developed countries? Or was it research that could only be conducted in an environment in which persons and their lives were neither adequately respected nor protected?

Another case of dubious and controversial research arose while this chapter was in galleys. It was also brought to light by Angell when she published an article by Peter Lurie and Sidney Wolfe (1997) followed by a very strong editorial criticizing quite severely research that was being done in sub-Saharan Africa, Thailand, and the Dominican Republic on pregnant women with AIDS. These trials attempt to establish the minimum dose of AZT in order to prevent vertical transmission from HIV-infected mothers to their fetuses. The main controversy originally emerged because of the use of placebo in the control group: AZT (ACTG 176) has been proven effective in blocking approximately two-thirds of transmission of HIV to the fetus (Connor et al. 1997), and it is the regimen given to women in industrialized countries. Was it justified to deny this treatment—by using a placebo—to pregnant women in these developing countries? Strong replies came from researchers in both developed and developing countries. Harold Varmus, director of the National Institutes of Health, and David Satcher, director of the Centers for Disease Control and Prevention, offered an early reply. They justified the importance of such trials for developing countries by differentiating this research from merely exploitative experiments, and they pointed to extensive in-country participation (Varmus and Satcher 1997). Later on, there were even stronger letters from the Medical Research Council Joint Ethical Committee of the Gambia Government (1998) and by Dr. Edward Mbidde (1998) of Uganda.

There are not overwhelming arguments for one side or the other (Resnik 1998; Schüklenk 1998; Thomas 1998; del Rio 1998; Luna forthcoming). Nevertheless, I think this kind of discussion airs the ethical problems involved and helps raise consciousness about the implications and risks of international multicentric research. It may also influence the implementation and design of AIDS vaccine trials in relation to questions of safety, standards of care, kind of treatment to be provided if the person gets sick during the trials, informed consent, and prevention.

Publishers today need to refuse to publish unethical research, not out of respect for the victims of the Nazi experiments or because of Beecher's whistle-blowing article about research that endangered the health or the life of the subjects in the 1960s (Beecher 1966) or in deference to the findings of the Advisory Committee on Human Radiation Experiments (1995) about experiments conducted during the Cold War. They need to enforce ethical standards because there is still a potential for researchers to abuse their subjects, especially in developing countries. In the absence of international standards for ethical scientific publication, it will become increasingly tempting to conduct experiments in the developing world that have been declared unethical in the United States and the European Community, simply because it is easier and subjects are more vulnerable in the developing world.

Collaborative International Efforts

I believe that the international bioethics community should be more active in assisting bioethicists in the developing world in promoting a change of attitudes toward respect for patients' rights both in the patient–physician relationship and in the subject–researcher relationship. In relation to the latter, there are several ways that the international bioethics community can assist in deterring unethical research. These include conducting educational programs, establishing procedural safeguards, and developing universal and unambiguous rules related to research.

For example, the requirement that ethics committees approve research protocols is beginning to change certain practices. Nowadays, there is international pressure to have research approved by local ethics committees and to require informed consent. This international requirement is promoting the creation of ethics committees—institutions that simply did not exist years ago—and raising awareness of international standards for ethical conduct in research.

International bioethics guidelines and international regulations for conducting ethical research are also helping to change attitudes. What is interesting and appealing about these policies is that they do not coerce, but instead they set standards—ethical guidelines that should be respected by all researchers who choose to participate in a multicenter international research. This kind of policy is promoting a slow but important change in the attitude toward ethical issues. Even in contexts where there are no systematic studies, the international pressure for having research protocols approved by local ethics committees is incorporating ethics "explicitly" into the practice of research. Requiring approval of ethics committees and informed consent may not be sufficient to protect against all forms of ethical abuse, and it may well run the risk of transforming ethical concerns into hollow legal exercises, but it nonetheless seems to be an appropriate first step toward a universal ethical consciousness in the conduct of human subjects research.

This change in attitudes is quite important and may be accelerated if we develop clear standards in related areas. I think there should be an internationally recognized policy that if research is to be published in reputable journals, their methodology section should incorporate not only scientific standards but also ethical standards so that these too can be assessed as part of the editorial evaluation and approval process. Although this requirement is suggested by the Helsinki Declaration, there is no such universally recognized standard at present. In this vein, Angell observes that the International Committee of Medical Journal Editors (ICMJE) emphasizes process rather than substance and avoids the issue of what editors should do when they believe a study unethical, if it has satisfied the procedural requirement of IRB's approval and informed consent (Angell 1992). I further believe that editors should explicitly explain ethical standards and that reference to international ethics codes should be made in the "Instructions to Authors."

Conclusion

In the first part of this chapter I tried to show the sort of bioethical problems that many developing countries face. In the case of the patient–physician relationship, the moral burden rests on locals to address these issues, especially since direct intervention by the international bioethics community may be viewed as intrusive. In the end, the responsibility for moral change must rest mainly with those who work in these developing countries. Like all other bioethicists, they must encourage bioethics education, identify conceptual bias and erroneous practices, and promote changes in the regulations and laws of their own countries that enhance patients' rights.

In the second part I privileged the international community effort. In the case of research, an active international role is easier to accept because of the multicentered nature of international projects. I also argued that a similar case can be outlined with respect to international journals. Researchers around the world wish to publish in prestigious international journals. By setting ethical guidelines, therefore, these journals will help the promotion of worldwide ethical standards.

I believe that the work local bioethicists can do in close cooperation with the international community is very important, and in this sense, setting international guidelines may help deter unethical practices. I have discussed just one case—not publishing morally tainted research—but I think an international and collaborative approach to ethical problems can be a fruitful way of meeting the challenges we must face to change the world for the better.

References

Advisory Committee on Human Radiation Experiments. 1995. Final Report. Washington D.C.: U.S. Government Printing Office.

Angell, Marcia. 1990. The Nazi Hypothermia Experiments and Unethical Research Today. *New England Journal of Medicine* 322:1463.

———. 1992. Editorial Responsibility: Protecting Human Rights by Restricting Publication of Unethical Research. In *The Nazi Doctors and the Nuremberg Code*, ed. G. Annas and M. Grodin, 283. New York: Oxford University Press.

———. 1997. The Ethics of Clinical Research in the Third World. *New England Journal of Medicine* 337(12):347–49.

Beauchamp, Tom, and Childress, James. 1994. *Principles of Biomedical Ethics*, 4th ed. New York: Oxford University Press.

Beecher, Henry. 1966. Ethics and Clinical Research. *New England Journal of Medicine* 274:1354–60.

Connor, E. M.; Sperling, R. S.; Gelber, R.; et al. 1994. Reduction of Maternal-Infant Transmission of Human Immunodeficiency Virus Type 1 with Zidovudine Treatment. *New England Journal of Medicine* 331:1173–80.

Luna, Florencia. 1995. Paternalism and the Argument from Illiteracy. *Bioethics* 9: 3–4.

———. 1997. Vulnerable Populations and Morally Tainted Experiments. *Bioethics* 9(3/4):283–90.

———. Forthcoming. Bioethics and Research in Argentina.

Lurie, P., and Wolfe, S. 1997. Unethical Trials of Interventions to Reduce Perinatal Transmission of the Human Immunodeficiency Virus in Developing Countries. *New England Journal of Medicine* 337(12):853–56.

Mbidde, Edward. 1998. Bioethics and Local Circumstances. *Science* 279:155.

Resnik, David. The Ethics of HIV in Developing Countries. *Bioethics* 12(4):286–306.

Schüklenk, Udo. 1998. Unethical Perinatal HIV Transmission Trials Establish Bad Precedent. *Bioethics* 12(4):312–19.

Thomas, Joe. 1998. Ethical Challenges of HIV Clinical Trials in Developing Countries. *Bioethics* 12(4):320–28.

Varmus, H., and Satcher, D. Ethical Complexities of Conducting Research in Developing Countries. *New England Journal of Medicine* 337(14):1003–5.

20

Medical Ethics and Human Rights

Reflections on the Fiftieth Anniversary of the Nuremberg Code

GEORGE J. ANNAS, J.D., M.P.H.

American bioethics draws both its strengths and its weaknesses from the fact that it is rooted in and dominated by American law. Its strengths are derived from the rich tradition of American constitutional law, which is founded on concepts of liberty, equality, and justice, and on the universal concept of inalienable rights. Its weaknesses stem from the fact that the multicultural American experience is unique in the world, and that its once famous "melting pot" is threatened with cultural fragmentation. This, combined with America's secular humanist liberalism, helps explain why its free-market economic system often seems to provide a more coherent value system for its citizens than any other creed.

Historian Arthur M. Schlesinger Jr. has captured and capsulized the American experience. Tocqueville, he notes, observed that immigrants to the United States became transformed into Americans "through the exercise of the political rights and civic responsibilities bestowed on them by the Declaration of Independence and the Constitution." More than a century later, in 1944, Gunnar Myrdal of Sweden wrote of Americans that "of all national origins, religions, creeds, and colors," they hold in common "the most explicitly expressed system of general ideals" of any country in the West. In Schlesinger's paraphrase, these ideals are "the essential dignity and equality of all human beings, of inalienable rights to freedom, justice and opportunity." Myrdal labeled these ideas "the American Creed" and properly observed that in trying to live up to them, "America is continuously struggling for its soul" (Schlesinger 1982).

It is probably too much to say that American bioethics is engaged in a struggle for the soul of American medicine. It is not, however, too much to say that the values and ideals of American law, including the concept of inalienable rights, as expressed in the Declaration of Independence and the Constitution, have consistently dominated the ethical discourse concerning both substantive and procedural approaches to medical practice. In this chapter I address the dominance of American bioethics by American law, the fiftieth anniversary of the Nuremberg Code, and the opportunity this anniversary presents for the world's doctors and lawyers to work together to promote human rights, the inalienable rights of all of the world's citizens.

The Dominance of American Bioethics by Law

The Declaration of Independence is the foundational document of the American Revolution and the American experience. At its core is the belief that all persons are endowed with "certain unalienable rights" including the rights of "life, liberty and the pursuit of happiness" (Wills 1978). The document that established our government, the U.S. Constitution, was almost immediately amended by the addition of the Bill of Rights, the first ten amendments. These specify individual rights, such as freedom of speech and freedom of religion, that the government cannot interfere with (at least not unless it can demonstrate a compelling state interest for such interference). Thus when we discuss Americans, we are talking about people with rights; and when we discuss the life and death of Americans, we cannot help but frame the discourse in terms of rights.

Rights talk dominates America, as it has dominated American bioethics discourse. The major issues in bioethics over the past two decades, for example, have involved abortion, care of the dying, and human experimentation. In all of these areas, the principles of American law, usually constitutional law, have defined and dominated the debate (Annas 1993). The abortion debate has been primarily a legal, and often a political, debate, at least since the 1973 case of *Roe v. Wade*. At the other end of life, "right to die" discourse has been dominated by law since the 1976 *Quinlan* case, which was about whether, and on what basis, life-sustaining ventilator treatment could be legally withdrawn from a permanently unconscious person. This debate continues to be dominated by legal concerns such as passing statutes to provide physicians with legal immunity for assisting patients to commit suicide. As with abortion, the

U.S. Supreme Court has had the last word regarding the attempt to constitutionalize the "right to physician-assisted suicide," an attempt that ultimately failed in June 1997 (Annas 1997).

In pragmatic America, where religious, cultural, and ethnic diversity have, along with the religious freedom and antiestablishment clauses of the First Amendment, precluded a single ethic, the law has often been seen as defining not only the nation's minimum morality, but its norms of conduct as well. This has been especially true in medicine, where the question "Can I get sued?" is much more likely to be heard than the question "What's the right thing to do?" The major challenge contemporary bioethics faces is to move its focus beyond defining the minimum morality that the law requires, and into the realm of the right and the good.

More generally, American bioethics developed as a reaction to medical paternalism, the practitioner's parentlike power to render patient wishes irrelevant, which has been intensified by medical technology. The legal reaction to paternalism, including the related Civil Rights and women's movements, made three major characteristics of contemporary bioethical discourse inevitable: the stress on self-determination, the use of paradigmatic cases, and the use of procedural mechanisms to resolve disputes. Self-determination or liberty is the fundamental concept enunciated in our Bill of Rights, our Declaration of Independence, and our common law history. The use of paradigmatic case examples parallels the history of the common law itself, which is based on using past judicial decisions (precedents) as the basis for deciding current controversies. Finally, much of the law is concerned with the use of procedural mechanisms to resolve disputes. So it is almost inevitable that when you get procedural decision making, you get lawyers, because lawyers are experts at procedure.

Nor is it only bioethicists who refer (and defer) to the law. American physicians have a long history of equating ethical obligations with legal obligations. This accounts for the consistent insistence of organized medicine, acting through groups such as the American Medical Association (AMA), that if society wants physicians to act in particular ethical ways, such as stopping to help accident victims, society must grant physicians legal immunity for these actions. Insistence on legal immunity pervades medicine and often displaces ethical discussion. It was at the heart of much of the right-to-die / right-to-refuse-treatment discussion. Thus, the Karen Ann Quinlan case came to the courts because physicians, who believed treatment termination was ethically appropriate, nonetheless would not act without legal immunity. This insistence on immunity continues to dominate the physician-assisted suicide debate, including the public referenda in California, Washington, and Oregon. The quest for prospective legal immunity in these instances makes no more sense than it would if heart or brain surgeons refused to operate on patients unless courts gave them prior legal immunity in case anything went wrong in surgery. The AMA should abandon its quest for legal immunity in all spheres and replace it with a program of quality assurance and accountability.

The lack of moral courage and self-policing in American medicine helps explain why the most important ethical development in medicine over the past two decades, informed consent, had to be imposed on medicine through the courts rather than adopted as a professionally developed ethical principle. Informed consent is a rejection of medical paternalism, since it requires physicians to share certain information with patients prior to obtaining their consent to treat them. It is remarkable that information sharing had to be imposed by law, and that many in the medical profession still view information sharing with patients as either optional or inappropriate.

Just as law was needed to counterbalance paternalism, it has also been needed to help bend technology to human purposes by taking informed consent seriously and letting patients decide whether or not to use advanced medical technologies. It should nonetheless be underlined that the courts are not attacking medicine or physicians by rejecting paternalism. Rather, the model has been to derive the legal obligation of obtaining informed consent from the fiduciary or trust nature of the doctor-patient relationship. In this view, shared information and shared decision making are critical elements to foster (rather than undermine) the relationship between doctor and patient. In the attack by managed care on the doctor-patient relationship (through gag clauses, treatment limitations, etc.), courts will thus likely seek to protect the valued doctor-patient relationship by limiting third-party interference with it that has the effect of limiting patient self-determination.

Human Rights and Medicine

If the argument of the previous section is correct, and bioethics in America—the country in which it was conceived—is the creature of American law and legalistic inclinations and of the proclivity of American physicians to substitute law for morality, how can bioethics apply outside of America? To explore this question we need to reconsider the issues that gave rise to bioethics. This is not only the 150th anniversary of the AMA Code of Ethics. It is also the fiftieth anniversary of the conclusion of the trial of Nazi physicians at Nuremberg, a trial that has been variously designated as the "Doctors' Trial" and the "Medical Case," and that is generally considered the inspiration for bioethics (Annas and Grodin 1992; *Trials* 1950). In addition to documenting atrocities committed by physicians and scientists during the war, the primary product of the trial has come to be known as the "Nuremberg Code," a judicial codification of ten prerequisites for the moral and legal use of human beings in medical experiments.

The 1946–47 trial of the Nazi doctors documented the most extreme example of physician participation in human rights abuses, criminal activities, and murder. Hitler called upon physicians not only to help justify his racial hatred policies with a "scientific" rationale (racial hygiene), but also to direct his sterilization and euthanasia programs, experimentation programs, and ultimately his death camps (Proctor 1987; Lifton 1986). Sixteen physicians and scientists were found guilty, and seven were executed. A universal standard of physician responsibility in human rights abuses involving experimentation on humans, the Nuremberg Code, was articulated and has been widely recognized, if not always followed, by the world community.

The Nuremberg Code was a response to the horrors of Nazi experimentation in the death camps—wide-scale experimentation, without consent, that often had the death of the prisoner-subjects as its planned endpoint (Katz 1993). The code has ten provisions—two designed to protect the rights of subjects of human experimentation, and eight designed to protect their welfare. The best known is its first, the consent requirement, which states in part:

> The voluntary consent of the human subject is absolutely essential. This means that the person involved should have legal capacity to give consent; should be so situated as to be able to exercise free power of choice, without the intervention of any element of force, fraud, deceit, duress, overreaching, or other ulterior form of constraint or coercion; and should have sufficient knowledge and comprehension of the elements of the subject matter involved as to enable him to make an understanding and enlightened decision.[1]

Although the Nuremberg Code has never been formally adopted as a whole by the United Nations, a statement related to torture appears as article 5 of the Universal Declaration of Human Rights. A second sentence added to the text of article 5, which reflects the concerns of the Nuremberg Code, also appears as article 7 in the United Nations International Covenant on Civil and Political Rights (adopted and opened for signature, ratification, and accession by the UN General Assembly in 1966, entered into force in 1976). Article 7 of the covenant states:

No one shall be subjected to torture or to cruel, inhuman or degrading treatment or punishment. In particular, no one shall be subjected without his free consent to medical or scientific experimentation.

The World Medical Association

In late 1946, one hundred delegates from thirty-two national medical associations met in London to form the world's first international medical organization. The World Medical Association (WMA) was created to promote ties between national medical organizations and doctors of the world. Its objectives were:

- To promote closer ties among the national medical organizations and among the doctors of the world by personal contact and all other means available.
- To maintain the honour and protect the interests of the medical profession.
- To study and report on the professional problems which confront the medical profession in the different countries.
- To organize an exchange of information on matters of interest to the medical profession.
- To establish relations with, and to present the views of the medical profession to the World Health Organization, UNESCO, and other appropriate bodies.
- To assist all peoples of the world to attain the highest possible level of health.
- To promote world peace (Routley 1949).

In September 1947, shortly after the final judgment at the Doctors' Trial, the first official meeting of the WMA was held in Paris. The WMA formulated a new physician oath to promote and serve the health of humanity. This was followed by a discussion of the "principles of social security." Key principles adopted included:

- Freedom of physician to choose his *[sic]* location and type of practice.
- All medical services to be controlled by physicians.
- That it is not in the public interest that doctors should be full-time salaried servants of government or social security bodies.
- Remuneration of medical services ought not to depend directly on the financial condition of the insurance organization.

• Freedom of choice of patient by doctor except in cases of emergency or humanitarian considerations.

To the WMA's credit, one of the first issues discussed by the 1947 general assembly was the "betrayal of the traditions of medicine" that had occurred in Germany. The assembly asked, "Why did these doctors lack moral or professional conscience and forget or ignore the humanitarian motives and ideals of medical service?" "How can a repetition of such crimes be averted?" and acknowledged the "widespread criminal conduct of the German medical profession since 1933." The WMA endorsed "the judicial action taken to punish those members of the medical profession who shared in the crimes," and it solemnly condemned "the crimes and inhumanity committed by doctors in Germany and elsewhere against human beings" (WMA 1949). The assembly continued: "We undertake to expel from our organization those members who have been personally guilty of the crimes. . . . We will exact from all our members a standard of conduct that recognizes the sanctity, moral liberty and personal dignity of every human being."

Nonetheless, consistent with its physician-protection goals, the WMA has consistently focused more on physicians' rights than on patients' rights. Through its Declaration of Helsinki in 1964, for example, it endorsed shifting the focus of protection of the human subjects in medical research from the protection of human rights through informed consent to the protection of patient welfare through physician responsibility. The 1964 Declaration, for example, divided research into two types: research combined with professional care, and nontherapeutic research. Consent was required for the latter. But as to the former, the subject was transformed into a patient, and consent was simply urged: "If at all possible, consistent with patient psychology, the doctor *should* obtain the patient's freely given consent after the patient has been given a full explanation." The Declaration of Helsinki thus attempted to undermine the primacy of subject consent in the Nuremberg Code and displace it with the paternalistic values of the traditional doctor-patient relationship (Annas 1992).

Although the WMA has also issued a number of noble statements, including condemning physician involvement in torture and capital punishment, it has largely acted like other professional trade associations. Its primary interest is the members' welfare, with a secondary objective of issuing "ethical" statements. With the exception of barring membership of Japanese and German physicians following World War II, the WMA has never sought or exercised any authority to identify, monitor, or punish either physicians or medical societies who violate their ethical principles. In fact, in 1992 the WMA irrevocably lost all claim to speak on behalf of the ethics of the world's physicians when it elected a Nazi physician as president.

The Sewering Affair

Hans-Joachim Sewering is a former member of the Nazi Party and the Nazi blackshirt troops known as the SS. During World War II he was a physician at the Schönbrunn Institute for the Handicapped in the city of Dachau. During his tenure at the institute, he transferred at least one fourteen-year-old girl with epilepsy to Eglfing-Haar Hospital. Three weeks later, in late 1943, this otherwise physically healthy girl was dead. Of 275 children who were admitted to Eglfing-Haar from 1940 to 1942, 213 were killed. Sewering's 1992 election to the presidency of the WMA provoked public protests. Andre Wynen, fellow German physician and the secretary general of the WMA, defended him, saying that "we must accept that the young people of that time had the right to make mistakes." Sewering later acknowledged his Nazi past, but claimed no knowledge of, or involvement in, the euthanasia program. In January 1993 four nuns still living at the Schönbrunn Institute, who had worked there during the war, substantiated that from 1940 to 1944 more than nine hundred mentally and physically handicapped patients were sent to specific "healing centers." The nuns said that they knew the patients would be exterminated at these centers as so-called unworthy lives, and that Sewering, despite his denials, must also have known.

Following receipt of information documenting Sewering's past, Dr. James Todd, executive vice-president of the American Medical Association (AMA), requested a full explanation from the German Federal Physician Chamber. The chamber responded that the charges against Sewering had been extensively covered in the European press and were so well known that they did not require further notification of WMA members. The AMA called on the WMA to amend the nominating form for all WMA officers to require "verification by the national medical association that the candidate is an individual of impeccable character signed by the Association President and Chief Executive Officer." The AMA also recommended that the WMA set up an ethics committee to help it address ethical issues. The AMA believes that such "strong measures" have brought "this issue to conclusion." I do not share this view. These events follow an earlier controversy regarding the WMA's admission of the Medical Association of South Africa and its refusal to take a strong stand against apartheid, a crime against humanity. I believe these actions require the conclusion that the WMA does not, and cannot be permitted to pretend to, represent and enforce the ethics of the world medical community (Grodin, Annas, and Glantz 1993). If electing a Nazi physician involved in the euthanasia program as president does not disqualify an organization to set the ethical standards for the world's physicians, what would? The WMA should be abolished.

British Medical Association Report

The 1992 report of the British Medical Association's working party on the participation of doctors in human rights abuses documents continued physician involvement in crimes against humanity throughout the world (BMA Working Party 1992). Physicians have been directly involved in the torture of prisoners as well as in indirect activities that facilitate torture. Physician involvement includes the examination and assessment of "fitness" of prisoners to be tortured, the monitoring of victims while being tortured, the resuscitation and medical treatment of prisoners during torture, and falsification of medical records and death certificates after torture.

The report documents examples of physician involvement in psychiatric "diagnosis" and commitment of political dissidents, forcible sterilizations, force feeding of hunger strikers, and supervision of amputation and other corporal punishments. Countries implicated span the globe and include the former Soviet Union, the United States, the United Kingdom, China, India, and South Africa, as well as countries in the Middle East and Central and South America. The working party notes the existence of international law and codes of ethics, but acknowledges the lack of enforcement and inability to monitor compliance. The theme of the report is that neither medical associations nor international law have been effective in preventing physician involvement in crimes against humanity.

A Permanent Nuremberg

In light of these problems and other ethical and human-rights issues involving physicians, many have argued that the world needs an international tribunal with authority to judge and punish the physician violators of international norms of medical conduct, as well as an independent body to conduct ongoing surveillance and to develop a rapid-response capacity. Without these, the world is as before Nuremberg: international norms of medical conduct are relegated solely to the domain of poorly defined medical ethics. In addition, the courts of individual countries, including the United States, for example, have consistently proven incapable either of punishing those engaged in unlawful or unethical human experimentation or of compensating the victims of such experimentation, primarily because such experimentation is often justified on the basis of national security or military necessity.

The International War Crimes Tribunal declared in 1946 that there were such things as war crimes and crimes against humanity, and that those who committed these crimes could be punished for them (the so-called Nuremberg Principles). The enumeration of these crimes followed from the concept of "inalienable rights" as expressed in such documents as the U.S. Declaration of Independence. The remaining or "subsequent" trials at Nuremberg, including the Doctors' Trial, were based on the legal precedent articulated by the International War Crimes Tribunal, but were held exclusively under the control and jurisdiction of the U.S. Army. M. Cherif Bassiouni, Robert Drinan, Telford Taylor, and others have argued eloquently and persuasively that a permanent international tribunal is needed to judge and punish those accused of war crimes and crimes against humanity (Taylor 1992; Bassiouni 1992).

In mid-1998, at a meeting held in Rome under the auspices of the United Nations, the countries in attendance voted overwhelmingly (120 to 7) to propose the establishment of a permanent International Criminal Court with jurisdiction over war crimes, crimes against humanity, genocide, and aggression. The United States refused to support the establishment of the court unless it could, among other things, veto trials of Americans, especially American troops operating abroad. This condition, of course, is incompatible with the entire purpose of the court: to punish violations of basic human rights regardless of the perpetrator. The court will be established without U.S. involvement if it is ratified by 60 nations by the end of the year 2000 (Annas 1998b).

An International Medical Tribunal

Medicine and law are often viewed as opponents, but in the promotion of human rights in health, they have a common agenda. One way for the world's physicians and lawyers to work together is to form and support an international medical tribunal. Ideally such a body should be established with the sanction and authority of the United Nations. However, given the competing political agendas of the member states, initial failure to win UN approval and support should not doom this project. Even if unable to punish with criminal sanctions, a tribunal could hear cases, develop an international code, and publicly condemn the actions of individual physicians who violate international standards of medical conduct. The establishment and support of such a tribunal is a worthy project for the world's physicians and lawyers.

The medical profession is the most promising candidate to take a leading role here because it has an apolitical history, has consistently argued for at least some neutrality in wartime to aid the sick and wounded, and has a basic humanitarian purpose for its existence, and because physician acts intended to destroy human health and life are a unique betrayal of both societal trust and the profession itself. It is also much easier for governments to adopt inherently evil and destructive policies if they are aided by the patina of legitimacy that physician participation provides.

To move forward, the establishment of such an international medical tribunal could be put on the agenda as an advocacy effort of all medical and legal associations around the world. Since such a tribunal must be both authoritative and politically neutral, no one country or political philosophy would be permitted to dominate it, either by having a disproportionate representation on the tribunal, or by disproportionately funding it. The tribunal itself would be composed of a large panel of distinguished judges. Recruiting such judges (without which the court would have little credibility) would require a commitment from governments to permit the selected judges to take time off from their full-time judicial duties to hear these cases.

Medical Ethics and Human Rights

International human rights law is similar to medical ethics in that both are universal and aspirational, and both have so far been unenforceable. A critical challenge is to make both meaningful, and this may be the most important legacy of the Nuremberg trials. For physicians, the challenge is to articulate and follow a universal medical ethics based on human rights, and to guard this ethic, for the sake of humanity, against its subversion and corruption by governments and corporations that would use medicine for their own purposes. Examples of the use of physicians for governmental purposes include the U.S. military and cold war radiation experiments, and the use of investigational drugs on U.S. soldiers in the Gulf War without consent, both done in direct violation of the Nuremberg Code. Other examples include the use of physicians in lethal injection executions, using psychiatrists to drug prisoners for easier control, and using physicians in the military for nonmedical purposes. This list could also include government-sanctioned use of physicians for "euthanasia" of incompetent persons (Grodin and Annas 1996).

Physicians need more than codes that proscribe putting their skills in the service of the nonmedical goals of governments, military establishments, and corporations. They also need support for upholding medical ethics and human rights, and mechanisms to punish those who would violate basic medical ethics and human rights in medicine. International human rights law and codes of medical ethics are necessary, but not sufficient, to prevent human rights abuses by physicians. Many physician groups, including International Physicians for the Prevention of Nuclear War and its U.S. affiliate, Physicians for Social Responsibility, and Physicians for Human Rights, are already active in promoting human rights globally. But physicians should not be expected to shoulder the cause of human rights alone.

Judges and lawyers were tried separately at Nuremberg in the "Justice Case," for engaging in "an unholy masquerade of brutish tyranny disguised as justice, and converting the German judicial system to an engine of despotism, conquest, pillage, and slaughter" (Taylor 1951). As Professor Lon Fuller has described the rise of the Nazi state, "The first attacks on the established order were on ramparts which, if they were manned by anyone, were manned by lawyers and judges. These ramparts fell almost without a struggle" (Fuller 1958). Just as it took lawyers and physicians working together to bring the Nazi physicians to justice at Nuremberg, it will take the world's lawyers and physicians working together not only to prevent wholesale violations of human rights but also to proactively support the growth of human rights worldwide. The world's physicians and lawyers, both because of their moral authority in defending life and justice and because of their privileged positions in society, have special obligations to humanity. To exercise these obligations more effectively, my physician colleague Dr. Michael Grodin and I have proposed joining together to promote and defend human rights through a new organization, Global Lawyers and Physicians (GLP), with the purpose of working together for human rights in all countries.[2]

The world's physicians and lawyers can, for example, work together transnationally to identify, publicize, and isolate physicians, lawyers, and judges involved in human rights abuses. Even if these abuses are tolerated in the country in which they work, professionals can be effectively isolated and "imprisoned" within their own outlaw countries. This can be done by refusing to license outlaw physicians or lawyers in any other country, by refusing to provide specialty or other training or access to professional meetings in any other country, and by refusing to publish any articles or research done by outlaw professional physicians in the world's professional literature. Lawyers should work with and defend physicians who resist subversion of their medical skills by representing them in court and other settings, including employment settings. Lawyers should also work to enact laws that protect physician autonomy in all cases in which physicians follow acceptable principles of medical ethics and protect and promote human rights, whether they act as healers or researchers.

The primary mission of GLP is to work collaboratively toward the global implementation of the health-related provisions of the Universal Declaration of Human Rights (1948) and the Covenant on Civil and Political Rights (1967) with a focus on healthcare ethics, patients' rights, medical research, and human experimentation. Specific goals of the organization include providing information and resources about human rights in health; serving as a network and referral source for professionals working on health-related human rights issues; and providing support and assistance in developing, implementing, and advocating public policies and legal remedies that protect and enhance human rights in health.

Conclusion

What lessons have we learned from the dominant role of law in American bioethics and the Doctors' Trial? Three stand out: (1) statements, even authoritative statements, of medical ethics are not self-enforcing and require active promulgation, education, and enforcement; (2) human experimentation and torture are important areas where violations of human rights and medical practice occur, but are too narrow in themselves to provide guidance for physicians and the public to the broad range of physician involvement in human rights abuses around the world; and (3) there is no effective mechanism to promulgate and enforce basic medical ethics and human rights principles in the world.

It is the legacy of Nuremberg and the Doctors' Trial that physicians have special obligations to use their power to protect human rights, and that medical ethics devoid of human rights become no more than hollow words. Bioethics must move beyond law and economics, and be challenging and even subversive. As Arthur Schlesinger has concluded: "The American identity will never be fixed and final; it will always be in the making" (Schlesinger 1982). American bioethics should also be actively involved "in the making." We should also be about fashioning a bioethics that moves beyond the laws of individual countries and into the realm of universal inalienable rights—the realm of human rights. A synthesis of medical ethics and human rights could tap into the reason most physicians and lawyers joined their professions in the first place: to help make the world a better place for everyone.

Acknowledgments

Portions of this chapter are adapted from Annas 1995 and Grodin and Annas 1996. See also Annas 1998a.

Endnotes

1. The Nuremberg Code:

1. The voluntary consent of the human subject is absolutely essential. This means that the person involved should have legal capacity to give consent; should be so situated as to be able to exercise free power of choice, without the intervention of any element of force, fraud, deceit, duress, overreaching, or other ulterior form of constraint or coercion; and should have sufficient knowledge and comprehension of the elements of the subject matter involved as to enable him to make an understanding and enlightened decision. This latter element requires that before the acceptance of an affirmative decision by the experimental subject there should be made known to him the nature, duration, and purpose of the experiment; the method and means by which it is to be conducted; all inconveniences and hazards reasonably to be expected; and the effects upon his health or person which may possibly come from his participation the experiment. The duty and responsibility for ascertaining the quality of the consent rests upon each individual who initiates, directs, or engages in the experiment. It is a personal duty and responsibility which may not be delegated to another with impunity.

2. The experiment should be such as to yield fruitful results for the good of society, unprocurable by other methods or means of study, and not random and unnecessary in nature.

3. The experiment should be so designed and based on the results of animal experimentation and a knowledge of natural history of the disease or other problem under study that the anticipated results will justify the performance of the experiment.

4. The experiment should be so conducted as to avoid all unnecessary physical and mental suffering and injury.

5. No experiment should be conducted where there is an a priori reason to believe that death or disabling injury will occur; except, perhaps, in those experiments where the experimental physicians also serve as subjects.

6. The degree of risk to be taken should never exceed that determined by the humanitarian importance of the problem to be solved by the experiment.

7. Proper preparations should be made and adequate facilities provided to protect the experimental subject against even remote possibilities of injury, disability, or death.

8. The experiment should be conducted only by scientifically qualified persons. The highest degree of skill and care should be required through all stages of the experiment of those who conduct or engage in the experiment.

9. During the course of the experiment the human subject should be at liberty to bring the experiment to an end if he has reached the physical or mental state where continuation of the experiment seems to him to be impossible.

10. During the course of the experiment the scientist in charge must be prepared to terminate the experiment at any stage, if he has probable cause to believe, in the exercise of the good faith, superior skill, and careful judgment required of him, that a continuation of the experiment is likely to result in injury, disability, or death to the experimental subject.

2. Current information on Global Lawyers and Physicians is available at http://www.glphr.org or by writing GLP at the Health Law Department, Boston University School of Public Health, 715 Albany Street, Boston, MA 02118.

References

Annas, G. J. 1992. The Changing Landscape of Human Experimentation: Nuremberg, Helsinki, and Beyond. *Health Matrix* 2:119–40.

———. 1993. *Standard of Care: The Law of American Bioethics.* New York: Oxford University Press.

———. 1995. The Dominance of American Law (and Market Values) Over American Bioethics. In *Meta Medical Ethics: The Philosophical Foundations of Bioethics,* ed. M. A. Grodin, 83–96. Dordrecht: Kluwer.

———. 1997. The Bell Tolls for a Constitutional Right to Physician-Assisted Suicide, *New England Journal of Medicine* 337:1098–103.

———. 1998. *Some Choice: Law, Medicine and the Market.* New York: Oxford University Press.

———. 1998b. Human Rights and Health: The Universal Declaration of Human Rights at 50. *New England Journal of Medicine* 339:1778–81.

Annas, G. J., and Grodin, M. A., eds. 1992. *The Nazi Doctors and the Nuremberg Code: Human Rights in Human Experimentation.* New York: Oxford University Press.

Bassiouni, M. C. 1992. *Crimes Against Humanity in International Criminal Law.* Dordrecht: Martinus Nijhoff Publisher.

British Medical Association Working Party ("BMA Working Party"). 1992. *Medicine Betrayed: The Participation of Doctors in Human Rights Abuses.* London: Zed Books.

Fuller, L. 1958. Positivism and Fidelity to Law—A Response to Professor Hart. *Harvard Law Review* 71:138–80.

Grodin, M. A., and Annas, G. J. 1996. Legacies of Nuremberg: Medical Ethics and Human Rights. *JAMA* 276:1682–83.

Grodin, M. A.; Annas, G. J.; and Glantz, L. H. 1993. Medicine and Human Rights: A Proposal for International Action. *Hastings Center Report* 2394:8–12.

Katz, J. 1993. Human Experimentation and Human Rights. *Saint Louis University Law Journal* 38(1):7–54.

Lifton, J. R. 1986. *The Nazi Doctors: Medical Killing and the Psychology of Genocide.* New York: Basic Books.

Proctor, R. 1987. *Racial Hygiene: Medicine Under the Nazis.* Cambridge: Harvard University Press.

Routley, T. C. 1949. Aims and Objects of the World Medical Association. *World Medical Association Bulletin* 1(1):18–19.

Schlesinger Jr., A. M. 1982. *The Disuniting of America: Reflections on a Multicultural Society.* New York: W. W. Norton.

Taylor, T. 1951. Opening Statement in the "Justice Case." In *Trials of War Criminals Before the Nuremberg Military Tribunals Under Control Council Law No. 10,* 3:30. Washington, D.C.: U.S. Government Printing Office.

———. 1992. *The Anatomy of the Nuremberg Trials.* New York: Knopf.

Trials of War Criminals Before the Nuremberg Military Tribunals Under Control Council 10 ("Trials"). 1950. Vol. 1 and 2. Washington, D.C.: U.S. Government Printing Office; Military Tribunal, Case 1, United States v. Karl Brandt, et al. October 1946–April 1949.

Wills, G. 1978. *Inventing America: Jefferson's Declaration of Independence.* New York: Vintage Books.

World Medical Association (WMA). 1949. Editorial. *World Medical Association Bulletin* 1:3–14.

Appendixes

AMA Codes and Principles of Medical Ethics, 1847–1997

Appendix A

Note to 1847 Convention

ISAAC HAYS

Doctor Hays, on presenting this report, stated that justice required some explanatory remarks should accompany it. The members of the Convention, he observed, would not fail to recognize in parts of it, expressions with which they were familiar. On examining a great number of codes of ethics adopted by different societies in the United States, it was found that they were all based on that by Dr. Percival, and that the phrases of this writer were preserved, to a considerable extent, in all of them. Believing that language which had been so often examined and adopted, must possess the greatest of merits for such a document as the present, clearness and precision, and having no ambition for the honours of authorship, the Committee which prepared this code have followed a similar course, and have carefully preserved the words of Percival wherever they convey the precepts it is wished to inculcate. A few of the sections are in the words of the late Dr. Rush, and one or two sentences are from other writers. But in all cases, wherever it was thought that the language could be made more explicit by changing a word, or even a part of a sentence, this has been unhesitatingly done; and thus there are but few sections which have not undergone some modification; while, for the language of many, and for the arrangement of the whole, the Committee must be held exclusively responsible.

Submission of Code of Ethics

The Committee appointed under the sixth resolution adopted by the Convention which assembled in New York, in May last, to prepare a Code of Ethics for the government of the medical profession of the United States, respectfully submit the following Code. Philadelphia, June 5, 1847.

Committee
John Bell
Isaac Hays
G. Emerson
W. W. Morris
T. C. Dunn
A. Clark
R. D. Arnold

Appendix B

Introduction to the 1847 Code of Ethics

JOHN BELL

Medical ethics, as a branch of general ethics, must rest on the basis of religion and morality. They comprise not only the duties, but, also, the rights of a physician: and, in this sense, they are identical with Medical Deontology—a term introduced by a late writer, who has taken the most comprehensive view of the subject.

In framing a code on this basis, we have the inestimable advantage of deducing its rules from the conduct of many eminent physicians who have adorned the profession by their learning and their piety. From the age of Hippocrates to the present time, the annals of every civilized people contain abundant evidences of the devotedness of medical men to the relief of their fellow creatures from pain and disease, regardless of the privation and danger, and not seldom obloquy, encountered in return; a sense of ethical obligation rising superior, in their minds, to considerations of personal advancement. Well and truly was it said by one of the most learned men of the last century: that the duties of a physician were never more beautifully exemplified than in the conduct of Hippocrates, nor more eloquently described in his writings.

We may here remark, that, if a state of probation be intended for moral discipline, there is, assuredly, much in the daily life of a physician to impart this salutary training, and to insure continuance in a course of self-denial, and, at the same time, of zealous and methodical efforts for the relief of the suffering and unfortunate, irrespective of rank or fortune, or of fortuitous elevation of any kind.

A few considerations on the legitimate range of medical ethics will serve as an appropriate introduction to the requisite rules for our guidance in the complex relations of professional life.

Every duty or obligation implies, both in equity and for its successful discharge, a corresponding right. As it is the duty of a physician to advise, so has he a right to be attentively and respectfully listened to. Being required to expose his health and life for the benefit of the community, he has a just claim, in return, on all its members, collectively and individually, for aid to carry out his measures, and for all possible tenderness and regard to prevent needlessly harassing calls on his services and unnecessary exhaustion of his benevolent sympathies.

His zeal, talents, attainments and skill are qualities which he holds in trust for the general good, and which can not be prodigally spent, either through his own negligence or the inconsiderateness of others, without wrong and detriment both to himself and to them.

The greater the importance of the subject and the more deeply interested all are in the issue, the more necessary is it that the physician—he who performs the chief part, and in whose judgment and discretion under Providence, life is secured and death turned aside—should be allowed the free use of his faculties, undisturbed by a querulous manner, and desponding, angry, or passionate interjections, under the plea of fear, or grief, or disappointment of cherished hopes, by the sick and their friends.

All persons privileged to enter the sick room, and the number ought to be very limited, are under equal obligations of reciprocal courtesy, kindness and respect; and, if any exception be admissible, it cannot be at the expense of the physician. His position, purposes and proper efforts eminently entitle him to, at least, the same respectful and considerate attentions that are paid, as a matter of course and apparently without constraint, to the clergyman, who is admitted to administer spiritual consolation, and to the lawyer, who comes to make the last will and testament.

Although professional duty requires of a physician, that he should have such a control over himself as not to betray strong emotion in the presence of his patient, nor to be thrown off his guard by the querulousness or even rudeness of the latter, or of his friends at the bedside, yet, and the fact ought to be generally known, many medical men, possessed of abundant attainments and resources, are so constitutionally timid and readily abashed as to lose much of their self-possession and usefulness at the critical moment, if opposition be abruptly interposed to any part of the plan which they are about devising for the benefit of their patients.

Medical ethics cannot be so divided as that one part shall obtain the full and proper force of moral obligations on physicians universally, and, at the same time, the other be construed in such a way as to free society from all restrictions in its conduct to them; leaving it to the caprice of the hour to determine whether the truly learned shall be overlooked in favor of ignorant pretenders—persons destitute alike of original talent and acquired fitness.

The choice is not indifferent, in an ethical point of view, besides its important bearing on the fate of the sick themselves, between the directness and sincerity of purpose, the honest zeal, the learning and impartial observations, accumulated from age to age for thousands of years, of the regularly initiated members of the medical profession, and the crooked devices and low arts, for evidently selfish ends, the unsupported promises and reckless trials of interloping empirics, whose very announcements of the means by which they profess to perform their wonders are, for the most part, misleading and false, and, so far, fraudulent.

In thus deducing the rights of a physician from his duties, it is not meant to insist on such a correlative obligation, that the withholding of the right exonerates from the discharge of the duty. Short of the formal abandonment of the practice of his profession, no medical man can withhold his services from the requisition either of an individual or of the community, unless under circumstances, of rare occurrence, in which his compliance would be not only unjust but degrading to himself, or to a professional brother, and so far diminish his future usefulness.

In the discharge of their duties to Society, physicians must be ever ready and prompt to administer professional aid to all applicants, without prior stipulation of personal advantages to themselves.

On them devolves, in a peculiar manner, the task of noting all the circumstances affecting the public health, and of displaying skill and ingenuity in devising the best means for its protection.

With them rests, also, the solemn duty of furnishing accurate medical testimony in all cases of criminal accusation of violence, by which health is endangered and life destroyed, and in those other numerous ones involving the question of mental sanity and of moral and legal responsibility.

On these subjects—Public Hygiene and Medical Jurisprudence—every medical man must be supposed to have prepared himself by study, observation, and the exercise of a sound judgment. They cannot be regarded in the light of accomplishments merely: they are an integral part of the science and practice of medicine.

It is a delicate and noble task, by the judicious application of Public Hygiene, to prevent disease and to prolong life; and thus to increase the productive industry, and, without assuming the office of moral and religious teaching, to add to the civilization of an entire people.

In the performance of this part of their duty, physicians are enabled to exhibit the close connection between hygiene and morals; since all the causes contributing to the former are nearly equally auxiliary to the latter.

Physicians, as conservators of the public health, are bound to bear emphatic testimony against quackery in all its forms; whether it appears with its usual effrontery, or masks itself under the garb of philanthropy and sometimes of religion itself.

By an anomaly in legislation and penal enactments, the laws, so stringent for the repression and punishment of fraud in general, and against attempts to sell poisonous substances for food, are silent, and of course inoperative, in the cases of both fraud and poisoning so extensively carried on by the host of quacks who infest the land.

The newspaper press, powerful in the correction of many abuses, is too ready for the sake of lucre to aid and abet the enormities of quackery. Honourable exceptions to the once general practice in this respect are becoming, happily, more numerous, and they might be more rapidly increased, if physicians, when themselves free from all taint, were to direct the intention of the editors and proprietors of newspapers, and of periodical works in general, to the moral bearings of the subject.

To those who, like physicians, can best see the extent of the evil, it is still more mortifying than in the instances already mentioned, to find members of other professions, and especially ministers of the Gospel, so prone to give their countenance, and, at times, direct patronage, to medical empirics, both by their use of nostrums, and by their certificates in favour of the absurd pretensions of the impostors.

The credulous, on these occasions, place themselves in the dilemma of bearing testimony either to a miracle or to an imposture: to a miracle, if one particular agent, and it often of known inertness or slight power, can cure all diseases, or even any one disease in all its stages; to an imposture, if the alleged cures are not made, as experiences shows that they are not.

But by no class are quack medicines and nostrums so largely sold and distributed as by apothecaries, whose position towards physicians, although it many not amount to actual affinity, is such that it ought, at least, to prevent them from entering into an actual, if not formally recognized, alliance with empirics of every grade and degree of pretention.

Too frequently we meet with physicians, who deem it a venial error, in ethics, to permit, and even to recommend, the use of quack medicine or secret compounds by their patients and friends. They forget that their toleration implies sanction of a recourse by the people generally to unknown, doubtful, and conjectural fashions of medication; and that the credulous in this way soon become the victims of an endless succession of empirics. It must have been generally noticed, also, that they, whose faith is strongest in the most absurd pretensions of quackery, entertain the greatest skepticism towards regular and philosophic medicine.

Adverse alike to ethical propriety and to medical logic, are the various popular delusions which, like so many epidemics, have, in successive ages, excited the imagination with extravagant expectations of the cure of all diseases and the prolongation of life beyond its customary limits, by means of a single substance. Although it is not in the power of physicians to prevent, or always to arrest, these delusions in their progress, yet it is incumbent on them, from their superior knowledge and better opportunities, as well as from their elevated vocation, steadily to refuse to extend to them the slightest countenance, still less support.

These delusions are sometimes manifested in the guise of a new and infallible system of medical practice—the faith in which, among the excited believers, is usually in the inverse ratio of the amount of common sense evidence in its favour. Among the volunteer missionaries for its dissemination, it is painful to see members of the sacred profession, who, above all others, ought to keep aloof from vagaries of any description, and especially of those medical ones which are allied to empirical imposture.

The plea of good intention is not an adequate reason for the assumption of so grave a responsibility as the propagation of a theory and practice of medicine, of the real foundation and nature of which the mere medical amateur must necessarily, from his want of opportunities for study, observation, and careful comparison, be profoundly ignorant.

In their relations with the sick, physicians are bound, by every consideration of duty, to exercise the greatest kindness with the greatest circumspection; so that, whilst they make every allowance for impatience, irritation, and inconsistencies of manner and speech of the sufferers, and do their utmost to soothe and tranquilize, they shall, at the same time, elicit from them, and the persons in their confidence, a revelation of all the circumstances connected with the probable origin of the diseases which they are called upon to treat.

Owing either to the confusion and, at times, obliquity of mind produced by the disease, or to considerations of false delicacy and shame, the truth is not always directly reached on these occasions; and hence the necessity, on the part of the physician, of a careful and minute investigation into both the physical and moral state of his patient.

A physician in attendance on a case should avoid expensive complications and tedious ceremonials, as being beneath the dignity of true science and embarrassing to the patient and his family, whose troubles are already great.

In their intercourse with each other, physicians will best consult and secure their own self-respect and consideration from society in general, by a uniform courtesy and high-minded conduct towards their professional brethren. The confidence in his intellectual and moral worth, which each member of the profession is ambitious of obtaining for himself among his associates, ought to make him willing to place the same confidence in the worth of others.

Veracity, so requisite in all the relations of life, is a jewel of inestimable value in medical description and narrative, the lustre of which ought never to be tainted for a moment, by even the breath of suspicion. Physicians are peculiarly enjoined, by every consideration of honour and of conscientious regard for the health and lives of their fellow beings, not to advance any statement unsupported by positive facts, nor to hazard an opinion or hypothesis that is not the result of deliberate inquiry into all the data and bearings of which the subject is capable.

Hasty generalization, paradox and fanciful conjectures, repudiated at all times by sound logic, are open to the severest reprehension on the still higher grounds of humanity and morals. Their tendency and practical operation cannot fail to be eminently mischievous.

Among medical men associated together for the performance of professional duties in public institutions, such as Medical Colleges, Hospitals and Dispensaries, there ought to exist, not only harmonious intercourse, but also a general harmony in doctrine and practice; so that neither students nor patients shall be perplexed, nor the medical community mortified by contradictory views of the theory of disease, if not of the means of curing it.

The right of free inquiry, common to all, does not imply the utterance of crude hypotheses, the use of figurative language, a straining after novelty for novelty's sake, and the involution of old truths, for temporary effect and popularity, by medical writers and teachers. If, therefore, they who are engaged in a common cause, and for the furtherance of a common object, could make an offering of the extreme, the doubtful, and the redundant, at the shrine of philosophical truth, the general harmony in medical teaching, now desired, would be of easy attainment.

It is not enough, however, that the members of the medical profession be zealous, well informed and self-denying, unless the social principle be cultivated by their seeking frequent intercourse with each other, and cultivating, reciprocally, friendly habits of acting in common.

By union alone can medical men hope to sustain the dignity and extend the usefulness of their profession. Among the chief means to bring this desirable end, are frequent social meetings and regularly organized Societies; a part of whose beneficial operation would be an agreement on a suitable standard of medical education, and a code of medical ethics.

Greatly increased influence, for the entire body of the profession, will be acquired by a union for the purposes of common benefit and the general good; while to its members, individually, will be insured a more pleasant and harmonious intercourse, one with another, and an avoidance of many heart burnings and jealousies, which originate in misconception, through misrepresentation on the part of individuals in general society, of each other's disposition, motives, and conduct.

In vain will physicians appeal to the intelligence and elevated feelings of the members of other professions, and of the better part of society in general, unless they be true to themselves, by a close adherence to their duties, and by firmly yet mildly insisting on their rights; and this not with a glimmering perception and faint avowal, but, rather with a full understanding and firm conviction.

Impressed with the nobleness of their vocation, as trustees of science and almoners of benevolence and charity, physicians should use unceasing vigilance to prevent the introduction into their body of those who have not been prepared by a suitably preparatory moral and intellectual training.

No youth ought to be allowed to study medicine, whose capacity, good conduct, and elementary knowledge are not equal, at least, to the common standard of academical requirements.

Human life and human happiness must not be endangered by the incompetency of presumptuous pretenders. The greater the inherent difficulties of medicine, as a science, and the more numerous the complications that embarrass in its practice, the more necessary is it that there should be minds of a high order and thorough cultivation, to unravel its mysteries and to deduce scientific order from apparently empirical confusion.

We are under the strongest ethical obligations to preserve the character which has been awarded, by the most learned men and best judges of human nature, to the members of the medical profession, for general and extensive knowledge, great liberality and dignity of sentiment, and prompt effusions of beneficence.

In order that we may continue to merit these praises, every physician, within the circle of his acquaintance, should impress both fathers and sons with the range and variety of medical study, and with the necessity of those who desire to engage in it, possessing, not only good preliminary knowledge, but, likewise, some habits of regular and systematic thinking.

If able teachers and writers, and profound inquirers, be still called for to expound medical science, and to extend its domain of practical application and usefulness, they cannot be procured by intuitive effort on their own part, nor by the exercise of the elective suffrage on the part of others. They must be the product of a regular and comprehensive system—members of a large class, from the great body of which they only differ by the course of fortuitous circumstances, that gives them temporary vantage ground for the display of qualities and attainments common to their brethren.

Appendix C

Code of Ethics (1847)

JOHN BELL AND ISAAC HAYS

Chapter I. Of the Duties of Physicians to Their Patients, and of the Obligations of Patients to Their Physicians

Art. I—*Duties of Physicians to their Patients*

1. A physician should not only be ever ready to obey the calls of the sick, but his mind ought also to be imbued with the greatness of his mission, and of the responsibility he habitually incurs in its discharge. Those obligations are the more deep and enduring, because there is no tribunal other than his own conscience, to adjudge penalties for carelessness or neglect. Physicians should, therefore, minister to the sick with due impressions of the importance of their office; reflecting that the ease, the health, and the lives of those committed to their charge, depend on their skill, attention and fidelity. They should study, also, in their deportment, so to unite *tenderness* with *firmness*, and *condescension* with *authority*, as to inspire the minds of their patients with gratitude, respect and confidence.

2. Every case committed to the charge of a physician should be treated with attention, steadiness and humanity. Reasonable indulgence should be granted to the mental imbecility and caprices of the sick. Secrecy and delicacy, when required by peculiar circumstances, should be strictly observed; and the familiar and confidential intercourse to which physicians are admitted in their professional visits, should be used with discretion, and with the most scrupulous regard to fidelity and honor. The obligation of secrecy extends beyond the period of professional services—none of the privacies of personal and domestic life, no infirmity of disposition or flaw of character observed during professional attendance, should ever be divulged by him except when he is imperatively required to do so. The force and necessity of this obligation are indeed so great, that professional men have, under certain circumstances, been protected in their observance of secrecy, by courts of justice.

3. Frequent visits to the sick are in general requisite, since they enable the physician to arrive at a more perfect knowledge of the disease—to meet promptly

every change which may occur, and also tend to preserve the confidence of the patient. But unnecessary visits are to be avoided, as they give useless anxiety to the patient, tend to diminish the authority of the physician, and render him liable to be suspected of interested motives.

4. A physician should not be forward to make gloomy prognostications, because they savor of empiricism, by magnifying the importance of his services in the treatment or cure of the disease. But he should not fail, on proper occasions, to give to the friends of the patient timely notice of danger, when it really occurs; and even to the patient himself, if absolutely necessary. This office, however, is so peculiarly alarming when executed by him, that it ought to be declined whenever it can be assigned to any other person of sufficient judgment and delicacy. For, the physician should be the minister of hope and comfort to the sick; that, by such cordials to the drooping spirit, he may smooth the bed of death, revive expiring life, and counteract the depressing influence of those maladies which often disturb the tranquility of the most resigned, in their last moments. The life of a sick person can be shortened not only by the acts, but also by the words or the manner of a physician. It is, therefore, a sacred duty to guard himself carefully in this respect, and to avoid all things which have a tendency to discourage the patient and to depress his spirits.

5. A physician ought not to abandon a patient because the case is deemed incurable; for his attendance may continue to be highly useful to the patient, and comforting to the relatives around him, even to the last period of a fatal malady, by alleviating pain and other symptoms, and by soothing mental anguish. To decline attendance, under such circumstances, would be sacrificing to fanciful delicacy and mistaken liberality, that moral duty, which is independent of, and far superior to all pecuniary consideration.

6. Consultations should be promoted in difficult or protracted cases, as they give rise to confidence, energy, and more enlarged views in practice.

7. The opportunity which a physician not unfrequently enjoys of promoting and strengthening the good resolutions of his patients, suffering under the consequences of vicious conduct, ought never to be neglected. His counsels, or even remonstrances, will give satisfaction, not offense, if they be proffered with politeness, and evince a genuine love of virtue, accompanied by a sincere interest in the welfare of the person to whom they are addressed.

Art. II—*Obligations of Patients to Their Physicians*

1. The members of the medical profession, upon whom are enjoined the performance of so many important and arduous duties towards the community, and who are required to make so many sacrifices of comfort, ease, and health, for the welfare of those who avail themselves of their services, certainly have a right to expect and require, that their patients should entertain a just sense of the duties which they owe to their medical attendants.

2. The first duty of a patient is, to select as his medical adviser one who has received a regular professional education. In no trade or occupation do mankind rely on the skill of an untaught artist; and in medicine, confessedly the most difficult and intricate of the sciences, the world ought not to suppose that knowledge is intuitive.

3. Patients should prefer a physician whose habits of life are regular, and who is not devoted to company, pleasure, or to any pursuit incompatible with his professional obligations. A patient should also confide the care of himself and family, as much as possible, to one physician, for a medical man who has become acquainted with the peculiarities of constitution, habits, and predispositions, of those he attends, is more likely to be successful in his treatment than one who does not possess that knowledge.

A patient who has thus selected his physician, should always apply for advice in whatever may appear to him trivial cases, for the most fatal results often supervene on the slightest accidents. It is of still more importance that he should apply for assistance in the forming stage of violent diseases; it is to a neglect of this precept that medicine owes much of the uncertainty and imperfection with which it has been reproached.

4. Patients should faithfully and unreservedly communicate to their physician the supposed cause of their disease. This is the more important, as many diseases of a mental origin simulate those depending on external causes, and yet are only to be cured by ministering to the mind diseased. A patient should never be afraid of thus making his physician his friend and adviser; he should always bear in mind that a medical man is under the strongest obligations of secrecy. Even the female sex should never allow feelings of shame and delicacy to prevent their disclosing the seat, symptoms and causes of complaints peculiar to them. However commendable a modest reserve may be in the common occurrences of life, its strict observance in medicine is often attended with the most serious consequences, and a patient may sink under a painful and loathsome disease, which might have been readily prevented had timely intimation been given to the physician.

5. A patient should never weary his physician with a tedious detail of events or matters not appertaining to his disease. Even as relates to his actual symptoms, he will convey much more real information by giving clear answers to interrogatories, than by the most minute account of his own framing. Neither should he obtrude the details of his business nor the history of his family concerns.

6. The obedience of a patient to the prescriptions of his physician should be prompt and implicit. He should never permit his own crude opinions as to their fitness, to influence his attention to them. A failure in one particular may render an otherwise judicious treatment dangerous, and even fatal. This remark is equally applicable to diet, drink, and exercise. As patients become convalescent, they are very apt to suppose that the rules prescribed for them may be disregarded, and the

consequence, but too often, is a relapse. Patients should never allow themselves to be persuaded to take any medicine whatever, that may be recommended to them by the self-constituted doctors and doctoresses, who are so frequently met with, and who pretend to possess infallible remedies for the cure of every disease. However simple some of their prescriptions may appear to be, it often happens that they are productive of much mischief, and in all cases they are injurious, by contravening the plan of treatment adopted by the physician.

7. A patient should, if possible, avoid even the *friendly visits of a physician* who is not attending him—and when he does receive them, he should never converse on the subject of his disease, as an observation may be made, without any intention of interference, which may destroy his confidence in the course he is pursuing, and induce him to neglect the directions prescribed to him. A patient should never send for a consulting physician without the express consent of his own medical attendant. It is of great importance that physicians should act in concert; for, although their modes of treatment may be attended with equal success when employed singly, yet conjointly they are very likely to be productive of disastrous results.

8. When a patient wishes to dismiss his physician, justice and common courtesy require that he should declare his reasons for so doing.

9. Patients should always, when practicable, send for their physician in the morning, before his usual hour of going out; for, by being early aware of the visits he has to pay during the day, the physician is able to apportion his time in such a manner as to prevent an interference of engagements. Patients should also avoid calling on their medical adviser unnecessarily during the hours devoted to meals or sleep. They should always be in readiness to receive the visits of their physician, as the detention of a few minutes is often of serious inconvenience to him.

10. A patient should, after his recovery, entertain a just and enduring sense of the value of the services rendered him by his physician; for these are of such a character, that no mere pecuniary acknowledgment can repay or cancel them.

Chapter II. Of the Duties of Physicians to Each Other and to the Profession at Large

Art. I *Duties for the Support of Professional Character*

1. Every individual, on entering the profession, as he becomes thereby entitled to all its privileges and immunities, incurs an obligation to exert his best abilities to maintain its dignity and honor, to exalt its standing, and to extend the bounds of its usefulness. He should therefore observe strictly, such laws as are instituted for the government of its members; should avoid all contumelious and sarcastic remarks relative to the faculty, as a body; and while, by unwearied dili-

gence, he resorts to every honorable means of enriching the science, he should entertain a due respect for his seniors, who have, by their labors, brought it to the elevated condition in which he finds it.

2. There is no profession, from the members of which greater purity of character and a higher standard of moral excellence are required, than the medical; and to attain such eminence, is a duty every physician owes alike to his profession, and to his patients. It is due to the latter, as without it he cannot command their respect and confidence; and to both, because no scientific attainments can compensate for the want of correct moral principles. It is also incumbent upon the faculty to be temperate in all things, for the practice of physic requires the unremitting exercise of a clear and vigorous understanding; and, on emergencies for which no professional man should be unprepared, a steady hand, an acute eye, and an unclouded head may be essential to the well-being, and even life, of a fellow creature.

3. It is derogatory to the dignity of the profession, to resort to public advertisements or private cards or handbills, inviting the attention of individuals affected with particular diseases—publicly offering advice and medicine to the poor gratis, or promising radical cures; or to publish cases and operations in the daily prints, or suffer such publications to be made;—to invite laymen to be present at operations—to boast of cures and remedies—to adduce certificates of skill and success, or to perform any other similar acts. These are the ordinary practices of empirics, and are highly reprehensible in a regular physician.

4. Equally derogatory to professional character is it, for a physician to hold a patent for any surgical instrument, or medicine; or to dispense a secret *nostrum,* whether it be the composition or exclusive property of himself or of others. For, if such nostrum be of real efficacy, any concealment regarding it is inconsistent with beneficence and professional liberality; and, if mystery alone give it value and importance, such craft implies either disgraceful ignorance, or fraudulent avarice. It is also reprehensible for physicians to give certificates attesting the efficacy of patent or secret medicines, or in any way to promote the use of them.

Art. II—*Professional Services of Physicians to Each Other*

1. All practitioners of medicine, their wives, and their children while under the paternal care, are entitled to the gratuitous services of any one or more of the faculty residing near them, whose assistance may be desired. A physician afflicted with disease is usually an incompetent judge of his own case; and the natural anxiety and solicitude which he experiences at the sickness of a wife, a child, or any one who by the ties of consanguinity is rendered peculiarly dear to him, tend to obscure his judgment, and produce timidity and irresolution in his practice. Under such circumstances, medical men are peculiarly dependent upon each other, and kind offices and professional aid should always be cheerfully and gratuitously afforded. Visits ought not, however, to be obtruded officiously; as such unasked civility may give rise to embarrassment, or interfere with that choice on which con-

fidence depends. But, if a distant member of the faculty, whose circumstances are affluent, request attendance, and an honorarium be offered, it should not be declined; for no pecuniary obligation ought to be imposed, which the party receiving it would wish not to incur.

Art. III—*Of the Duties of Physicians as Respects Vicarious Offices*

1. The affairs of life, the pursuit of health, and the various accidents and contingencies to which a medical man is peculiarly exposed, sometimes require him temporarily to withdraw from his duties to his patients, and to request some of his professional brethren to officiate for him. Compliance with this request is an act of courtesy, which should always be performed with the utmost consideration for the interest and character of the family physician, and when exercised for a short period, all the pecuniary obligations for such service should be awarded to him. But if a member of the profession neglect his business in quest of pleasure and amusement, he cannot be considered as entitled to the advantages of the frequent and long-continued exercise of this fraternal courtesy, without awarding to the physician who officiates the fees arising from the discharge of his professional duties.

In obstetrical and important surgical cases, which give rise to unusual fatigue, anxiety and responsibility, it is just that the fees accruing therefrom should be awarded to the physician who officiates.

Art. IV—*Of the Duties of Physicians in Regard to Consultations*

I. A regular medical education furnishes the only presumptive evidence of professional abilities and acquirements, and ought to be the only acknowledged right of an individual to the exercise and honors of his profession. Nevertheless, as in consultations, the good of the patient is the sole object in view, and this is often dependent on personal confidence, no intelligent regular practitioner, who has a license to practise from some medical board of known and acknowledged respectability, recognised by this association, and who is in good moral and professional standing in the place in which he resides, should be fastidiously excluded from fellowship, or his aid refused in consultation when it is requested by the patient. But no one can be considered as a regular practitioner, or fit associate in consultation, whose practice is based on an exclusive dogma, to the rejection of the accumulated experience of the profession, and of the aids actually furnished by anatomy, physiology, pathology, and organic chemistry.

2. In consultations, no rivalship or jealousy should be indulged; candor, probity, and all due respect, should be exercised towards the physician having charge of the case.

3. In consultations, the attending physician should be the first to propose the necessary questions to the sick; after which the consulting physician should have the opportunity to make such farther inquiries of the patient as may be necessary

to satisfy him of the true character of the case. Both physicians should then retire to a private place for deliberation; and the one first in attendance should communicate the directions agreed upon to the patient or his friends, as well as any opinions which it may be thought proper to express. But no statement or discussion of it should take place before the patient or his friends, except in the presence of all the faculty attending, and by their common consent; and no *opinions* or *prognostications* should be delivered, which are not the result of previous deliberation and concurrence.

4. In consultations, the physician in attendance should deliver his opinion first; and when there are several consulting, they should deliver their opinions in the order in which they have been called in. No decision, however, should restrain the attending physician from making such variations in the mode of treatment, as any subsequent unexpected change in the character of the case may demand. But such variation and the reasons for it ought to be carefully detailed at the next meeting in consultation. The same privilege belongs also to the consulting physician if he is sent for in an emergency, when the regular attendant is out of the way, and similar explanations must be made by him, at the next consultation.

5. The utmost punctuality should be observed in the visits of physicians when they are to hold consultation together, and this is generally practicable, for society has been considerate enough to allow the plea of a professional engagement to take precedence of all others, and to be an ample reason for the relinquishment of any present occupation. But as professional engagements may sometimes interfere, and delay one of the parties, the physician who first arrives should wait for his associate a reasonable period, after which the consultation should be considered as postponed to a new appointment. If it be the attending physician who is present, he will of course see the patient and prescribe; but if it be the consulting one, he should retire, except in case of emergency, or when he has been called from a considerable distance, in which latter case he may examine the patient, and give his opinion in *writing* and *under seal,* to be delivered to his associate.

6. In consultations, theoretical discussions should be avoided, as occasioning perplexity and loss of time. For there may be much diversity of opinion concerning speculative points, with perfect agreement in those modes of practice which are founded, not on hypothesis, but on experience and observation.

7. All discussions in consultation should be held as secret and confidential. Neither by words nor manner should any of the parties to a consultation assert or insinuate, that any part of the treatment pursued did not receive his assent. The responsibility must be equally divided between the medical attendants—they must equally share the credit of success as well as the blame of failure.

8. Should an irreconcilable diversity of opinion occur when several physicians are called upon to consult together, the opinion of the majority should be considered as decisive; but if the numbers be equal on each side, then the decision should rest with the attending physician. It may, moreover, sometimes happen, that two

physicians cannot agree in their views of the nature of a case, and the treatment to be pursued. This is a circumstance much to be deplored, and should always be avoided, if possible, by mutual concessions, as far as they can be justified by a conscientious regard for the dictates of judgment. But in the event of its occurrence, a third physician should, if practicable, be called to act as umpire; and if circumstances prevent the adoption of this course, it must be left to the patient to select the physician in whom he is most willing to confide. But as every physician relies upon the rectitude of his judgment, he should, when left in the minority, politely and consistently retire from any further deliberation in the consultation, or participation in the management of the case.

9. As circumstances sometimes occur to render a *special consultation* desirable, when the continued attendance of two physicians might be objectionable to the patient, the member of the faculty whose assistance is required in such cases, should sedulously guard against all future unsolicited attendance. As such consultations require an extraordinary portion both of time and attention, at least a double honorarium may be reasonably expected.

10. A physician who is called upon to consult, should observe the most honorable and scrupulous regard for the character and standing of the practitioner in attendance: the practice of the latter, if necessary, should be justified as far as it can be, consistently with a conscientious regard for truth, and no hint or insinuation should be thrown out, which could impair the confidence reposed in him, or affect his reputation. The consulting physician should also carefully refrain from any of those extraordinary attentions or assiduities, which are too often practised by the dishonest for the base purpose of gaining applause, or ingratiating themselves into the favor of families and individuals.

Art. V—*Duties of a Physician in Cases of Interference*

1. Medicine is a liberal profession, and those admitted into its ranks should found their expectations of practice upon the extent of their qualifications, not on intrigue or artifice.

2. A physician in his intercourse with a patient under the care of another practitioner, should observe the strictest caution and reserve. No meddling inquiries should be made; no disingenuous hints given relative to the nature and treatment of his disorder; nor any course of conduct pursued that may directly or indirectly tend to diminish the trust reposed in the physician employed.

3. The same circumspection and reserve should be observed, when, from motives of business or friendship, a physician is prompted to visit an individual who is under the direction of another practitioner. Indeed, such visits should be avoided, except under peculiar circumstances; and when they are made, no particular inquiries should be instituted relative to the nature of the disease, or the remedies employed, but the topics of conversation should be as foreign to the case as circumstances will admit.

4. A physician ought not to take charge of, or prescribe for a patient who has recently been under the care of another member of the faculty in the same illness, except in cases of sudden emergency, or in consultation with the physician previously in attendance, or when the latter has relinquished the case or been regularly notified that his services are no longer desired. Under such circumstances, no unjust and illiberal insinuations should be thrown out in relation to the conduct or practice previously pursued, which should be justified as far as candor, and regard for truth and probity will permit; for it often happens, that patients become dissatisfied when they do not experience immediate relief, and, as many diseases are naturally protracted, the want of success, in the first stage of treatment, affords no evidence of a lack of professional knowledge and skill.

5. When a physician is called to an urgent case, because the family attendant is not at hand, he ought, unless his assistance in consultation be desired, to resign the care of the patient to the latter, immediately on his arrival.

6. It often happens, in cases of sudden illness, or of recent accidents and injuries, owing to the alarm and anxiety of friends, that a number of physicians are simultaneously sent for. Under these circumstances courtesy should assign the patient to the first who arrives, who should select from those present, any additional assistance that he may deem necessary. In all such cases, however, the practitioner who officiates should request the family physician, if there be one, to be called, and, unless his further attendance be requested, should resign the case to the latter on his arrival.

7. When a physician is called to the patient of another practitioner, in consequence of the sickness or absence of the latter, he ought, on the return or recovery of the regular attendant, and with the consent of the patient, to surrender the case.

8. A physician, when visiting a sick person in the country, may be desired to see a neighboring patient who is under the regular direction of another physician, in consequence of some sudden change or aggravation of symptoms. The conduct to be pursued on such an occasion is to give advice adapted to present circumstances; to interfere no farther than is absolutely necessary with the general plan of treatment; to assume no future direction, unless it be expressly desired; and, in this last case, to request an immediate consultation with the practitioner previously employed.

9. A wealthy physician should not give advice *gratis* to the affluent; because his doing so is an injury to his professional brethren. The office of a physician can never be supported as an exclusively beneficent one; and it is defrauding, in some degree, the common funds for its support, when fees are dispensed with, which might justly be claimed.

10. When a physician who has been engaged to attend a case of midwifery is absent, and another is sent for, if delivery is accomplished during the attendance of the latter, he is entitled to the fee, but should resign the patient to the practitioner first engaged.

Art. VI—*Of Differences between Physicians*

1. Diversity of opinion, and opposition of interest, may, in the medical, as in other professions, sometimes occasion controversy and even contention. Whenever such cases unfortunately occur, and cannot be immediately terminated, they should be referred to the arbitration of a sufficient number of physicians, or a *court-medical*.

As peculiar reserve must be maintained by physicians towards the public, in regard to professional matters, and as there exist numerous points in medical ethics and etiquette through which the feelings of medical men may be painfully assailed in their intercourse with each other, and which cannot be understood or appreciated by general society, neither the subject-matter of such differences nor the adjudication of the arbitrators should be made public, as publicity in a case of this nature may be personally injurious to the individuals concerned, and can hardly fail to bring discredit on the faculty.

Art. VII—*Of Pecuniary Acknowledgments*

1. Some general rules should be adopted by the faculty, in every town or district, relative to *pecuniary acknowledgments* from their patients; and it should be deemed a point of honour to adhere to these rules with as much uniformity as varying circumstances will admit.

Chapter III. Of the Duties of the Profession to the Public, and of the Obligations of the Public to the Profession

Art. I—*Duties of the Profession to the Public*

1. As good citizens, it is the duty of physicians to be ever vigilant for the welfare of the community, and to bear their part in sustaining its institutions and burdens: they should also be ever ready to give counsel to the public in relation to matters especially appertaining to their profession, as on subjects of medical police, public hygiene, and legal medicine. It is their province to enlighten the public in regard to quarantine regulations—the location, arrangement, and dietaries of hospitals, asylums, schools, prisons, and similar institutions—in relation to the medical police of towns, as drainage, ventilation, &c.—and in regard to measures for the prevention of epidemic and contagious diseases; and when pestilence prevails, it is their duty to face the danger, and to continue their labors for the alleviation of the suffering, even at the jeopardy of their own lives.

2. Medical men should also be always ready, when called on by the legally constituted authorities, to enlighten coroners' inquests and courts of justice, on subjects strictly medical—such as involve questions relating to sanity, legitimacy, murder by poisons or other violent means, and in regard to the various other subjects embraced in the science of Medical Jurisprudence. But in these cases, and es-

pecially where they are required to make a post-mortem examination, it is just, in consequence of the time, labor and skill required, and the responsibility and risk they incur, that the public should award them a proper honorarium.

3. There is no profession, by the members of which, eleemosynary services are more liberally dispensed, than the medical; but justice requires that some limits should be placed to the performance of such good offices. Poverty, professional brotherhood, and certain public duties referred to in section 1 of this chapter, should always be recognised as presenting valid claims for gratuitous services; but neither institutions endowed by the public or by rich individuals, societies for mutual benefit, for the insurance of lives or for analogous purposes, nor any profession or occupation, can be admitted to possess such privilege. Nor can it be justly expected of physicians to furnish certificates of inability to serve on juries, to perform militia duty, or to testify to the state of health of persons wishing to insure their lives, obtain pensions, or the like, without a pecuniary acknowledgment. But to individuals in indigent circumstances, such professional services should always be cheerfully and freely accorded.

4. It is the duty of physicians, who are frequent witnesses of the enormities committed by quackery, and the injury to health and even destruction of life caused by the use of quack medicines, to enlighten the public on these subjects, to expose the injuries sustained by the unwary from the devices and pretensions of artful empirics and impostors. Physicians ought to use all the influence which they may possess, as professors in Colleges of Pharmacy, and by exercising their option in regard to the shops to which their prescriptions shall be sent, to discourage druggists and apothecaries from vending quack or secret medicines, or from being in any way engaged in their manufacture and sale.

Art. II—*Obligations of the Public to Physicians*

1. The benefits accruing to the public directly and indirectly from the active and unwearied beneficence of the profession, are so numerous and important, that physicians are justly entitled to the utmost consideration and respect from the community. The public ought likewise to entertain a just appreciation of medical qualifications—to make a proper discrimination between true science and the assumption of ignorance and empiricism—to afford every encouragement and facility for the acquisition of medical education—and no longer to allow the statute books to exhibit the anomaly of exacting knowledge from physicians, under liability to heavy penalties, and of making them obnoxious to punishment for resorting to the only means of obtaining it.

Appendix D

Principles of Medical Ethics (1903)

AMERICAN MEDICAL ASSOCIATION

Preface

At the annual meeting of the American Medical Association, held in New Orleans, the House of Delegates unanimously adopted, on May 7, 1903, the "Principles of Medical Ethics" recommended by its committee, and ordered that the following extract from the report of the Special Committee on Revision of the Code of Medical Ethics be printed as an explanatory preface to these "Principles":

"The caption 'Principles of Medical Ethics' has been substituted for 'Code of Medical Ethics.' Inasmuch as the American Medical Association may be conceived to hold a relation to the constituent state associations analogous to that of the United States through its constitution to the several states, the committee deemed it wiser to formulate the principles of medical ethics without definite reference to code or penalties. Large discretionary powers are thus left to the respective state and territorial societies to form such codes and establish such rules for the professional conduct of their members as they may consider proper, provided, of course, that there shall be no infringement of the established ethical principles of this Association."

The American Medical Association promulgates as a suggestive and advisory document the following:

Chapter I. The Duties of Physicians to Their Patients

The Physician's Responsibility

Section 1. Physicians should not only be ever ready to obey the calls of the sick and the injured, but should be mindful of the high character of their mis-

American Medical Association Press, Chicago, 1911; copyright 1903.

sion and of the responsibilities they must incur in the discharge of momentous duties. In their ministrations they should never forget that the comfort, the health and the lives of those entrusted to their care depend on skill, attention and fidelity. In deportment they should unite tenderness, cheerfulness and firmness, and thus inspire all sufferers with gratitude, respect and confidence. These observations are the more sacred because, generally, the only tribunal to adjudge penalties for unkindness, carelessness or neglect is their own conscience.

Humanity, Delicacy and Secrecy Needed

Sec. 2. Every patient committed to the charge of a physician, should be treated with attention and humanity, and reasonable indulgence should be granted to the caprices of the sick. Secrecy and delicacy should be strictly observed; and the familiar and confidential intercourse to which physicians are admitted, in their professional visits, should be guarded with the most scrupulous fidelity and honor.

Secrecy to Be Inviolate

Sec. 3. The obligation of secrecy extends beyond the period of professional services; none of the privacies of individual or domestic life, no infirmity of disposition or flaw of character observed during medical attendance, should ever be divulged by physicians, except when imperatively required by the laws of the state. The force of the obligation of secrecy is so great that physicians have been protected in its observance by courts of justice.

Frequency of Visits

Sec. 4. Frequent visits to the sick are often requisite, since they enable the physician to arrive at a more perfect knowledge of the disease, and to meet promptly every change which may occur. Unnecessary visits are to be avoided, as they give undue anxiety to the patient; but to secure the patient against irritating suspense and disappointment the regular and periodical visits of the physician should be made as nearly as possible at the hour when they may be reasonably expected by the patient.

Honesty and Wisdom in Prognosis

Sec. 5. Ordinarily, the physician should not be forward to make gloomy prognostications, but should not fail, on proper occasions, to give timely notice of dangerous manifestations to the friends of the patient; and even to the patient, if absolutely necessary. This notice, however, is at times so peculiarly alarming when given by the physician, that its deliverance may often be preferably assigned to another person of good judgment.

Encouragement of Patients

Sec. 6. The physician should be a minister of hope and comfort to the sick, since life may be lengthened or shortened not only by the acts, but by the words or manner of the physician, whose solemn duty is to avoid all utterances and actions having a tendency to discourage and depress the patient.

Incurable Cases Not to Be Neglected

Sec. 7. The medical attendant ought not to abandon a patient because deemed incurable; for continued attention may be highly useful to the sufferer and comforting to the relatives, even in the last period of the fatal malady, by alleviating pain and by soothing mental anguish.

Judicious Counsel to Patients

Sec. 8. The opportunity which a physician has of promoting and strengthening the good resolutions of patients suffering under the consequences of evil conduct ought never to be neglected. Good counsels, or even remonstrances, will give satisfaction, not offense, if they be tactfully proffered and evince a genuine love of virtue, accompanied by a sincere interest in the welfare of the person to whom they are addressed.

Chapter II. The Duties of Physicians to Each Other and to the Profession at Large

Article I.—Duties for the Support of Professional Character

Obligation to Maintain the Honor of the Profession

Section 1. Everyone on entering the profession, and thereby becoming entitled to full professional fellowship, incurs an obligation to uphold its dignity and honor, to exalt its standing and to extend the bounds of its usefulness. It is inconsistent with the principles of medical science and it is incompatible for physicians to designate their practice as based on an exclusive dogma or sectarian system of medicine.

Observation of Professional Rules

Sec. 2. The physician should observe strictly such laws as are instituted for the government of the members of the profession; should honor the fraternity as a body; should endeavor to promote the science and art of medicine, and should entertain a due respect for those seniors who, by their labors, have contributed to its advancement.

Duty to Join Medical Organization

Sec. 3. Every physician should identify himself with the organized body of his profession as represented in the community in which he resides. The organization of local or county medical societies, where they do not exist, should be effected, so far as practicable. Such county societies, constituting as they do the chief element of strength in the organization of the profession, should have the active support of their members and should be made instruments for the cultivation of fellowship, for the exchange of professional experience, for the advancement of medical knowledge, for the maintenance of ethical standards, and for the promotion in general of the interests of the profession and the welfare of the public.

County Societies to Affiliate with Higher Organizations

Sec. 4. All county medical societies thus organized ought to place themselves in affiliation with their respective state association, and these, in turn, with the American Medical Association.

Purity of Character and Morality Required

Sec. 5. There is no profession from the members of which greater purity of character and a higher standard of moral excellence are required than the medical; and to attain such eminence is a duty every physician owes alike to the profession and to patients. It is due to the patients, as without it their respect and confidence can not be commanded; and to the profession, because no scientific attainments can compensate for the want of correct moral principles.

Temperance in All Things

Sec. 6. It is incumbent on physicians to be temperate in all things, for the practice of medicine requires the unremitting exercise of a clear and vigorous understanding; and in emergencies—for which no physician should be unprepared—a steady hand, an acute eye, and an unclouded mind are essential to the welfare and even to the life of a human being.

Advertising Methods to Be Avoided

Sec. 7. It is incompatible with honorable standing in the profession to resort to public advertisement or private cards inviting the attention of persons affected with particular diseases; to promise radical cures; to publish cases or operations in the daily prints, or to suffer such publication to be made; to invite laymen (other than relatives who may desire to be at hand) to be present at operations; to boast of cures and remedies; to adduce certificates of skill and success, or to employ any of the other methods of charlatans.

Patents and Secret Nostrums

Sec. 8. It is equally derogatory to professional character for physicians to hold patents for any surgical instruments or medicines; to accept rebates on prescriptions or surgical appliances; to assist unqualified persons to evade legal restrictions governing the practice of medicine; or to dispense, or promote the use of, secret medicines, for if such nostrums are of real efficacy, any concealment regarding them is inconsistent with beneficence and professional liberality, and if mystery alone give them public notoriety, such craft implies either disgraceful ignorance or fraudulent avarice. It is highly reprehensible for physicians to give certificates attesting the efficacy of secret medicines, or other substances used therapeutically.

Article II.—Professional Services of Physicians to Each Other

Physicians Dependent on Each Other

Section 1. Physicians should not, as a general rule, undertake the treatment of themselves, nor of members of their family. In such circumstances they are peculiarly dependent on each other; therefore, kind offices and professional aid should always be cheerfully and gratuitously afforded. These visits should not, however, be obtrusively made; as they may give rise to embarrassment or interfere with that free choice on which such confidence depends.

Gratuitous Services to Fellow Physicians

Sec. 2. All practicing physicians and their immediate family dependents are entitled to the gratuitous services of any one or more of the physicians residing near them.

Compensation for Expenses

Sec. 3. When a physician is summoned from a distance to the bedside of a colleague in easy financial circumstances, a compensation, proportionate to traveling expenses and to the pecuniary loss entailed by absence from the accustomed field of professional labor, should be made by the patient or relatives.

One Physician to Take Charge

Sec. 4. When more than one physician is attending another, one of the number should take charge of the case, otherwise the concert of thought and action so essential to wise treatment can not be assured.

Attention to Absent Physician's Patients

Sec. 5. The affairs of life, the pursuit of health, and the various accidents and contingencies to which a physician is peculiarly exposed, sometimes require the temporary withdrawal of this physician from daily professional labor and the appointment of a colleague to act for a specified time. The colleague's compliance is an act of courtesy which should always be performed with the utmost consideration for the interest and character of the family physician.

Article III.—The Duties of Physicians in Regard to Consultations

The Broadest Humanity in Emergencies Required

Section 1. The broadest dictates of humanity should be obeyed by physicians whenever and wherever their services are needed to meet the emergencies of disease or accident.

Consultations Should Be Promoted

Sec. 2. Consultations should be promoted in difficult cases, as they contribute to confidence and more enlarged views of practice.

Punctuality in Consultations

Sec. 3. The utmost punctuality should be observed in the visits of physicians whey they are to hold consultations, and this is generally practicable, for society has been so considerate as to allow the plea for a professional engagement to take precedence over all others.

Necessary Delays

Sec. 4. As professional engagements may sometimes cause delay in attendance, the physician who first arrives should wait for a reasonable time, after which the consultation should be considered as postponed to a new appointment.

Good Feeling and Candor in Consultations

Sec. 5. In consultations no insincerity, rivalry or envy should be indulged; candor, probity and all due respect should be observed toward the physician in charge of the case.

Unauthorized Statements or Discussions

Sec. 6. No statement or discussion of the case should take place before the patient or friends, except in the presence of all the physicians attending, or by their common consent; and no opinions or prognostications should be delivered which are not the result of previous deliberation and concurrence.

Attending Physician May Vary Treatment

Sec. 7. No decision should restrain the attending physician from making such subsequent variations in the mode of treatment as any unexpected change in the character of the case may demand. But at the next consultation reasons for the variations should be stated. The same privilege, with its obligation, belongs to the consultant when sent for in an emergency during the absence of the family physician.

Attending Physician to Prescribe

Sec. 8. The attending physician, at any time, may prescribe for the patient; not so the consultant, when alone, except in a case of emergency or when called from a considerable distance. In the first instance the consultant should do what is needed, and in the second should do no more than make an examination of the patient and leave a written opinion, under seal, to be delivered to the attending physician.

Discussions in Consultation Confidential

Sec. 9. All discussions in consultation should be held as confidential. Neither by words nor by manner should any of the participants in a consultation assert or intimate that any part of the treatment pursued did not receive his assent.

Conflicts of Opinion

Sec. 10. It may happen that two physicians can not agree in their views of the nature of a case and of the treatment to be pursued. In the event of such disagreement, a third physician should, if practicable, be called in. None but the rarest and most exceptional circumstances would justify the consultant in taking charge of the case. He should not do so merely on the solicitation of the patient or friends.

Consultant to Scrupulously Regard Rights of Attending Physician

Sec. 11. A physician who is called in consultation should observe the most honorable and scrupulous regard for the character and standing of the attending physician, whose conduct of the case should be justified, as far as can be, consistently with a conscientious regard for truth, and no hint or insinuation should be thrown out which would impair the confidence reposed in the attending physician.

Article IV.—Duties of Physicians in Cases of Interference

Qualifications the Only Basis of Practice

Section 1. Medicine being a liberal profession, those admitted to its ranks should found their expectations of practice especially on the character and extent of their medical education.

Intercourse with Patients of Other Physicians

Sec. 2. The physician, in his intercourse with a patient under the care of another physician, should observe the strictest caution and reserve; should give no disingenuous hints relative to the nature and treatment of the patient's disorder, nor should the course of conduct of the physician, directly or indirectly, tend to diminish the trust reposed in the attending physician.

Circumspection as Regards Visits

Sec. 3. The same circumspection should be observed when, from motives of business or friendship, a physician is prompted to visit a person who is under the direction of another physician. Indeed, such visits should be avoided, except under peculiar circumstances; and when they are made, no inquiries should be instituted relative to the nature of the disease, or the remedies employed, but the topics of conversation should be as foreign to the case as circumstances will admit.

Duty as to Calls to Patients of Other Physicians

Sec. 4. A physician ought not to take charge of, or prescribe for, a patient who has recently been under the care of another physician, in the same illness, except in case of a sudden emergency, or in consultation with the physician previously in attendance, or when that physician has relinquished the case or has been dismissed in due form.

Criticisms to Be Avoided

Sec. 5. The physician acting in conformity with the preceding section should not make damaging insinuations regarding the practice adopted, and, indeed, should justify it if consistent with truth and probity; for it often happens that patients become dissatisfied when they are not immediately relieved, and, as many diseases are naturally protracted, the seeming want of success, in the first stage of treatment, affords no evidence of a lack of professional knowledge or skill.

Emergency Cases

Sec. 6. When a physician is called to an urgent case, because the family attendant is not at hand, unless assistance in consultation is desired, the former should resign the care of the patient immediately on the arrival of the family physician.

Duty When Called with Other Physicians

Sec. 7. It often happens, in cases of sudden illness, and of accidents and injuries, owing to the alarm and anxiety of friends, that several physicians are simultaneously summoned. Under these circumstances, courtesy should assign the patient to the first who arrives, and who, if necessary, may invoke the aid of some of those present. In such case, however, the acting physician should request that the family physician be called, and should withdraw unless requested to continue in attendance.

Cases to Be Relinquished to Regular Attendant

Sec. 8. Whenever a physician is called to the patient of another physician during the enforced absence of that physician the case should be relinquished on the return of the latter.

Emergency Attention and Advice

Sec. 9. A physician, while visiting a sick person in the country, may be asked to see another physician's patient because of a sudden aggravation of the disease. On such an occasion, the immediate needs of the patient should be attended to and the case relinquished on the arrival of the attending physician.

Substitute Obstetric Work

Sec. 10. When a physician who has been engaged to attend an obstetric case is absent and another is sent for, delivery being accomplished during the vicarious attendance, the acting physician is entitled to the professional fee, but must resign the patient on the arrival of the physician first engaged.

Article V.—Differences between Physicians

Arbitration of Differences

Section 1. Diversity of opinion and opposition of interest may, in the medical as in other professions, sometimes occasion controversy and even contention. Whenever such unfortunate cases occur and can not be immediately adjusted, they should be referred to the arbitration of a sufficient number of impartial physicians.

Reserve Toward Public on Certain Professional Questions

Sec. 2. A peculiar reserve must be maintained by physicians toward the public in regard to some professional questions, and as there exist many points in medical ethics and etiquette through which the feelings of physicians may be painfully assailed in their intercourse, and which can not be understood or appreciated by general society, neither the subject-matter of their differences nor the adjudication of the arbitration should be made public.

Article VI.—Compensation

The Limits of Gratuitous Service

Section 1. By the members of no profession are eleemosynary services more liberally dispensed than by the medical, but justice requires that some limits should be placed to their performance. Poverty, mutual professional obligations, and certain of the public duties named in Sections 1 and 2 of Chapter III, should always be recognized as presenting valid claims for gratuitous services; but neither institutions endowed by the public or the rich, or by societies for mutual benefit, for life insurance, or for analogous purposes, nor any profession or occupation, can be admitted to possess such privilege.

Certifying or Testifying to Be Paid For

Sec. 2. It can not be justly expected of physicians to furnish certificates of inability to serve on juries, or to perform militia duty; to testify to the state of health of persons wishing to insure their lives, obtain pensions, or the like, without due compensation. But to persons in indigent circumstances such services should always be cheerfully and freely accorded.

Fee Bills

Sec. 3. Some general rules should be adopted by the physicians in every town or district relative to the minimum pecuniary acknowledgment from their patients; and it should be deemed a point of honor to adhere to these rules with as much uniformity as varying circumstances will admit.

Giving or Receiving of Commissions Condemned

Sec. 4. It is derogatory to professional character for physicians to pay or offer to pay commissions to any person whatsoever who may recommend to them patients requiring general or special treatment or surgical operations. It is equally derogatory to professional character for physicians to solicit or to receive such commissions.

Chapter III. The Duties of the Profession to the Public

Duties as to Public Hygiene, etc.

Section 1. As good citizens it is the duty of physicians to be very vigilant for the welfare of the community, and to bear their part in sustaining its laws, institutions and burdens; especially should they be ready to cooperate with the proper authorities in the administration and the observance of sanitary laws and regulations, and they should also be ever ready to give counsel to the public in relation to subjects especially appertaining to their profession, as on questions of sanitary police, public hygiene and legal medicine.

Enlightenment of Public on Sanitary Matters. Duties in Epidemics

Sec. 2. It is the province of physicians to enlighten the public in regard to quarantine regulations; to the location, arrangement and dietaries of hospitals, asylums, schools, prisons and similar institutions; in regard to measures for the prevention of epidemic and contagious diseases; and when pestilence prevails, it is their duty to face the danger, and to continue their labors for the alleviation of the suffering people, even at the risk of their own lives.

Physicians as Witnesses

Sec. 3. Physicians, when called on by legally constituted authorities, should always be ready to enlighten inquests and courts of justice on subjects strictly medical, such as involve questions relating to sanity, legitimacy, murder by poison or other violent means, and various other subjects embraced in the science of medical jurisprudence. It is but just, however, for them to expect due compensation for their services.

Enlightenment of the Public as to Charlatans

Sec. 4. It is the duty of physicians who are frequent witnesses of the great wrongs committed by charlatans and of the injury to health and even destruction of life caused by the use of their treatment, to enlighten the public on these subjects and to make known the injuries sustained by the unwary from the devices and pretensions of artful impostors.

Relations to Pharmacists

Sec. 5. It is the duty of physicians to recognize and by legitimate patronage to promote the profession of pharmacy, on the skill and proficiency of which depends the reliability of remedies, but any pharmacist who, although educated in his own profession, is not a qualified physician, and who assumed to prescribe for the sick, ought not to receive such countenance and support. Any druggist or pharmacist who dispenses deteriorated or sophisticated drugs or who substitutes one remedy for another designated in a prescription ought thereby to forfeit the recognition and influence of physicians.

Appendix E

Principles of Medical Ethics (1912)

AMERICAN MEDICAL ASSOCIATION

Chapter I. The Duties of Physicians to Their Patients

The Physician's Responsibility

Section 1. The profession has for its prime object the service it can render to humanity; reward or financial gain should be a subordinate consideration. The practice of medicine is a profession. In choosing this profession an individual assumes an obligation to conduct himself in accord with its ideals.

Patience, Delicacy and Secrecy

Sec. 2. Patience and delicacy should characterize all the acts of a physician. The confidences concerning individual or domestic life entrusted by a patient to a physician and the defects of disposition or flaws of character observed in patients during medical attendance should be held as a trust and should never be revealed except when imperatively required by the laws of the state. There are occasions, however, when a physician must determine whether or not his duty to society requires him to take definite action to protect a healthy individual from becoming infected because the physician has knowledge, obtained through the confidences entrusted to him as a physician, of a communicable disease to which the healthy individual is about to be exposed. In such a case, the physician should act as he would desire another to act toward one of his own family under like circumstances. Before he determines his course, the physician should know the civil law of his commonwealth concerning privileged communications.

Adopted by the House of Delegates at Atlantic City, New Jersey, June 4, 1912.

Prognosis

Sec. 3. A physician should give timely notice of dangerous manifestations of the disease to the friends of the patient. He should neither exaggerate nor minimize the gravity of the patient's condition. He should assure himself that the patient or his friends will have such knowledge of the patient's condition as will serve the best interests of the patient and the family.

Patients Must Not Be Neglected

Sec. 4. A physician is free to choose whom he will serve. He should, however, always respond to any request for his assistance in an emergency or whenever temperate public opinion expects the service. Once having undertaken a case, a physician should not abandon or neglect the patient because the disease is deemed incurable; nor should he withdraw from the case for any reason until a sufficient notice of a desire to be released has been given the patient or his friends to make it possible for them to secure another medical attendant.

Chapter II. The Duties of Physicians to Each Other and to the Profession at Large

Article I.—Duties to the Profession

Uphold Honor of Profession

Section 1. The obligation assumed on entering the profession requires the physician to comport himself as a gentleman and demands that he use every honorable means to uphold the dignity and honor of his vocation, to exalt its standards and to extend its sphere of usefulness. A physician should not base his practice on an exclusive dogma or sectarian system, for "sects are implacable despots; to accept this thraldom is to take away all liberty from one's action and thought." (Nicon, father of Galen.)

Duty of Medical Societies

Sec. 2. In order that the dignity and honor of the medical profession may be upheld, its standards exalted, its sphere of usefulness extended, and the advancement of medical science promoted, a physician should associate himself with medical societies and contribute his time, energy and means in order that these societies may represent the ideals of the profession.

Deportment

Sec. 3. A physician should be "an upright man, instructed in the art of healing." Consequently, he must keep himself pure in character and conform to a high standard of morals, and must be diligent and conscientious in his studies. "He should also be modest, sober, patient, prompt to do his whole duty without anxiety; pious without going so far as superstition, conducting himself with propriety in his profession and in all the actions of his life." (Hippocrates.)

Advertising

Sec. 4. Solicitation of patients by circulars or advertisements, or by personal communications or interviews, not warranted by personal relations, is unprofessional. It is equally unprofessional to procure patients by indirection through solicitors or agents of any kind, or by indirect advertisement, or by furnishing or inspiring newspaper or magazine comments concerning cases in which the physician has been or is concerned. All other like self-laudations defy the traditions and lower the tone of any profession and so are intolerable. The most worthy and effective advertisement possible, even for a young physician, and especially with his brother physicians, is the establishment of a well-merited reputation for professional ability and fidelity. This cannot be forced, but must be the outcome of character and conduct. The publication or circulation of ordinary simple business cards, being a matter of personal taste or local custom, and sometimes of convenience, is not *per se* improper. As implied, it is unprofessional to disregard local customs and offend recognized ideals in publishing or circulating such cards.

It is unprofessional to promise radical cures; to boast of cures and secret methods of treatment or remedies; to exhibit certificates of skill or of success in the treatment of diseases; or to employ any methods to gain the attention of the public for the purpose of obtaining patients.

Patents and Perquisites

Sec. 5. It is unprofessional to receive remuneration from patents for surgical instruments or medicines; to accept rebates on prescriptions or surgical appliances, or perquisites from attendants who aid in the care of patients.

Medical Laws—Secret Remedies

Sec. 6. It is unprofessional for a physician to assist unqualified persons to evade legal restrictions governing the practice of medicine; it is equally unethical to prescribe or dispense secret medicines or other secret remedial agents, or manufacture or promote their use in any way.

Safeguarding the Profession

Sec. 7. Physicians should expose without fear or favor, before the proper medical or legal tribunals, corrupt or dishonest conduct of members of the profession. Every physician should aid in safeguarding the profession against the admission to its ranks of those who are unfit or unqualified because deficient either in moral character or education.

Article II.—Professional Services of Physicians to Each Other

Physicians Dependent on Each Other

Section 1. Experience teaches that it is unwise for a physician to treat members of his own family or himself. Consequently, a physician should always cheerfully and gratuitously respond with his professional services to the call of any physician practicing in his vicinity, or of the immediate family dependents of physicians.

Sec. 2. When a physician from a distance is called on to advise another physician or one of his family dependents, and the physician to whom the service is rendered is in easy financial circumstances, a compensation that will at least meet the traveling expenses of the visiting physician should be proffered. When such a service requires an absence from the accustomed field of professional work of the visitor that might reasonably be expected to entail a pecuniary loss, that loss should, in part at least, be provided for in the compensation offered.

One Physician to Take Charge

Sec. 3. When a physician or a member of his dependent family is seriously ill, he or his family should select a physician from among his neighboring colleagues to take charge of the case. Other physicians may be associated in the care of the patient as consultants.

Article III.—Duties of Physician in Consultations

Consultations Should Be Required

Section 1. In serious illness, especially in doubtful or difficult conditions, the physician should request consultations.

Consultation for Patient's Benefit

Sec. 2. In every consultation, the benefit to be derived by the patient is of first importance. All the physicians interested in the case should be frank and candid with the patient and his family. There never is occasion for insincerity, rivalry or envy and these should never be permitted between consultants.

Punctuality

Sec. 3. It is the duty of a physician, particularly in the instance of a consultation, to be punctual in attendance. When, however, the consultant or the physician in charge is unavoidably delayed, the one who first arrives should wait for the other for a reasonable time, after which the consultation should be considered postponed. When the consultant has come from a distance, or when for any reason it will be difficult to meet the physician in charge at another time, or if the case is urgent, or if it be the desire of the patient, he may examine the patient and mail his written opinion, or see that it is delivered under seal, to the physician in charge. Under these conditions, the consultant's conduct must be especially tactful; he must remember that he is framing an opinion without the aid of the physician who has observed the course of the disease.

Patient Referred to Specialist

Sec. 4. When a patient is sent to one specially skilled in the care of the condition from which he is thought to be suffering, and for any reason it is impracticable for the physician in charge of the case to accompany the patient, the physician in charge should send to the consultant by mail, or in the care of the patient under seal, a history of the case, together with the physician's opinion and an outline of the treatment, or so much of this as may possibly be of service to the consultant; and as soon as possible the consultant should address the physician in charge and advise him of the results of the consultant's investigation of the case. Both these opinions are confidential and must be so regarded by the consultant and by the physician in charge.

Discussions in Consultation

Sec. 5. After the physicians called in consultation have completed their investigations of the case, they may meet by themselves to discuss conditions and determine the course to be followed in the treatment of the patient. No statement or discussion of the case should take place before the patient or friends, except in the presence of all the physicians attending, or by their common consent; and no opinions or prognostications should be delivered as a result of the deliberations of the consultants, which have not been concurred in by the consultants at their conference.

Attending Physician Responsible

Sec. 6. The physician in attendance is in charge of the case and is responsible for the treatment of the patient. Consequently, he may prescribe for the patient at any time and is privileged to vary the mode of treatment outlined and agreed on at a consultation whenever, in his opinion, such a change is warranted. However, at the next consultation, he should state his reasons for departing from the course decided on at the previous conference. When an emergency occurs during the absence of the attending physician, a consultant may provide for the emergency and the subsequent care of the patient until the arrival of the physician in charge, but should do no more than this without the consent of the physician in charge.

Conflict of Opinion

Sec. 7. Should the attending physician and the consultant find it impossible to agree in their view of a case another consultant should be called to the conference or the first consultant should withdraw. However, since the consultant was employed by the patient in order that his opinion might be obtained, he should be permitted to state the result of his study of the case to the patient, or his next friend in the presence of the physician in charge.

Consultant and Attendant

Sec. 8. When a physician has attended a case as a consultant, he should not become the attendant of the patient during that illness except with the consent of the physician who was in charge at the time of the consultation.

Article IV.—Duties of Physicians in Cases of Interference

Criticism to Be Avoided

Section 1. The physician, in his intercourse with a patient under the care of another physician, should observe the strictest caution and reserve; should give no disingenuous hints relative to the nature and treatment of the patient's disorder; nor should the course of conduct of the physician, directly or indirectly, tend to diminish the trust reposed in the attending physician.

Social Calls on Patient of Another Physician

Sec. 2. A physician should avoid making social calls on those who are under the professional care of other physicians without the knowledge and consent of the attendant. Should such a friendly visit be made, there should be no inquiry relative to the nature of the disease or comment upon the treatment of the case, but the conversation should be on subjects other than the physical condition of the patient.

Services to Patient of Another Physician

Sec. 3. A physician should never take charge of or prescribe for a patient who is under the care of another physician, except in an emergency, until after the other physician has relinquished the case or has been properly dismissed.

Criticism to Be Avoided

Sec. 4. When a physician does succeed another physician in the charge of a case, he should not make comments or insinuations regarding the practice of the one who preceded him. Such comments or insinuations tend to lower the esteem of the patient for the medical profession and so react against the critic.

Emergency Cases

Sec. 5. When a physician is called in an emergency and finds that he has been sent for because the family attendant is not at hand, or when a physician is asked to see another physician's patient because of an aggravation of the disease, he should provide only for the patient's immediate need and should withdraw from the case on the arrival of the family physician after he has reported the condition found and the treatment administered.

When Several Physicians Are Summoned

Sec. 6. When several physicians have been summoned in a case of sudden illness or of accident, the first to arrive should be considered the physician in charge. However, as soon as the exigencies of the case permit, or on the arrival of the acknowledged family attendant or the physician the patient desires to serve him, the first physician should withdraw in favor of the chosen attendant; should the patient or his family wish some one other than the physician known to be the family physician to take charge of the case the patient should advise the family physician of his desire. When, because of sudden illness or accident, a patient is taken to a hospital, the patient should be returned to the care of his known family physician as soon as the condition of the patient and the circumstances of the case warrant this transfer.

A Colleague's Patient

Sec. 7. When a physician is requested by a colleague to care for a patient during his temporary absence, or when, because of an emergency, he is asked to see a patient of a colleague, the physician should treat the patient in the same manner and with the same delicacy as he would have one of his own patients cared for under similar circumstances. The patient should be returned to the care of the attending physician as soon as possible.

Relinquishing Patient to Regular Attendant

Sec. 8. When a physician is called to the patient of another physician during the enforced absence of that physician, the patient should be relinquished on the return of the latter.

Substituting in Obstetric Work

Sec. 9. When a physician attends a women in labor in the absence of another who has been engaged to attend, such physician should resign the patient to the one first engaged, upon his arrival; the physician is entitled to compensation for the professional services he may have rendered.

Article V.—Differences between Physicians

Arbitration

Section 1. Whenever there arises between physicians a grave difference of opinion which cannot be promptly adjusted, the dispute should be referred for arbitration to a committee of impartial physicians, preferably the Board of Censors of a component county society of the American Medical Association.

Article VI.—Compensation

Limits of Gratuitous Service

Section 1. The poverty of a patient and the mutual professional obligation of physicians should command the gratuitous services of a physician. But institutions endowed by societies, the organizations for mutual benefit, or for accident, sickness and life insurance, or for analogous purposes, should be accorded no such privileges.

Contract Practice

Sec. 2. It is unprofessional for a physician to dispose of his services under conditions that make it impossible to render adequate service to his patient or which interfere with reasonable competition among the physicians of a community. To do this is detrimental to the public and to the individual physician, and lowers the dignity of the profession.

Secret Division of Fees Condemned

Sec. 3. It is detrimental to the public good and degrading to the profession, and therefore unprofessional, to give or to receive a commission. It is also unprofessional to divide a fee for medical advice or surgical treatment, unless the patient or his next friend is fully informed as to the terms of the transaction. The patient should be made to realize that a proper fee should be paid the family physician for the service he renders in determining the surgical and medical treatment suited to the condition, and in advising concerning those best qualified to render any special service that may be required by the patient.

Chapter III. The Duties of the Profession to the Public

Physicians as Citizens

Section 1. Physicians, as good citizens and because their professional training specially qualifies them to render this service, should give advice concerning the public health of the community. They should bear their full part in enforcing its laws and sustaining the institutions that advance the interests of humanity. They should coöperate especially with the proper authorities in the administration of sanitary laws and regulations. They should be ready to counsel the public on subjects relating to sanitary police, public hygiene and legal medicine.

Physicians Should Enlighten Public—Duties in Epidemics

Sec. 2. Physicians, especially those engaged in public health work, should enlighten the public regarding quarantine regulations; on the location, arrangement and dietaries of hospitals, asylums, schools, prisons and similar institutions; and concerning measures for the prevention of epidemic and contagious diseases. When an epidemic prevails, a physician must continue his labors for the alleviation of suffering people, without regard to the risk to his own health or life or to financial return. At all times, it is the duty of the physician to notify the properly constituted public health authorities of every case of communicable disease under his care, in accordance with the laws, rules and regulations of the health authorities of the locality in which the patient is.

Public Warned

Sec. 3. Physicians should warn the public against the devices practiced and the false pretensions made by charlatans which may cause injury to health and loss of life.

Pharmacists

Sec. 4. By legitimate patronage physicians should recognize and promote the profession of pharmacy; but any pharmacist, unless he be qualified as a physician, who assumes to prescribe for the sick, should be denied such countenance and support. Moreover, whenever a druggist or pharmacist dispenses deteriorated or adulterated drugs, or substitutes one remedy for another designated in a prescription, he thereby forfeits all claims to the favorable consideration of the public and physicians.

Conclusion

While the foregoing statements express in a general way the duty of the physician to his patients, to other members of the profession and to the profession at large, as well as of the profession to the public, it is not to be supposed that they cover the whole field of medical ethics, or that the physician is not under many duties and obligations besides these herein set forth. In a word, it is incumbent on the physician that under all conditions, his bearing toward patients, the public and fellow practitioners should be characterized by a gentlemanly deportment and that he constantly should behave toward others as he desires them to deal with him. Finally, these principles are primarily for the good of the public, and their enforcement should be conducted in such a manner as shall deserve and receive the endorsement of the community.

Appendix F

Principles of Medical Ethics (1957)

AMERICAN MEDICAL ASSOCIATION

Until 1957 the American Medical Association's Code of Ethics had been basically that adopted in 1847, although there were revisions in 1903, 1912, and 1947. A major change in the code's format occurred when the current Principles of Medical Ethics were adopted in 1957. These ten principles, which replace the forty-eight sections of the older code, are intended as expressions of the fundamental concepts and requirements of the earlier code, unencumbered by easily outdated practical codifications. From time to time the Association's principles are interpreted and applied to contemporary ethical and professional problems, usually in the form of Opinions and Reports of the Judicial Council. In justifying the change from the original Percivalean format, the Council on Constitution and Bylaws remarked that "every basic principle has been preserved; on the other hand, as much as possible of the prolixity and ambiguity which in the past obstructied ready explanation, practical codification and particular selection of basic concepts has been eliminated."

From time to time the AMA's principles are interpreted and applied to contemporary ethical and professional problems, usually in the form of Opinions and Reports from the AMA's Council on Ethical and Judicial Affairs (CEJA). The collected opinions, together with annotations noting their use by courts and academic journals, fill over 200 pages. The rationales behind new opinions (and changes to old opinions) are published biannually in detailed reports; from 1984 to 1999 over 70 of these reports were published. (See Appendix I, Selected Opinions and Reports.)

These principles are intended to aid physicians individually and collectively in maintaining a high level of ethical conduct. They are not laws but standards by which a physician may determine the propriety of his conduct in his re-

Reprinted with the permission of the American Medical Association.

lationship with patients, with colleagues, with members of allied professions, and with the public.

Section 1. The principal objective of the medical profession is to render service to humanity with full respect for the dignity of man. Physicians should merit the confidence of patients entrusted to their care, rendering to each a full measure of service and devotion.

Section 2. Physicians should strive continually to improve medical knowledge and skill, and should make available to their patients and colleagues the benefits of their professional attainments.

Section 3. A physician should practice a method of healing founded on a scientific basis; and he should not voluntarily associate professionally with anyone who violates this principle.

Section 4. The medical profession should safeguard the public and itself against physicians deficient in moral character or professional competence. Physicians should observe all laws, uphold the dignity and honor of the profession and accept its self-imposed disciplines. They should expose, without hesitation, illegal or unethical conduct of fellow members of the profession.

Section 5. A physician may choose whom he will serve. In an emergency, however, he should render service to the best of his ability. Having undertaken the care of a patient, he may not neglect him; and unless he has been discharged he may discontinue his services only after giving adequate notice. He should not solicit patients.

Section 6. A physician should not dispose of his services under terms or conditions which tend to interfere with or impair the free and complete exercise of his medical judgment and skill or tend to cause a deterioration of the quality of medical care.

Section 7. In the practice of medicine a physician should limit the source of his professional income to medical services actually rendered by him, or under his supervision, to his patients. His fee should be commensurate with the services rendered and the patient's ability to pay. He should neither pay nor receive a commission for referral of patients. Drugs, remedies or appliances may be dispensed or supplied by the physician provided it is in the best interests of the patient.

Section 8. A physician should seek consultation upon request; in doubtful or difficult cases; or whenever it appears that the quality of medical service may be enhanced thereby.

Section 9. A physician may not reveal the confidences entrusted to him in the course of medical attendance, or the deficiencies he may observe in the character of patients, unless he is required to do so by law or unless it becomes necessary in order to protect the welfare of the individual or of the community.

Section 10. The honored ideals of the medical professional imply that the responsibilities of the physician extend not only to the individual, but also to society where these responsibilities deserve his interest and participation in activities which have the purpose of improving both the health and the well-being of the individual and the community.

Appendix G

Principles of Medical Ethics (1980)

AMERICAN MEDICAL ASSOCIATION

The medical profession has long subscribed to a body of ethical statements developed primarily for the benefit of the patient. As a member of this profession, a physician must recognize responsibility not only to patients, but also to society, to other health professionals, and to self. The following Principles adopted by the American Medical Association are not laws, but standards of conduct which define the essentials of honorable behavior for the physician.

I. A physician shall be dedicated to providing competent medical service with compassion and respect for human dignity.

II. A physician shall deal honestly with patients and colleagues, and strive to expose those physicians deficient in character or competence, or who engage in fraud or deception.

III. A physician shall respect the law and also recognize a responsibility to seek changes in those requirements which are contrary to the best interests of the patient.

IV. A physician shall respect the rights of patients, of colleagues, and of other health professionals, and shall safeguard patient confidences within the constraints of the law.

V. A physician shall continue to study, apply and advance scientific knowledge, make relevant information available to patients, colleagues, and the public, obtain consultation, and use the talents of other health professionals when indicated.

VI.   A physician shall, in the provision of appropriate patient care, except in emergencies, be free to choose whom to serve, with whom to associate, and the environment in which to provide medical services.

VII. A physician shall recognize a responsibility to participate in activities contributing to an improved community.

Appendix H

Fundamental Elements of the Patient-Physician Relationship (1990; Updated 1994)

AMA COUNCIL ON ETHICAL AND JUDICIAL AFFAIRS

From ancient times, physicians have recognized that the health and well-being of patients depends upon a collaborative effort between physician and patient. Patients share with physicians the responsibility for their own health care. The patient-physician relationship is of greatest benefit to patients when they bring medical problems to the attention of their physicians in a timely fashion, provide information about their medical condition to the best of their ability, and work with their physicians in a mutually respectful alliance. Physicians can best contribute to this alliance by serving as their patients' advocates and by fostering these rights:

1. The patient has the right to receive information from physicians and to discuss the benefits, risks, and costs of appropriate treatment alternatives. Patients should receive guidance from their physicians as to the optimal course of action. Patients are also entitled to obtain copies or summaries of their medical records, to have their questions answered, to be advised of potential conflicts of interest that their physicians might have, and to receive independent professional opinions.

2. The patient has the right to make decisions regarding the health care that is recommended by his or her physician. Accordingly, patients may accept or refuse any recommended medical treatment.

3. The patient has the right to courtesy, respect, dignity, responsiveness, and timely attention to his or her needs.

Originally adopted June 1990. Updated June 1994.

4. The patient has the right to confidentiality. The physician should not reveal confidential communications or information without the consent of the patient, unless provided for by law or by the need to protect the welfare of the individual or the public interest.

5. The patient has the right to continuity of health care. The physician has an obligation to cooperate in the coordination of medically indicated care with other health care providers treating the patient. The physician may not discontinue treatment of a patient as long as further treatment is medically indicated, without giving the patient reasonable assistance and sufficient opportunity to make alternative arrangements for care.

6. The patient has a basic right to have available adequate health care. Physicians, along with the rest of society, should continue to work toward this goal. Fulfillment of this right is dependent on society providing resources so that no patient is deprived of necessary care because of an inability to pay for the care. Physicians should continue their traditional assumption of a part of the responsibility for the medical care of those who cannot afford essential health care. Physicians should advocate for patients in dealing with third parties when appropriate.

Appendix I

Selected Opinions and Reports

AMA COUNCIL ON ETHICAL AND JUDICIAL AFFAIRS

Opinion

7.03 Records of Physicians upon Retirement or Departure from a Group. A patient's records may be necessary to the patient in the future not only for medical care but also for employment, insurance, litigation, or other reasons. When a physician retires or dies, patients should be notified and urged to find a new physician and should be informed that upon authorization, records will be sent to the new physician. Records which may be of value to a patient and which are not forwarded to a new physician should be retained, either by the treating physician, another physician, or such other person lawfully permitted to act as a custodian of the records.

The patients of a physician who leaves a group practice should be notified that the physician is leaving the group. Patients of the physician should also be notified of the physician's new address and offered the opportunity to have their medical records forwarded to the departing physician at his or her new practice. It is unethical to withhold such information upon request of a patient. If the responsibility for notifying patients falls to the departing physician rather than to the group, the group should not interfere with the discharge of these duties by withholding patient lists or other necessary information. (IV)

Issued prior to April 1977.

Updated June 1994 and June 1996.

Opinion

8.061 Gifts to Physicians from Industry. Many gifts given to physicians by companies in the pharmaceutical, device, and medical equipment industries serve an important and socially beneficial function. For example, companies have long provided funds for educational seminars and conferences. However, there has been growing concern about certain gifts from industry to physicians. Some gifts that reflect customary practices of industry may not be consistent with the Principles of Medical Ethics. To avoid the acceptance of inappropriate gifts, physicians should observe the following guidelines:

(1) Any gifts accepted by physicians individually should primarily entail a benefit to patients and should not be of substantial value. Accordingly, textbooks, modest meals, and other gifts are appropriate if they serve a genuine educational function. Cash payments should not be accepted. The use of drug samples for personal or family use is permissible as long as these practices do not interfere with patient access to drug samples. It would not be acceptable for non-retired physicians to request free pharmaceuticals for personal use or use by family members.

(2) Individual gifts of minimal value are permissible as long as the gifts are related to the physician's work (e.g., pens and notepads).

(3) Subsidies to underwrite the costs of continuing medical education conferences or professional meetings can contribute to the improvement of patient care and therefore are permissible. Since the giving of a subsidy directly to a physician by a company's representative may create a relationship that could influence the use of the company's products, any subsidy should be accepted by the conference's sponsor who in turn can use the money to reduce the conference's registration fee. Payments to defray the costs of a conference should not be accepted directly from the company by the physicians attending the conference.

(4) Subsidies from industry should not be accepted directly or indirectly to pay for the costs of travel, lodging, or other personal expenses of physicians attending conferences or meetings, nor should subsidies be accepted to compensate for the physicians' time. Subsidies for hospitality should not be accepted outside of modest meals or social events held as a part of a conference or meeting. It is appropriate for faculty at conferences or meetings to accept reasonable honoraria and to accept reimbursement for reasonable travel, lodging, and meal expenses. It is also appropriate for consultants who provide genuine services to receive reasonable compensation and to accept reimbursement for reasonable travel, lodging, and meal expenses. Token consulting or advisory arrangements cannot be used to justify the compensation of physicians for their time or their travel, lodging, and other out-of-pocket expenses.

(5) Scholarship or other special funds to permit medical students, residents, and fellows to attend carefully selected educational conferences may be permissible as long as the selection of students, residents, or fellows who will receive the funds is made by the academic or training institution. Carefully selected educational conferences are generally defined as the major educational, scientific, or policymaking meetings of national, regional, or specialty medical associations.

(6) No gifts should be accepted if there are strings attached. For example, physicians should not accept gifts if they are given in relation to the physician's prescribing practices. In addition, when companies underwrite medical conferences or lectures other than their own, responsibility for and control over the selection of content, faculty, educational methods, and materials should belong to the organizers of the conferences or lectures. (II)

Issued December 1990 with companion report "Gifts to Physicians from Industry" (*JAMA*. 1991; 265: 501 and *Food and Drug Law Journal*. 1992; 47: 445–458).

Updated June 1996.

Report 1-I-97   Financial Incentives and the Practice of Medicine

Introduction*

Several past Council reports and opinions have addressed, whether directly or indirectly, the ethical implications of practicing medicine in an environment that provides financial rewards and penalties to physicians.[i] The House of Delegates has also examined the issues surrounding financial incentives, and has produced a number of policy statements relating generally to the application of monetary inducements to the practice of medicine.[ii] Despite the wide variety of issues these past statements address, they are all based on a fundamental appreciation of the patient-physician relationship and the role of the profession in advocating for the medical needs of each patient. Maintaining a focus on this ethical foundation is increasingly important as the nation's health care system continues to evolve and the methods of physician reimbursement continue to change. Although it is impossible to provide a discrete ethical analysis of each model of physician reimbursement, the Council presents this report in an effort to highlight the fundamental ethical concerns of any health care payment regime.

Background

There are numerous types of financial incentives including bonuses attached to specific patterns of practice or utilization goals, payments made out of a pool of

---

*In accordance with the Joint Report of the Council on Ethical and Judicial Affairs and the Council on Constitution and Bylaws (I-91), this report may be adopted, not adopted, or referred. It may be amended, with the concurrence of the Council, to clarify its meaning.
[i]See for example Opinions 4.01, 4.03, 6.01, 6.02, 6.03, 6.04, 6.05, 6.10, 8.03, 8.031, 8.032, 8.035, 8.06, 8.061, 8.13, 8.132, 8.134, 9.011.
[ii]See for example HOD Policies 140.978, 285.982, and also CMS Rep. 3-I-96.

withheld funds used to cover the cost of referral services, and fee-for-service payments. The many forms and combinations of incentive payments are often divided into two categories according to the "direction" they encourage physicians to move along the spectrum of utilization. This simple system distinguishes between incentives to provide care and incentives to limit resource use. For example, paying physicians on a fee-for-service basis provides an inducement to provide more services. On the other hand, paying physicians a portion of whatever balance remains in a pool of funds used first to cover referral services strongly encourages physicians to reduce utilization.

Although the system of categorization described above can be a useful model for discussion, it has important shortcomings. The choice of "direction" as the defining characteristic of a particular incentive is often not value-neutral. It is often assumed that providing more care is preferable to providing less, and that incentives to limit care are necessarily worse than those that encourage resource utilization. This assumption persists despite the lack of conclusive data linking different incentives to reductions in quality of care. Identifying the "direction" of an incentive also does little to reflect the underlying goal or goals of a particular payment regime, focusing instead exclusively on levels of utilization. Finally, such a system of labeling incentives has no category for those incentives which are not directly related to providing or limiting services, such as incentives which target improvements in quality and patient satisfaction.

This report resists separating incentive plans into these two categories. It attempts instead to find the elements common to all, and to provide general guidance on the ethical implications of introducing the financial interest of the physician into the treatment relationship. Having established the ethical parameters governing the universe of incentives, it will be possible to provide more specific guidelines to ensure that the goals of the profession are protected and in fact actualized.

One element common to different financial incentive plans is that they encourage specific behaviors by penalizing or rewarding physicians on the basis of their patterns of clinical practice. Although fee-for-service medicine was not introduced as an explicit incentive, several studies have shown that providing a financial return for each service rendered can have an impact on the decision-making process of some physicians.[iii–v] Noting the effectiveness of incentives at modifying clinical behavior, managed care organizations have developed a wide variety of payment mechanisms that target either specific practices or general patterns of care in an effort to reduce the cost of providing care to plan patients.

[iii]Clancy CM and Hillner, BE. Physicians as Gatekeepers: The Impact of Financial Incentives. *Archives of Internal Medicine.* Vol. 149, April 1989: 917–920.

[iv]Epstein AM, Begg CB, McNeil BJ. The Use of Ambulatory Testing in Prepaid and Fee-For-Service Group Practices. *NEJM.* April 24, 1986. 314;17:1089–1094.

[v]Hemenway D, et al. Physicians' Responses to Financial Incentives. *NEJM.* 1990; 322: 1059–1063.

Financial incentive plans also share the same general hazards. Regardless of the specific behavior targeted for a monetary inducement, the potential exists to create a conflict of interest involving the needs of the patient and the personal financial interests of the treating physician. For instance, a sufficiently large bonus tied to reducing the length of hospital stays could force a physician to choose between a substantial portion of his or her income and potentially beneficial care for a patient. Although the ethic of the profession demands that physicians provide their patients with all necessary care regardless of the personal reward or penalty involved,[vi] the conflict becomes particularly acute in cases of marginal need or when the benefits of treatment are uncertain. Fee-for-service medicine creates a similar conflict, except that the physician is inclined by his or her financial interests to provide care that is only marginally indicated.

Although medicine has a long tradition requiring physicians to resolve these conflicts to the benefit of the patient, avoiding or minimizing these conflicts is important both to the patient's perception of clinical objectivity and to the physician's ability to practice medicine as an advocate for the patient. It is appropriate and important, therefore, for the profession to establish the goals upon which incentive plans should be based and to provide basic parameters that will protect the system of fundamental values governing physician behavior.

Goals for the Application of Incentives

The most fundamental goal of the medical profession is to provide for the health of patients. Applied broadly, this objective encompasses a commitment to safeguard the public health through the provision of quality, cost-effective care and to extend access to adequate health care to every individual.[vii] Applied in the context of clinical care, this requires physicians to place the health interests of their individual patients before all other concerns and to facilitate access to all necessary treatments. Financial incentives should be designed around this principle and ultimately judged according to their success or failure at fostering improvements in patient care.

Incentives should also be judged according to the extent to which they foster the treatment relationship between patient and physician by allowing physicians to assume their role as advocates for the health of individual patients. Physicians should never be discouraged by incentives from fulfilling their obligations to disclose all treatment options, to appeal any denials of coverage for necessary care, to

[vi]See Opinions 8.03, 8.13.
[vii]See for example: Council on Ethical and Judicial Affairs of the American Medical Association. Report 53: "Ethical Issues in Health Care Systems Reform: The Provision of Adequate Health Care." See also Opinion 2.095 and HOD Policy 165.960 (1).

make referrals on the basis of individual patient needs, and to provide to each patient those treatments which they believe will be of material benefit. Individual patients do not behave according to statistics and physicians must have the freedom to recognize and to accommodate the specific medical, financial, and psychosocial needs of the individuals in their practices.

Potential Benefits of Employing Financial Incentives

One of the strongest potential benefits financial incentives can provide is a reduction of waste in the application of medical resources, thereby effectively increasing the pool of resources for care. Fee-for-service medicine provides no incentive for physicians to economize use, and abuses of that system are manifest in cases of overutilization. Incentives can be applied to eliminate inefficiencies and defensive practices that may lead to artificial inflation of health care costs. Such incentives can be tailored to encourage the conservative but appropriate provision of medical care, thus maximizing the benefit gained from limited resources. For example, assuming appropriate utilization could be established by objective means, bonuses could be paid to physicians on the basis of their success at applying resources in an effective and efficient manner.

Applying incentives to specific patterns of care allows health plans to encourage a shift in practice towards preventive medicine and ambulatory care. Not only can such a shift produce cost savings, it can encourage physicians to become more involved in the health-related lifestyle choices of their patients. Ultimately, it can also improve the long-term health of patients. Additionally, incentives can be used to reward the integration and coordination of services, benefiting patients by providing more convenient access to care at a variety of levels.

A final advantage afforded by many incentive programs is the increased attention paid on a system level to patient satisfaction. Many managed care entities tie bonuses or reimbursement to patient surveys critiquing the performance of physicians and the managed care organization itself. Such plans encourage physicians to provide quality care and give patients the opportunity to voice any concerns they have regarding the level or type of care available through their plan.

Potential Risks Associated with Financial Incentives

Financial incentives operate by involving the personal interests of the physician in the therapeutic relationship. Physicians have a long-established obligation to put the interests of patients before all others, and in the majority of treatment circumstances, the appropriate manifestation of this obligation is clear. No physician can justify denying a patient absolutely necessary care or providing clearly unnecessary care, regardless of the incentive involved. However, there are certainly cases in which multiple treatment options exist, and in which the best among them is not abundantly clear. The physician must then exercise his or her judgment and weigh the probabilities of benefit against potential harms, taking into consideration factors including efficacy and cost in an effort to identify the treatment (or lack of treatment) most likely to benefit the patient.

The effect of financial incentives is felt most acutely in situations such as this, when the clinical imperfections of medicine become apparent and the physician is called upon to render an objective analysis of several complex considerations. It is exceedingly difficult to maintain true objectivity when a monetary reward or penalty is associated with a specific course of action. While this inducement will have little if any effect when the best treatment course is clear, its influence will grow as the gap separating different clinical options shrinks and the effects of each become similar. It is not reasonable to expect that all physicians can resist completely the influence of a financial incentive on true borderline cases. It is therefore critical to place limits on financial incentives to ensure that clinical objectivity is protected.

The potential to affect the objectivity of physicians is not the only cause for concern associated with financial incentives. Inducements that are based on the use of resources across physicians' practices compound the conflict between the interests of the physician and those of the patient by introducing conflicts between patients. When physicians are provided with incentives to meet specific levels of utilization, they are encouraged to consider the needs of the individual patient relative to the needs of other patients. For instance, bonuses attached to patterns of reduced use encourage physicians to consider which patients need certain services most rather than simply which patients need certain services. Such an incentive would not, in all likelihood, have any noticeable impact on the cases of clear patient need. Again, however, these incentives would have a greater impact on the care offered in cases of potential but unclear benefit.

Incentives that encourage physicians to consider the needs of patients in relation to one another could impact the ability of physicians to carry out their fundamental obligation of individual patient advocacy. Whether or not physicians are ever forced by incentives into a form of circumstantial or "bedside" rationing, patients may feel as though they must compete for scarce resources in a forum lacking significant oversight or consistent structure. The essential premise that physicians act wholly in the interests of each individual, constrained only by publicly determined limits on resources, allows patients to trust their physicians. Any incentive plan that challenges or appears to challenge this fundamental notion could have a far-reaching impact on the patient-physician relationship.

Even the appearance of rationing hints at perhaps the most troubling side-effect of incentive programs, namely their potential to disrupt the trust that exists between patients and physicians. No consequence of applying financial incentives would be more destructive to patient care than a widespread degradation of the public trust in the medical profession. While perceived competition between patients for resources could cast doubt on the ability of the treating physician to act as an individual advocate, the simple fact that a physician could stand to reap significant financial gain by providing (or not providing) a specific form of care may raise fundamental questions about the therapeutic relationship. This challenge to the patient's conception of medical practice could arise regardless of the actual effect any given incentive has, or does not have, on the clinical decision-making process.

Disclosure of Financial Incentives

Since the existence of financial incentives alone could impact the patient-physician relationship, developing an appropriate strategy to disclose those incentives is not a straightforward task. Patients have a right to be informed of all factors that could impact their care, including the payment system under which their physician practices. Disclosure is also necessary because the sense of betrayal and suspicion that would result from the independent discovery of a system capable of affecting clinical judgment would far outweigh the impact of full disclosure.

A much more difficult question to answer than whether or not to disclose incentives is where the responsibility for providing such information lies. A compelling argument can be made for disclosure prior to enrollment in a health plan, as the structure of financial inducements could influence the patient's decision to purchase a specific form of coverage.[viii] However, if disclosure of the nature of financial arrangements between payer and physician does not occur at the level of the payer, some obligation exists on the part of the physician to provide that information.

Effects of Financial Incentives on the Profession

The biggest concern associated with financial incentives is the conflict of interest they generate and the possible impact of that conflict on clinical objectivity and patient care. However, the ramifications of monetary inducements are by no means limited to the health of patients; they extend to physicians' perceptions of the profession and their role in caring for patients. The reaction of many physicians to the increasingly prevalent tension between personal economic interests and the therapeutic relationship has been one of discontent. In many ways, the application of

[viii]See Council on Ethical and Judicial Affairs of the American Medical Association. "Ethical Issues in Managed Care." *JAMA*. 1995; 273:330–335. (Opinion 8.13)

financial incentives to reduce or limit utilization has changed the manner in which physicians are being asked to treat patients. The bottom line requires constant attention, breeding resentment towards those patients who require the most care and resources. Physicians are implicitly or even explicitly encouraged to shorten office visits and to reduce the use of certain services. Many recognize the inherent conflict of interest created through the use of financial incentives, but feel they have few options available to alleviate that conflict. The effect of this discontent on the patient-physician relationship and ultimately on the practice of medicine is not yet clear, but is cause for some concern.

Another sentiment common among physicians is that many financial incentives are transforming their station in the health care system. Physicians have defined themselves as a profession by their dedication to the principles of ethical practice, their dedication to the individual patient, and their ability to weigh these and other factors in determining the appropriate course of treatment for the sick. In many ways, the increased use and specificity of financial incentives is challenging this definition. The practice of medicine is not an exact science and relies heavily upon the ability of physicians to interpret a number of conditions other than physiological symptoms when recommending treatment. And yet, some financial incentive plans tied directly to average utilization rates encourage physicians to treat in exactly the same way all patients presenting the same or similar symptoms. In this way, many plans attempt to define rigidly what has for years been the purview of professional judgment and expert interpretation of nonquantifiable factors. The end result may be that physicians question their status as professionals in the face of increased micromanagement through utilization review and bonus schedules.

Limiting the Influence of Incentives to Preserve the Goals of the Profession

The Council has long recognized the primacy of patient interests, stating in part, "If a conflict develops between the physician's financial interest and the physician's responsibilities to the patient, the conflict must be resolved to the patient's benefit."[ix] This broad statement applies equally to all financial conflicts engendered by incentives. There is also an obligation on the part of the medical profession to protect medical resources against waste and thereby to minimize the costs borne by patients. The intersection of these obligations provides a standard with which to judge the ethical propriety of various incentive plans. Well-designed plans encourage the appropriate use of medical resources without creating conflicts of interest that could impact individual, clinical care. Poorly-designed plans

[ix]See Opinion 8.03.

are either ineffective at encouraging efficiency, or intrusive on the independent judgment of patient and physician. In light of this standard, the task before the profession is to provide a framework identifying the factors that influence the degree to which different incentive plans allow physicians to uphold their ethical commitments.

The size of the financial reward or penalty associated with certain practices can help distinguish appropriate from inappropriate incentives. All other factors being equal, a direct correlation exists between the size of a financial inducement and the degree of influence it exercises. Large bonuses are more likely to affect objectivity than smaller ones, and placing a large portion of a physician's income at risk for treatment decisions creates a more substantial conflict of interest than placing a small percentage of potential earnings at risk.

Although the size of the incentive is important, it is not the sole determinant of ethical propriety and often works in conjunction with other factors. For instance, the proximity of an incentive to an individual act is crucial in predicting its eventual influence on services rendered. Proximity is a function of the degree to which physicians can reap personal benefit from individual treatment decisions rather than broader patterns of practice. The closer the proximity of an incentive to individual clinical encounters, the more likely it is to be given undue consideration.

Perhaps the most direct incentive is provided by a system of fee-for-service in which a direct correlation is established between individual service and payment. Unethical conduct under such circumstances can come in a variety of forms, including the provision of unnecessary services, self-referral, and fee-splitting. It is difficult to create systemic limitations which can eliminate these abuses; however, the individual acts themselves are readily identified and proscribed.[x] In addition to prohibiting these specific abuses, the Council has issued guidelines governing the establishment of appropriate fees in an effort to ensure that physicians charge rates commensurate with their skill and training.[xi]

The influence on clinical practice of most other forms of financial incentives can be limited by altering the proximity of the incentive to specific clinical encounters. Spreading the risks can dilute incentives and benefits accrued through individual treatment decisions across panels of physicians. Because the savings generated by one individual physician will benefit a group, the amount the individual stands to gain from any single act is dramatically reduced. Likewise, in those situations where personal income is placed at risk, physicians who share that risk stand to lose substantially less potential income as a result of any single clinical decision. In either case, an incentive to practice in accordance with standards of efficiency exists; however, the immediacy of that incentive to individual treatment options is dramatically reduced.

[x]See endnote i.
[xi]Opinion 6.05.

Similar to applying incentives across broad physician groups, the proximity of incentives to single decisions can also be reduced by tying inducements to experience related to a large patient pool. As the laws of probability dictate, larger patient populations are more likely to have stable and predictable health care needs. When considering the care offered to a large number of patients, it becomes clear that expensive or extensive treatments for one patient will be balanced by the relatively minor or non-existent needs of others. Because the physician whose incentive plan applies to a large group can rely upon other cases to balance the needs of even exceptional patients, the freedom to exercise clinical judgment is preserved.

Following the same laws of probability, it becomes clear that incentives attached to utilization can also be limited by calculating patterns of use over longer rather than shorter periods of time. Despite potentially wide variations in individual care, the mean rates of resource consumption more closely approximate a consistent average as the time period over which they are calculated expands. Therefore, lengthening the time frame over which incentive payments are calculated reduces the risk that any one treatment decision will have a significant impact on the physician's financial reward or penalty.

It is important to note that some incentive plans that appear on their face to incentivize treatment patterns rather than individual decisions may in fact create circumstances in which enormous and unintended inducements result. Incentives that are awarded when a discrete point of utilization is achieved may satisfy the requirement to consider the use of resources across broad patterns of care. In some situations, though, they may create untenable conflicts. For instance, a bonus attached to an increased number of patient-visits may be awarded in its entirety when the physician reaches a specific number of clinical encounters. As the end of the fiscal period approaches, if the physician is within striking distance of that goal, an enormous incentive is created to see enough patients to realize what might be a substantial bonus.

Consider the case of a physician who stands to be awarded a $15,000 bonus if he can conduct 8,000 patient visits in a year. If, on the other hand, he conducts 7,999 visits, he receives nothing. In the last week of the year, $15,000 may ride on his ability to see 200 patients and a coercive incentive is established. In general, it is necessary to guard against the possibility that an incentive intended for annual or broadly calculated patterns could effectively ride on a much smaller number of individual cases. Consequently, incentives that are established on a continuum of utilization rather than a system of bracketed cutoff points will be more likely to prevent potentially severe conflicts of interest.

Even with safeguards in place, catastrophic care for a single patient can in many instances have a significant impact on the incentive payment that a physician receives. It is important, therefore, to provide some further protection from the potentially significant impact any treatment for a single patient could have on the income of a physician. The best means to achieve this protection is through the provision of a stop-loss plan. When the costs of treatment for a single patient climb above a fixed level, an insurance policy or an overflow pool of funds pays the majority of the balance. This allows physicians to recommend and provide treatment that would otherwise deplete a pool of withheld money or skew the appearance of their utilization rate.

A final means through which the potentially negative effects of financial incentives can be avoided is to include among other specific mechanisms rewards and penalties tied to quality measures. This will reinforce the importance of establishing efficient but effective practice patterns. It also provides a simple check against any movement to view reductions in utilization rather than the provision of optimal care as the primary goal.

Conclusion

The purpose of incentive plans is to motivate physicians to eliminate waste and to provide optimal levels of care. The specific mechanisms used to achieve this goal should therefore be tailored in accordance with predictions of utilization dictated by medical necessity rather than by market economics and a plan's competitive standing. Physicians should not be offered monetary incentives that are designed to reduce costs below levels compatible with the provision of all necessary care. Such inducements introduce conflicts of interest that encroach upon the therapeutic relationship and threaten individual as well as public trust in the profession. To protect against such eventualities, the health needs of each patient and the ability of physicians to act as individual advocates must remain the principal considerations of any reimbursement plan.

Recommendations

In order to achieve the necessary goals of patient care and to protect the role of physicians as advocates for individual patient needs, the Council recommends the following:

1. Although physicians have an obligation to consider the needs of broader patient populations within the context of the physician-patient relationship, their first duty must be to the individual patient.

This obligation must override considerations of the reimbursement mechanism or specific financial incentives applied to a physician's clinical practice.

2. Physicians, individually or through their representatives, should evaluate the financial incentives associated with participation in a health plan before contracting with that plan. The purpose of the evaluation is to ensure that quality of patient care is not compromised by unrealistic expectations for utilization or by plac-

ing that physician's payments for care at excessive risk. In the process of making judgments about the ethical propriety of such reimbursement systems, physicians should refer to the following general guidelines:

a) Monetary incentives may be judged in part on the basis of their size. Large incentives may create conflicts of interest that can in turn compromise clinical objectivity. While an obligation has been established to resolve financial conflicts of interest to the benefit of patients, it is important to recognize that sufficiently large incentives can create an untenable position for physicians.

b) The proximity of large financial incentives to individual treatment decisions should be limited in order to prevent physicians' personal financial concerns from creating a conflict with their role as individual patient advocates. When the proximity of incentives cannot be mitigated, as in the case of fee-for-service payments, physicians must behave in accordance with prior Council recommendations limiting the potential for abuse. This includes the Council's prohibitions on fee-splitting arrangements, the provision of unnecessary services, unreasonable fees, and self-referral. For incentives that can be distanced from clinical decisions, the following factors should be considered in order to evaluate the correlation between individual act and monetary reward or penalty.

i) In general, incentives should be applied across broad physician groups. This dilutes the effect any one physician can have on his or her financial situation through clinical recommendations, thus allowing physicians to provide those services they feel are necessary in each case. Simultaneously, however, physicians are encouraged by the incentive to practice efficiently.

ii) The size of the patient pool considered in calculations of incentive payments will affect the proximity of financial motivations to individual treatment decisions. The laws of probability dictate that in large populations of patients, the overall level of utilization remains relatively stable and predictable. Physicians practicing in plans with large numbers of patients in a risk pool therefore have greater freedom to provide the care they feel is necessary based on the likelihood that the needs of other plan patients will balance out decisions to provide extensive care.

iii) The time period over which incentives are determined should be long enough to accommodate fluctuations in utilization resulting from the random distribution of patients and illnesses. For example, basing incentive payments on an annual analysis of resource utilization is preferable to basing them on monthly review.

iv) Financial rewards or penalties that are triggered by specific points of utilization may create enormous incentives as a physician's practice approaches the established level. Incentives should therefore be calculated on a continuum of utilization rather than a bracketed system with tiers of widely varied bonuses or penalties.

v) A stop-loss plan should be in place to prevent the costs of treating a single patient from significantly impacting the reward or penalty offered to a physician.

3. Incentives should be designed to promote efficient practice, but should not be designed to realize cost savings beyond those attainable through efficiency. As a counterbalance to the focus on utilization reduction, incentives should also be based upon measures of quality of care and patient satisfaction.

4. Patients must be informed of financial incentive that could impact the level or type of care they receive. This responsibility should be assumed by the health plan to ensure that patients are aware of such incentives prior to enrollment. Physicians, individually or through their representative, must be prepared to discuss with patients any financial arrangements that could impact patient care. Physicians should avoid reimbursement systems that cannot be disclosed to patients without negatively affecting the physician-patient relationship.

Council Report: Sexual Misconduct in the Practice of Medicine

The American Medical Association's Council on Ethical and Judicial Affairs recently reviewed the ethical implications of sexual or romantic relationships between physicians and patients. The Council has concluded that (1) sexual contact or a romantic relationship concurrent with the physician-patient relationship is unethical; (2) sexual contact or a romantic relationship with a former patient may be unethical under certain circumstances; (3) education on the ethical issues involved in sexual misconduct should be included throughout all levels of medical training; and (4) in the case of sexual misconduct, reporting offending colleagues is especially important.

There is a long-standing consensus within the medical profession that sexual contact or sexual relations between physicians and patients are unethical. The prohibition against sexual relations with patients was incorporated into the Hippocratic oath: ". . . I will come for the benefit of the sick, remaining free of all intentional injustice, of all mischief and in particular of sexual relations with both female and male persons. . . ."[1]

Current ethical thought uniformly condemns sexual relations between patients and physicians.[2-4] In addition, the laws of many states prohibit sexual contact between psychiatrists or other physicians and their patients.[5-9] The ban on physi-

JAMA. 1991;266:2741–2745.

Members of the Council on Ethical and Judicial Affairs include the following: Richard J. McMurray, MD, Flint, Mich, Chair; Oscar W. Clarke, MD, Gallipolis, Ohio, Vice Chair; John A. Barrasso, MD, Casper, Wyo; Dexanne B. Clohan, Arlington, Va; Charles H. Epps, Jr, MD, Washington, DC; John Glasson, MD, Durham, NC; Robert McQuillan, MD, Kansas City, Mo; Charles W. Plows, MD, Anaheim, Calif; Michael A. Puzak, MD, Arlington, Va; David Orentlicher, MD, JD, Chicago, Ill, Secretary and staff author; Kristen A. Halkola, Chicago, Ill, Associate Secretary and staff author.

cian–patient sexual contact is based on the recognition that such contact jeopardizes patients' medical care.

Physician–Patient Sexual Contact

Incidence

A number of studies have tried to establish the incidence of physician–patient sexual contact. Much of the research done on the prevalence of physician–patient sexual contact is based on studies that survey physicians about their own behavior.[10–13] The general stigma attached to sexual contact with patients and the professional repercussions that may result from admitting to such contact have led many researchers to believe that the occurrence of patient–physician sexual contact is underreported.[10,14,15]

Studies indicate that there is a small minority of physicians who have reported having sexual contact with patients.[10,11,16,17] Psychiatrists have been particularly diligent in examining the phenomenon of sexual contact with patients. Consequently, the majority of existing studies on physician–patient sexual contact examine sexual contact between psychiatrists and their patients. Studies of psychiatrists indicate that between 5% and 10% reported having sexual contact with patients.[10,11,16,18] Data for all specialties are not available, but a 1976 study suggested that the percentages may be comparable for other specialties.[11] While much of the discussion in this report centers on sexual misconduct by psychiatrists, it is clear that sexual misconduct is a problem not confined to any particular specialty.

Sexual contact between physician and patient can occur in a variety of ways: (1) physicians may become involved in personal relationships with patients that are concurrent with but independent of treatment[10]; (2) some physicians may use their position to gain sexual access to their patients by representing sexual contact as part of care or treatment[19]; and (3) others may assault patients by engaging in sexual contact with incompetent or unconscious patients. There seems to be little or no data indicating the prevalence of each type of sexual misconduct.

Physicians Who Engage in Sexual Contact with Patients

Failure to Handle the Emotional Content of the Therapeutic Relationship

For some physicians, sexual contact with a patient is a result of a temporary failure to constructively manage the emotions arising from the physician–patient relationship. The professional physician–patient relationship frequently evokes strong and complicated emotions in both the physician and the patient.[20–22] It is not unusual for sexual attraction to be one of these emotions. Many commentators agree that sexual or romantic attraction to patients is not uncommon or abnormal.[2,23]

However, sexual attraction to a patient, while not necessarily detrimental to the physician-patient relationship, can also lead to sexual contact or a sexual relationship between the patient and physician. The emotions of admiration, affection, and caring that are a part of the physician-patient relationship can become particularly powerful when either party is experiencing intense pressures or traumatic or major life events. The usual professional restraint exhibited by physicians may falter under such profound emotional influences, resulting in the transformation of sexual attraction into sexual contact.

Currently, the research on sexual misconduct is insufficient to determine how many sexual interactions between physicians and patients occur under these circumstances. Although figures vary widely, one nationwide study of psychiatrists showed that 67% of psychiatrists who reported sexual contact with a patient indicated that the contact occurred with only one patient.[10] This study showed that approximately 50% of psychiatrists who reported sexual contact with only one patient sought help or consultation for the matter.[10] However, engaging in sexual contact with a patient because of temporary impairment of proper judgment or perspective is not ethically excusable or condonable.

Sexual Contact Under Exploitative Conditions

For some physicians, sexual misconduct is the conscious (and usually repeated) use of their professional positions in order to manipulate or exploit their patients' vulnerabilities for their own gratification. Presumably, most physicians who represent sexual contact to patients as part of treatment would belong to this category. Certainly, self-gratification is the only basis for the behavior of physicians who engage in sexual contact with incompetent or unconscious patients.

Several researchers have compared the occurrence of sexual misconduct with sexual assault and incest.[16,19,24,35] It is clear that, for at least some offenders, sexual misconduct with patients results from an impulse to assert power over or to humiliate another person.[26(pp60–61)] Masters and Johnson[27] advocated that therapists who exploit their power in order to have sexual intercourse with their patients should be charged with rape.[23] Four states classify sexual exploitation by a psychotherapist as sex offenses under criminal statutes.[4,6,8,9]

The comparison with sexual assault is most easily understood when a physician represents sexual contact to the patient as being an appropriate medical or therapeutic procedure or an appropriate part of the therapeutic relationship. For health professionals engaged in a therapeutic relationship with patients, sexual misconduct is also often a manifestation of the health professional's own need to control or subjugate the patient or the sexual relationship.[28(pp60–61)] In such situations, a physician uses his or her status as a physician to influence or coerce the patient into accepting sexual contact. For instance, one researcher examined the responses of 16 women who had been sexually molested during routine gynecological examinations by the same physician.[19] The majority of the women did not stop the physician even after becoming uncomfortable with the length and nature of his examination since they trusted that their physician would not conduct an unethical examination.[19]

Several elements of the physician-patient relationship can combine to give the physician disproportionate influence over the patient. Within the physician-patient relationship, the physician possesses considerable knowledge, expertise, and status. A person is often most vulnerable, both physically and emotionally, when seeking medical care.[1,26] When a physician acts in a way that is not to the patient's benefit, the relative position of the patient within the professional relationship is such that it is difficult for the patient to give meaningful consent to such behavior, including sexual contact or sexual relations.[15,26] It is the lack of reliable or true consent on the part of the patient that has led researchers to compare physician-patient sexual contact with other sexually exploitative situations such as sexual assault and incest.[15,24,26(p47)] It is noteworthy that several states specify that consent of the patient or client cannot be used as a defense to charges of sexual misconduct.[6,7]

In fact, instances of sexual contact with patients do seem to occur most commonly where there is considerable disparity in power, status, and emotional vulnerability between physician and patient. Physicians who engage in sexual contact with patients are typically older and male, while patients are typically younger and female. Studies among psychiatrists indicate that approximately 85% to 90% of sexual contact involves a male psychiatrist and a female patient.[10] In one study of psychiatrists, a majority admitted that sexual contact with a patient was for their own emotional or sexual gratification.[10] Other studies of patient-psychiatrist sexual contact showed that the patients who were involved in sexual contact with their psychiatrists were also the ones most likely to be particularly vulnerable emotionally.[16] Patients who had sexual contact with psychiatrists were more likely than other patients to consider exploitative relations with an authority figure to be normal.[15]

A significant amount of sexual contact with patients does not seem to be an isolated instance of mismanaging the emotions of the professional relationship.[10,19] In one study, 33% of psychiatrists who reported sexual contact with patients also reported repeated instances of sexual contact with patients.[10] Despite considerable evidence to the contrary, repeat offenders were the most likely of all psychiatrists to claim that their conduct was beneficial to patients. These repeat offenders were also the least likely to seek help or consultation regarding the sexual contact.[10]

Effects of Sexual Contact Between Patients and Physicians

Some early attempts were made to show that sexual contact between patient and physician is or could be beneficial to the patient.[28,29] However, most researchers agree that the effects of physician-patient contact are almost universally negative or damaging to the patient.[15,19,24,26(pp24,38–45),30,31] (and *Boston Globe.* June 18, 1990:29, health science section). Studies show that 85% to 90% of patients experience such sexual contact as damaging.[22] Similar to the reactions of women who have been sexually assaulted, female patients tended to feel angry, abandoned, humiliated, mistreated, or exploited by their physicians.[14,26(p206),30,31] Victims have been reported to experience guilt, severe distrust of their own judgment, and mistrust of both men and physicians.[15,25(pp41,48,205),18] Patients who have been involved in therapist-patient sexual relationships can suffer from depression, anxiety, sexual disorders, sleeping disorders, and cognitive dysfunctions and are at risk for substance abuse.[15,26(pp18,45,208),34] While most researchers agree that sexual contact between patient and physician is potentially deleterious, it is important to note that most research has been based on patients who have initiated disciplinary action against physicians or on patients whom subsequent psychiatrists or therapists have identified as being harmed by the sexual contact with a physician. Patients not harmed by sexual contact with a physician may have escaped the attention of researchers. Also, assessing damage to patients may be complicated by the existence of preexisting conditions that are exacerbated by sexual involvement with the physician.[26(pp48,53,206)]

Most studies that have examined the effects of physician-patient sexual contact have focused on psychiatrists or therapists and their patients. However, one study found that the psychological impact of physician-patient sexual contact was negative for the patient regardless of the type of practitioner involved.[30] The study suggests that it is at least in part the betrayal of the patient's trust in the physician that produces negative psychological consequences for the patient. In addition, the risks posed to patient well-being due to loss of professional objectivity are equal regardless of the physician's specialty.

Ethical Considerations

Serving the Needs of the Patient

The satisfaction or gratification that a physician derives from treating patients is a fortunate benefit of the physician-patient alliance. However, the physician's professional obligation to serve the needs of the patient means that the physician's own needs or gratification cannot become a consideration in decisions about the patient's medical care. Regard for the physician's needs or gratifications may interfere with efforts to address the needs of the patient. At the very least, the emotional factors that accompany sexual involvement may affect or obscure the physician's medical judgment, thus jeopardizing the patient's diagnosis or treatment. Sexual contact or relationships between patient and physician are unethical because the physician's gratification inappropriately becomes part of the professional relationship.[16,30,35]

Trust Integral to the Physician-Patient Relationship

From ancient times, members of the medical profession have accepted the special responsibility that is accorded them by virtue of their unique skills of healing. The degree of knowledge, training, and expertise required to practice the art of medicine is highly sophisticated and complex. Physicians recognize that the health of individuals and society depends on their willingness to employ their knowledge, expertise, and influence solely for the welfare of patients. Patients who seek medical care must, in turn, be able to trust in the physician's dedication to the patient's welfare in order for the physician-patient alliance to succeed.[25]

A physician who engages in sexual contact with a patient seriously compromises the patient's welfare. The patient's trust that the physician will work only for the patient's welfare is violated. Consequently, sexual contact and sexual relationships between physicians and their patients are unethical.

Ethical Implications of Nonsexual Physical Contact with Patients

The ethical prohibition against romantic relationships or sexual contact with patients is not meant to bar nonsexual touching of patients by physicians. In addition to its role in physical examination, nonsexual touching may be therapeutic or comforting to patients. However, even nonsexual contact with patients should be approached with caution. It may be difficult to identify a strict boundary between nonsexual and sexual touching. Either the patient or the physician may misinterpret the touching behavior of the other.[32] There is also some concern that what may begin as benign, nonsexual contact may eventually lead to sexual contact.[11,12]

If a physician feels that a patient may misinterpret the nature of physical contact or if a physician's nonsexual touching behavior may be leading to sexual contact, then the contact should be avoided.

Termination of the Professional Relationship

It is of course possible for a physician and a patient to be genuinely attracted to or have genuine romantic affection for each other. However, any relationship in which a physician is (or risks) taking advantage of a patient's emotional or psychological vulnerability would be unethical. Therefore, before initiating a dating, romantic, or sexual relationship with a patient, a physician's minimum duty would be to terminate his or her professional relationship with the patient.[16] In addition, it would be advisable for a physician to seek consultation with a colleague before initiating a relationship with the former patient. Termination of the professional relationship would also be appropriate if a sexual or romantic attraction to (as opposed to contact with) a patient threatens to interfere with the judgment of the physician or to jeopardize the patient's care.

Sexual Contact After Termination of the Relationship

Posttermination Relationship May Also Be Unethical

Termination of the physician–patient relationship does not eliminate the possibility that sexual contact between a physician and a former patient might be unethical. Sexual contact between a physician and a patient with whom professional relations had been terminated would be unethical if the sexual contact occurred as a result of the use or exploitation of trust, knowledge, influence, or emotions derived from the former professional relationship. The ethical propriety of a sexual relationship between a physician and a former patient, then, may depend substantially on the nature and context of the former relationship.

In most patient–psychiatrist relationships, the intense and emotional nature of treatment makes it difficult for a romantic relationship between a psychiatrist and a former patient not to be affected by the previous professional relationship. The American Psychiatric Association has accordingly stated that "sexual involvement with one's former patients generally exploits emotions deriving from treatment and is therefore almost always unethical."[4]

Relationships between patients and other types of physicians may also include considerable trust, intimacy, or emotional dependence. The length of the former professional relationship, the extent to which the patient has confided personal or private information to the physician, the nature of the patient's medical problem, and the degree of emotional dependence that the patient has on the physician, all may contribute to the intimacy of the relationship. In addition, the extent of the physician's general knowledge about the patient (ie, the patient's past, the patient's family situation, and the patient's current emotional state) is also a factor that may render a sexual or romantic relationship with a former patient unethical.

Prohibiting Sexual Contact with Former Patients

Some commentators have suggested that the amount of time that has elapsed since the termination of the professional relationship and the initiation of the sexual or romantic relationship may be pertinent to the ethical propriety of physician-former patient relationships.[24]

It may be that a sexual or romantic relationship that immediately follows the termination of the physician–patient relationship may be more suspect than one that occurs after considerable time has passed. Yet, some emotions and dependencies that were created during the professional relationship may not disappear even after a considerable amount of time has passed. Research on psychotherapists has shown that patients experience strong feelings about their therapists for 5 to 10 years after the termination of treatment.[26(pp116–118),32]

For these reasons, it is not useful to determine the appropriateness of a sexual relationship between a physician and a former patient based on the amount of time that has elapsed since the termination of the professional relationship. Rather, the relevant standard is the potential for misuse of emotions derived from the former professional relationship.

Prevention and Discipline of Sexual Misconduct

Education

There is evidence that the issue of sexual misconduct and sexual or romantic attraction to patients is not adequately covered in many medical training programs.[23,36] However, almost all commentators agree that the issues surrounding sexual misconduct need attention during medical education.[23,33,37,38]

Education may serve to distinguish sexual or romantic attraction to patients, which is a common and normal experience, from inappropriate behavior, such as acting on the attraction or allowing the attraction to jeopardize the care of the patient. Education may also promote appropriate responses to sexual attraction to patients, such as seeking consultation with colleagues or counseling, when patient care is potentially jeopardized.[23] Obviously education about sexual misconduct would also inform physicians and medical students about the ethical implications of physician–patient sexual contact as well as the potential harm to patient well-being.

Detection and Reporting of Sexual Misconduct of Colleagues

Sexual misconduct is unlikely to be brought to the attention of the proper authorities by many of the usual means of exposing deficiencies in the practice of medicine. Other transgressions can be detected through the analysis of records or may be brought to the attention of the authorities by hospital staff or peer review processes. However, the discovery and investigation of sexual misconduct is unlikely unless victims of sexual misconduct initiate and pursue disciplinary or ethical review procedures.[37]

Unfortunately, patients who have had sexual contact with their physicians may be hindered from reporting the misconduct. There is some evidence that offenders tend to refer patients to colleagues whom they know to be sympathetic to their actions.[37] Patients may thus be discouraged from reporting instances of sexual misconduct. Also, while the rate of dismissals of cases alleging sexual intimacy between psychologists and clients is decreasing, many psychiatrists continue to express misgivings about the effectiveness of disciplinary bodies in this area.[26(pp24–25),37]

Further, some patients may not be able emotionally to report instances of sexual misconduct or to undergo the process of review and investigation required to discipline an offending physician. When the sexual relationship was a result of the physician's mishandling of the emotional influences of the professional relationship, the patient may not be able to recognize that the physician's behavior was improper or inappropriately motivated. Victims of sexual misconduct through medical deception may be incapable of reporting the offense because of the emotions of shame, humiliation, degradation, and blame that also often make it difficult for victims of sexual assault to report their assaults.

One of the few remaining avenues for identifying offending physicians is reporting by colleagues. Consequently, reporting of transgressions by peers is especially important in the case of sexual misconduct. Unfortunately, physicians are often reluctant to report instances of sexual transgression by their colleagues. A 1987 survey of 1423 practicing psychiatrists (a response rate of 26%) revealed that 65% of them reported treating patients who had been sexually involved with previous therapists, and 87% of those psychiatrists believed that the previous involvement was harmful to the patient. However, only 8% of them reported their colleagues' behavior to a professional organization or legal authority.[37]

Literature that has studied the reporting practices of physicians indicates that reluctance to report may involve concerns over confidentiality, either in the physician-patient relationship or among colleagues. Reluctance to take action contrary to a patient's wishes or concern that a patient's recovery process may be damaged also may affect the reporting practices. Some physicians may also regard the patient's allegations as hearsay and therefore unreportable.[37] Other physicians may feel that reporting laws lack sufficient clarity or immunity for good-faith reporting.

The American Medical Association includes among its Principles of Medical Ethics the standard that "[a] physician shall . . . strive to expose those physicians deficient in character or competence, or who engage in fraud or deception." Because the nature of sexual misconduct is such that most victims are rendered reluctant or unable to report the misconduct on their own, physicians should be particularly vigilant in exposing colleagues who commit sexual misconduct. Presently, four states have mandatory reporting laws specific to the reporting of sexual misconduct by colleagues.[32] The Council on Ethical and Judicial Affairs believes that physicians who learn of sexual misconduct by a colleague must report the misconduct to the local medical society, the state licensing board, or other appropriate authorities. Exception may be made if a physician learns of the misconduct while treating the offending physician for the misconduct, provided that the offending physician is not continuing the misconduct and does not resume the misconduct in the future. An exception may also be made in cases in which a patient refuses to consent to reporting or in cases where the treating physician believes that reporting would significantly harm the patient's treatment. Physicians who make good-faith reports of the sexual misconduct of a colleague should be protected from potential legal, professional, or personal repercussions.

Discipline

Some commentators have expressed concern that existing disciplinary bodies have not been sufficiently effective in dealing with sexual misconduct.[37] While the frequency of false accusations of sexual misconduct seems to be extremely low[32,38] (and *Boston Globe.* June 18, 1990:29, health science section), the rate at which practitioners are disciplined for ethical violations of this kind does not seem commensurate with the number of accusations.[37,39] There may be myriad concerns that limit the efficiency of investigative and disciplinary bodies, including the difficulties inherent in ensuring procedural fairness to the accused physician while remaining sensitive to the needs of the patient who reports physician sexual misconduct. For instance, procedural mechanisms must be in place that would prevent the leveling of baseless accusations against innocent physicians. However, procedures must also be flexible and sensitive enough so that victims are not so daunted or intimidated by the procedural requirements that they decline to proceed with complaints.

There are some ways, however, to structure disciplinary bodies that would maximize both effectiveness in detecting and disciplining offenders and sensitivity to patients who report sexual misconduct. For instance, some research has shown that women who experienced sexual contact with male psychotherapists showed an increased distrust both of men and of psychotherapists.[37] Patients should therefore be given the option of a preliminary interview with a member of the disciplinary board with whom or with whose gender they feel most comfortable. In addition, it is important that a disciplinary panel hearing sexual misconduct charges have equal gender distribution among its members.

Members of disciplinary bodies that deal with reports of sexual misconduct should undergo training and education specific to the problem.[37] Patents may face greater obstacles in reporting and pursuing legal action in the case of sexual misconduct than with other medical transgressions. Some institutions may consider establishing a special disciplinary body to handle allegations of sexual misconduct, one whose members are educated and sensitized to the particular difficulties facing victims of sexual misconduct.[32] Alternatively, an institution might establish special procedures for handling sexual misconduct complaints.

Finally, physicians who commit sexual misconduct must be able to get help. Physicians are subject to many pressures and influences, including attraction to patients, the emotional influences of the physician-patient interaction, and the effect of their own emotional problems or conflicts on their professional lives. Many physicians who commit sexual misconduct may benefit from rehabilitation for their problem. Currently, there is virtually no research regarding the efficacy of therapy for physicians who engage in sexual misconduct. However, programs similar to those that help other kinds of physician impairments, such as alcohol and drug addiction, should be developed and made available for sexual misconduct offenders.[23,33]

Conclusions

The Council on Ethical and Judicial Affairs concludes that sexual contact or a romantic relationship with a patient concurrent with the physician-patient relationship is unethical. Sexual or romantic relationships with former patients are also unethical if the physician uses or exploits trust, knowledge, emotions, or influence derived from the previous professional relationship.

In addition, education on the issue of sexual attraction to patients and sexual misconduct should be included throughout all levels of medical training. Disciplinary bodies must be structured to maximize effectiveness in dealing with the problem of sexual misconduct. Physicians who learn of sexual misconduct by a colleague must report the misconduct to the local medical society, the state licensing board, or other appropriate authorities. Exceptions to reporting may be made in order to protect patient welfare. It should be noted that many states have legal prohibitions against relationships between physicians and current or former patients.

References

1. Campbell M. The oath: an investigation of the injunction prohibiting physician-patient sexual relations. *Perspect Biol Med.* 1989;32:300–308.
2. Gartell N, Herman J, Olarte S, Localio R, Feldstein M. Psychiatric residents' sexual contact with educators and patients: results of a national survey. *Am J Psychiatry.* 1988;145:690–694.
3. Council on Ethical and Judicial Affairs, American Medical Association. *Current Opinions of the Council on Ethical and Judicial Affairs 1989, Opinion 8.14, Sexual Misconduct.* Chicago, Ill: American Medical Association; 1989.
4. American Psychiatric Association. *The Principles of Medical Ethics With Annotations Especially Applicable to Psychiatry.* Washington, DC: American Psychiatric Association; 1989.
5. Minn Stat Ann §609.344 (1990).
6. SD Codified Laws Ann §36-4-30 (1989).
7. Fla Stat §458.331 (1988).
8. Colo Rev Stat §18-3-405.5 (1989).
9. Wis Stat §940.22 (1986).
10. Gartrell N, Herman J, Olarte S, Feldstein M, Localio R. Psychiatrist-patient sexual contact: results of a national survey, I: prevalence. *Am J Psychiatry.* 1986;143:1126–1231.
11. Kardener S H, Fuller M, Mensh I N. Characteristics of 'erotic' practitioners. *Am J Psychiatry.* 1976;133:1324–1325.
12. Perry J A. Physicians' erotic and nonerotic physical involvement with patients. *Am J Psychiatry.* 1976;133:838–840.
13. Kardener S H, Fuller M, Mensh I N. A survey of physicians' attitudes and prac-

tices regarding erotic and nonerotic contact of patients. *Am J Psychiatry.* 1973;130:1077–1081.

14. Holroyd J C, Brodsky A M. Psychologists' attitudes and practices regarding erotic and nonerotic physical contact with patients. *Am Psychologist.* 1977;32: 843–849.

15. Kluft R P. Treating the patient who has been exploited by a previous therapist. *Psychiatr Clin North Am.* 1989;12:483–500.

16. Rapp M S. Sexual misconduct. *Can Med Assoc J.* 1987;137:193–194.

17. Derosis H, Hamilton J A, Morrison E, Strauss M. More on psychiatrist-patient sexual contact. *Am J Psychiatry.* 1987;144:688–689.

18. Belote B. *Sexual Intimacy Between Female Clients and Male Psychotherapists: Masochistic Sabotage.* San Francisco: California School of Professional Psychology; 1974. Unpublished doctoral dissertation.

19. Burgess A. Physician sexual misconduct and patients' responses. *Am J Psychiatry.* 1981;138:1355–1342.

20. Zinn W M. Doctors have feelings too. *JAMA.* 1988;259:3296–3298.

21. Groves J E. Taking care of the hateful patient. *N Engl J Med.* 1978;298:883–887.

22. Gorlin R, Zucker H D. Physicians' reactions to patients. *N Engl J Med* 1983;308:1059–1063.

23. Pope K S, Keith-Speigel P, Tabachnick B G. Sexual attraction to clients: the human therapist and (sometimes) inhuman training system. *Am Psychologist.* 1986;41:147–158.

24. Herman J L, Gartrell N, Olarte S, Feldstein M, Localio R. Psychiatrist-patient sexual contact: results of a national survey, II: psychiatrists' attitudes. *Am J Psychiatry.* 1987;144:164–169.

25. Kardener S H. Sex and physician-patient relationship. *Am J Psychiatry.* 1974;131:1134–1136.

26. Gabbard G O. *Sexual Exploitation in Professional Relationships.* Washington, DC: American Psychiatric Press; 1989.

27. Masters W H, Johnson V E. Principles of the new sex therapy. *Am J Psychiatry.* 1976;133:548–554.

28. McCartney J. Overt transference. *J Sex Res.* 1966;2:227–237.

29. Shepard M. *The Love Treatment: Sexual Intimacy Between Patients and Psychotherapists.* New York, NY: Peter Wyden; 1971.

30. Feldman-Summers S, Jones G. Psychological impacts of sexual contact between therapists or other health care practitioners and their clients. *J Consult Clin Psychol.* 1984;52:1054–1061.

31. Bouhoutsos J, Holroyd J, Lerman H, Forer B, Greenberg M. Sexual intimacy between psychotherapists and patients. *Professional Psychol Res Pract.* 1983;14:185–196.

32. Bemmann K C, Goodwin J. New laws about sexual misconduct by therapists: knowledge and attitudes among Wisconsin psychiatrists. *Wis Med J.* 1989;88(5):11–16.

33. Zelen S L. Sexualization of therapeutic relationships: the dual vulnerability of patient and therapist. *Psychotherapy.* 1985;22:178–185.
34. California Legislature. *Report of the California Senate Task Force on Psychotherapist and Patients Sexual Relations.* Prepared for the California Senate Rules Committee, March 1987.
35. Seeman M V. Sexual misconduct. *Can Med Assoc J.* 1987;137:699–700.
36. Glaser R D, Thorpe J S. Unethical intimacy: a survey of sexual contact and advances between psychology educators and female graduate students. *Am Psychol.* 1986;41:43–51.
37. Gartrell N, Herman J, Olarte S, Feldstein M, Localio R. Reporting practices of psychiatrists who knew of sexual misconduct by colleagues. *Am J Orthopsychiatry.* 1987;57:287–295.
38. Gutheil T G. Borderline personality disorder, boundary violations, and patient-therapist sex: medicolegal pitfalls. *Am J Psychiatry.* 1989; 146:597–602.
39. Moore R A. Ethics in the practice of psychiatry update on the results of enforcement of the code. *Am J Psychiatry.* 1985;142:1043–1046.

Index

Boldfaced numbers indicate pages in the appendices.

Library of Congress Cataloging-in-Publication Data
The American medical ethics revolution : how the AMA's code of ethics
    has transformed physicians' relationships to patients,
    professionals, and society / edited by Robert B. Baker . . . [et al.].
        p.   cm.
    Includes bibliographical references and index.
    ISBN 0–8018–6170–5 (alk. paper)
        1. Medical ethics— United States.   2. Medical ethics—Social
    aspects—United States.   I. Baker, Robert, 1937–   .
    R725.A56   1999
    174′.2′0973—dc21   99–29636
                                                                            CIP